MEDICAL ECONOMICS
AND HEALTH FINANCE

MEDICAL ECONOMICS AND HEALTH FINANCE

STEVEN R. EASTAUGH
Cornell University

 Auburn House Publishing Company
Boston, Massachusetts

Library of Congress Cataloging in Publication Data

Eastaugh, Steven R., 1952–
   Medical economics and health finance.

   Includes index.
   1. Medical economics—United States. I. Title.
[DNLM: 1. Economics, Hospital—United States. 2. Cost
benefit analysis. 3. Cost control. WX 157 E12m]
RA410.53.E17   338.4'73621'0973   81-3450
ISBN 0-86569-065-0   AACR2

Printed in the United States of America

PREFACE

In preparing this book, I have intentionally cast a wide net. This book is intended for managers, policy makers, health care providers, and students who are unfamiliar with many technical concepts (a glossary is provided in the back). It is anticipated that this wide audience is interested in a synthesis of currently available study results and potential policy ramifications, rather than new research methods. However, the footnotes and portions of four chapters (2, 8, 9, and 12) are intended for functional specialists and scholars with interests in technical issues. My hope is that the reader will come away with a better understanding of the medical economics and financial management literature and a renewed appreciation of the fact that the behavior of consumers and medical providers is only partially understood at this time.

In this text the various cost containment proposals that have been advanced in the 1970s will be examined against the backdrop of the empirical research available to date. In Part One of the text we shall define the elements that make up the medical cost inflation problem and survey a number of models of physician and hospital behavior. We conclude Part One with a review of the techniques and potential applications of cost-benefit and cost-effectiveness evaluation, although the determination of indirect and intangible benefits is often an imprecise matter in medical technology assessment.

In Part Two we shall discuss the alleged merits and demerits of the following: competition health plans, health marketing, health planning, rate regulation, promotion of increased information disclosure on price and quality to the consumer, and expansion of the supply of physician assistants and nurse practitioners. In Part Three our concerns shift to the viewpoint of the institutional manager and the impact that cost containment has had on all hospitals, large teaching hospitals, medical schools, and HMOs. Most of the emphasis will be on hospital finance. Hospitals have an excessive reliance on debt rela-

v

tive to other sectors of the economy, for example, three quarters of total new capitalization is debt financed. Public utilities borrow on the average about one half of new capitalization and manufacturing firms borrow only one third. A number of financing alternatives are evaluated, including two types of leasing options. Part Four summarizes a number of future policy options and concludes that no single cost containment strategy will be sufficient. A number of mixed strategies are suggested, and an innovative double-capitation reimbursement experiment is surveyed.

The title of this text is derived from two courses I have taught for five and three years, respectively: Medical Economics and Health Finance. The phrase "health finance" is intended to denote the study of financial management in health service institutions, such as hospitals, HMOs, and medical schools. As an alumnus of two graduate schools of public health, I cannot resist pointing out that health care can be conceived of as either a final output of our industry or an intermediate input in the production of "good health." Consequently, health finance could have been misinterpreted by some readers as the study of how society finances improved health in the population. However, many studies reviewed in this text have posed the tougher basic question regarding the minimal marginal impact that increased health services delivery has had on improving the health status of our citizens.

I have depended upon the ideas and assistance of others in writing this book and credit is due them. The final stages of manuscript were reviewed by James Begun, Roger Battistella, Thomas Rundall, and John McClain. Parts of the manuscript were reviewed in the early stages of development by Duncan Neuhauser, Charles Flagle, Robert Smiley, Richard Bailey, Mark Schaefer, and David Salkever. Four former research assistants, David Dranove, Nancy Bohn, James Lake, and Sandra Yeater, deserve special thanks for their help in the original data analysis for Chapters 4 and 8–11. For errors that remain I am responsible.

Finally, this book is dedicated to my parents, who provided moral support and an appreciation of good scholarship.

S.R.E.

CONTENTS

Part One

BROAD ECONOMIC ISSUES

Chapter 1

MEDICAL COST INFLATION

> *Cost inflation is important because it reflects the serious misallocation of resources and the failure of the health-care system to reflect individual preferences. . . . There are really only two ingredients to understanding the rise in costs: The changing nature of the hospital, and the impact of insurance.*
>
> —Martin S. Feldstein

Hospitals have priced themselves into the public eye. During the past twelve years annual hospital inflation has averaged 15 percent, more than double the inflation rate that has bedeviled the rest of the economy. Prior to beginning a discussion of hospital cost inflation, it is essential first to explain how it is known that costs are in fact increasing each year. In other words, it is necessary to identify the indexes of cost inflation being used and to understand their implications. Most of the statistical evidence cited in this chapter pertains to hospital care, because the other components of medical care have had a cost inflation rate more in line with the general economy—for example, annual inflation rates in physician expenditures have averaged five points above the general economy and drug costs one percentage point above the nonhealth sectors of the economy.

There are two generally used indexes of the cost of hospital care. The first is used in the medical care component of the consumer price index. Published by the Bureau of Labor Statistics and called the "Index of Hospital Service Charges" (IHSC), it is a weighted average of the price indexes for several common components of

3

hospital care. These components include room charge, use of the operating room, and eight common services such as a diagnostic x-ray and a laboratory test. The purpose of this index is to measure the change in price of a fixed basket of common services. The success of the IHSC in measuring changes in price—not quality and intensity—is limited by the extent to which improvements in the quality of care are built into the basic charges.

The second index, the Average Cost Per Patient Day (ACPPD), is published by the American Hospital Association. The intention of the ACPPD is to account for the change in the volume and mix of hospital services as well as the change in prices. This index is calculated by taking the figure for total hospital expenditures (excluding capital investment) and dividing it by the number of patient days. Total hospital expenditures include outpatient as well as inpatient care, and the AHA has therefore recently begun to publish an "adjusted" ACPPD which excludes outpatient care. However, Feldstein and Taylor (1981), who generally quote the ACPPD, view the adjustment as somewhat arbitrary and rely on the original ACPPD figure as a measure of total hospital cost inflation.

It is important to keep in mind that the IHSC and ACPPD are *not* measures of productivity, efficiency, or price increases. These two measures are only very broad indicators of the rapidly expanding amount of resources spent on medical care each year, and indicate in part the willingness of Americans to buy more and better hospital services than ever before.

Magnitude of the Cost Problem

How much has the ACPPD actually increased? Since 1950 the ACPPD has gone from $15.62 to $251.02, a sixteen-fold increase, and it has nearly doubled since 1974 (see line B, Table 1.1). Yet prices for other goods and services have increased as well. Line D gives the ACPPD in constant dollars, illustrating that, even accounting for inflation, the ACPPD is five times what it was in 1950 and has more than doubled since 1966. One indicator of the *relative* quantity of resources devoted to health care is the percentage of the GNP devoted to health expenditures. National health expenditures rose from 4.5 percent of the GNP in 1950, to 7.2 percent in 1970, and 9.5 percent in 1980 (see Table 1.2) (Gibson, 1979).

Table 1.1 Insurance and the Net Cost of Hospital Care. Short-Term Non-Federal General Hospitals, Selected Years 1950–1979

	1950	1955	1960	1966	1970	1972	1974	1975	1976	1977	1978	1979
A. Percentage of Costs Paid by:												
1. Private Insurance	29.3	44.7	52.5	51.4	45.6	45.4	45.4	43.6	44.9	42.8	42.7	43.0
2. Government	21.1	19.9	18.8	25.5	37.8	41.1	42.8	44.5	44.0	43.6	43.0	43.0
3. Direct Consumer Spending	49.6	35.2	28.7	23.1	16.6	13.5	11.8	11.9	11.1	13.5	14.2	14.0 est.
B. Average Cost per Patient Day[1]	15.62	23.12	32.23	48.15	81.01	105.21	128.05	151.53	175.08	200.29	224.53	251.02
C. 1. Net Consumer Cost per Diem[2]	7.75	8.14	9.25	11.12	13.53	14.20	15.11	18.03	19.43	27.04	31.88	35.14
2. Net Consumer Cost per Diem[3]	9.82	10.19	11.38	12.41	21.71	24.09	26.38	32.43	34.70	47.94	55.93	61.65
D. Average Cost per Patient Day (1967 dollars)	21.66	28.83	36.34	49.54	69.66	83.97	86.70	94.00	102.33	110.35	114.90	115.46

Table 1.1 (continued)

	1950	1955	1960	1966	1970	1972	1974	1975	1976	1977	1978	1979
E. 1. Net Consumer Cost per Diem (1967 dollars)[2]	10.75	10.15	10.43	11.44	11.63	11.34	10.23	11.18	11.36	14.90	16.32	16.16
2. Net Consumer Cost per Diem (1967 dollars)[3]	13.62	12.71	12.83	12.77	18.67	19.22	17.86	20.11	20.35	26.41	28.62	28.35
F. Average Cost per Day Relative to CPI Annual Percentage Change	—	5.9	4.7	5.3	9.2	10.3	0.6	8.4	8.9	7.8	4.1	0.5
G. CPI (1967 = 100)	0.721	0.802	0.887	0.972	1.163	1.253	1.477	1.612	1.705	1.815	1.954	2.174

SOURCES: Gibson, R. M. (1980) "National Health Expenditures, 1979," *Health Care Financing Review*, Summer 1980. *Handbook of Basic Economic Statistics* (1980), 24:5 (May), Economic Statistics Bureau, Washington, D.C.

NOTE: These percentages and the corresponding figures for later years are calculated on the basis of data published by the Social Security Administration and the American Hospital Association. The Social Security Administration estimates total expenditure on hospital care and the proportions financed by government, private insurance, and direct consumer spending. All of these amounts refer to care in all types of hospitals, including long-term and psychiatric institutions, and not just the short-term hospitals that are the subject of the current report. To develop estimates for short-term hospitals, we subtracted the American Hospital Association's measures of the cost of care in federal, long-term, tuberculosis, and psychiatric hospitals from the Social Security values for total and government spending. An alternative estimating procedure that started with the American Hospital Association data to estimate private expenditure directly produced almost the exact estimates as those presented here.

[1] ACPPD
[2] ACPPD × (Direct Consumer Expenditures/Total Expenditures).
[3] ACPPD × (Direct Consumer Expenditures/Private Expenditures).

Table 1.2   National Health Expenditures (aggregate and per capita)

Year Ending June 30	GNP (in billions)	Health Expenditures (in millions)	Health Expenses per capita	Health as a Percentage of GNP	Hospital Care as a Percentage of GNP[1]
1929	$ 101.3	$ 3,589	$ 29.16	3.5	0.7
1935	68.9	2,846	22.04	4.1	0.9
1940	95.4	3,883	28.98	4.1	0.9
1950	264.8	12,027	78.35	4.5	1.0
1955	381.0	17,330	103.76	4.5	1.1
1960	498.3	25,856	141.63	5.2	1.5
1965	688.0	38,892	197.75	5.9	1.9
1966	722.4	42,109	211.56	5.8	1.9
1967	773.5	47,897	237.93	6.2	2.2
1968	830.2	53,765	264.37	6.5	2.3
1969	904.2	60,617	295.20	6.7	2.4
1970	960.2	69,201	333.57	7.2	2.7
1971	1,019.8	77,162	368.25	7.6	2.9
1972	1,111.8	86,687	409.71	7.8	3.0
1973	1,238.6	95,383	447.31	7.7	3.0
1974	1,361.2	106,321	495.01	7.8	3.1
1975	1,451.5	123,716	571.21	8.5	3.3

Year Ending September 30

1975	1,487.1	127,719	588.48	8.6	3.4
1976	1,667.4	145,102	663.06	8.7	3.5
1977	1,838.0	162,627	736.92	8.8	3.5
1978	2,107.6	192,400	863.01	9.1	3.6

Projections

1980	2,572.0	244.6	1,078.0	9.5	3.8
1985	4,168.7	438.2	1,846.0	10.5	4.4
1990	6,562.5	757.9	3,057.0	11.5	5.1

SOURCE: Health Care Financing Administration (DHHS), and Freeland *et al.* (1980).

[1] This is an underestimate of the hospital sector's share of GNP because the figure does not include services provided by nonsalaried physicians within hospitals. Because physicians have increasingly pursued subspecialty careers that demand increased reliance on the hospital, the magnitude of the hospital sector underestimation bias has undoubtedly increased since the 1950s.

Increased Intensity

Aggregate expenditures on hospital care* rose from $27.799 billion in 1970 to $76.025 billion in 1978 (estimated). On a per capita basis, hospital care expenditures rose from $133.39 in 1970 to $340.93 in 1978 (estimated). These aggregate figures can be broken down into various components in order to facilitate discussion of hospital cost inflation. Accordingly, inflation accounts for 63 percent of the increase from 1970–1978, population growth for 7 percent, and increased "intensity" for 30 percent of the increase. "Intensity" refers to changes in the nature and quantity of services rendered (Gibson, 1979). Although the average number of days per stay in hospitals has declined, the resources utilized during each day have increased and the number of inpatient days overall has increased 8 percent since 1970. As an example of increased utilization of resources, from 1972 to 1977 the number of hospital laboratory tests nearly doubled and the number of surgical operations grew 18 percent (Gibson 1979). The data surveyed in Chapter 12 suggest that the intensity of services per case may be increasing without any concomitant increase in quality of care.

Increased expenditures on labor in the hospital setting is an example of the fact that the increase in the cost of hospital care reflects partly inflation (an increase in the *prices* of the resources employed) and partly an increase in intensity (an increase in the *amount* of resources employed). The argument is frequently made that because hospital personnel have traditionally been paid less than personnel in other professions, hospitals went through a catch-up phase in the 1950s and 1960s during which wages came to be on a par with wages in other industries. Over the 20-year period 1955–1975, earnings per employee increased on an average annual basis by 6.3 percent, but in addition the number of employees per patient day increased by an average of 2.6 percent per year, accounting for some 30 percent of the total increase in the cost of labor. Spending on nonlabor inputs increased so rapidly, however, that the fraction of costs accounted for by labor actually decreased (Feldstein and Taylor, 1981).

---

* Hospital care includes inpatient and outpatient care in all hospitals and all services and supplies provided by hospitals. Services provided by non-staff physicians are excluded.

Insurance and the Demand for Care

How, then, does the tremendous increase in expenditures on hospital care relate to the out-of-pocket costs borne by the consumer of hospital care at the time of illness? In other words, how is it that consumers are willing to bear the costs of such an increase in the intensity of hospital care without an equivalent return in the form of better health? Part of the answer lies in the fact that although there has been a great increase in the amount of national resources devoted to hospital care, there has been very little change in the cost of hospital care to the consumer at the time of illness.

In 1950 approximately 50 percent of the cost of hospital care (short-term, non-federal) was paid directly by the consumer and 50 percent was paid by third parties, including government and private insurance. By 1979 the proportion of the costs paid directly by the consumer had dropped to 14 percent (see line A.3, Table 1.1). The result of this growth in third-party coverage is that the average cost of a patient day to the consumer has only doubled in constant dollars since 1950, whereas the ACPPD is more than five times what it was in constant dollar terms in 1950 (see lines D and E, Table 1.1). The Net Consumer Cost figure just quoted excludes government assistance, since most families do not receive the benefit of such assistance. However, if government payments are included in the calculations, then the net consumer cost of a patient day would have only increased by 60 percent in constant dollars since 1950.

There is substantial evidence to indicate that when a large proportion of medical costs are offset by insurance, doctors will recommend more and better services, and consumers in turn will demand more and better services. Thus as insurance increases, a higher quality of care is demanded. At this juncture, it is important to make the point that the increase in demand is for greater intensity of care per diem, rather than for more bed days.* Hospitals, as they work to fill the demand for increased services, raise prices in order to raise revenue which can be used to provide the more expensive form of care demanded. Since most consumers do not pay out-of-pocket for medical care because they are heavily insured, they are shielded from the resulting increase in prices and do not respond in the normal way by curtailing demand. On the contrary, as consumers

---

* This is not to say that there was not a dramatic expansion in the demand for days of hospitalization prior to 1975, but the demand for days abated in the 1970s (Table 1.3).

Table 1.3   Growth Rates in the Demand Supply of Non-Federal Short-Term Hospitals, Selected Years 1950–1980

Year	FTE Personnel per Adjusted[1] Patient Day	Patient Days per Year		Admissions per Year (in thousands)	Number of Hospitals	Number of Beds	Bed Occupancy (percent)
		Days (millions)	Annual Growth (percent)				
1950	1.62	136	2.2	16,663	5,031	505,000	73.7
1955	1.85	149	1.9	19,100	5,237	568,000	71.5
1960	2.06	174	3.1	22,970	5,407	639,000	74.7
1965	2.24	205	3.3	26,463	5,736	741,000	76.0
1966	2.37	215	4.9	26,897	5,812	768,000	76.5
1967	2.41	223	3.7	26,988	5,850	788,000	77.6
1970	2.65	242	2.8	29,252	5,859	848,000	78.0
1974	2.89	256	1.4	32,943	5,977	931,000	75.3
1978	3.23	263	1.7	34,575	5,935	980,000	73.5
1979	3.28	267	1.7	35,160	5,923	988,000	73.8
1980	3.43	279	4.2	37,562	5,945	990,000	75.9

SOURCE: *American Hospital Association Guide: 1981 Edition*, Chicago: A.H.A., 1981.
[1] Full-Time Equivalent (FTE) personnel adjusted for outpatient visits rendered.

observe the higher prices, or cost, of medical care, their desire for insurance increases and likewise the demand for medical care increases, so the inflationary cycle continues. This six-step medical cost inflationary cycle is illustrated in Figure 1.1. The rate limiting step, the stage in the cycle at which intervention is most effective, is between A and B, the point at which insurance stimulates demand.

It is easy to see why individuals would want to insure themselves against the risk of a very large medical bill; it is not so readily apparent why they are willing to pay the additional actuarial charges associated with insurance for small bills when these extra charges could be avoided if the small bills were paid out-of-pocket. The reasons for the proliferation of comprehensive "first-dollar" insurance policies are two-fold. First, the present tax structure encourages such policies. Second, these insurance policies can be seen as a form of precommitment on the part of policy holders.

The current tax structure encourages comprehensive health insurance in the following way. Employer-paid health insurance may be deducted from the employing company's taxable income. At the same time, employees need not include the value of health insurance policies in their taxable income, nor are the premiums subject to social security or state income tax. Thus health insurance can be considered to be a form of tax-exempt extra income. In addition,

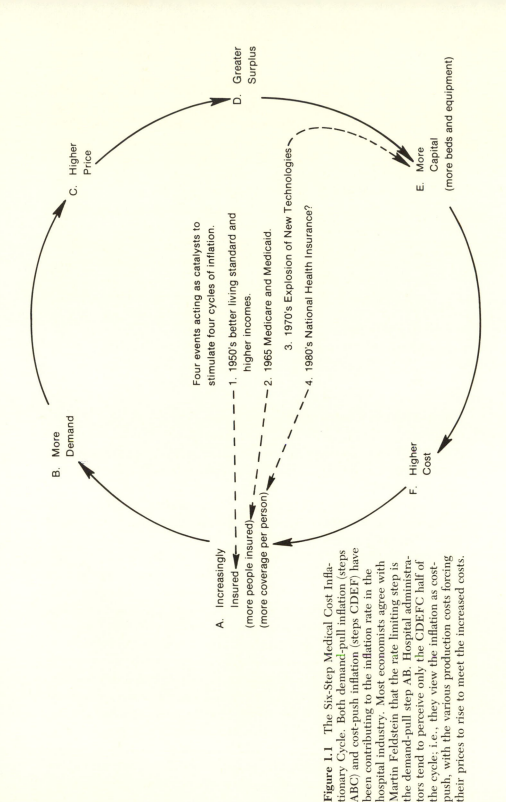

Figure 1.1 The Six-Step Medical Cost Inflationary Cycle. Both demand-pull inflation (steps ABC) and cost-push inflation (steps CDEF) have been contributing to the inflation rate in the hospital industry. Most economists agree with Martin Feldstein that the rate limiting step is the demand-pull step AB. Hospital administrators tend to perceive only the CDEFC half of the cycle; i.e., they view the inflation as cost-push, with the various production costs forcing their prices to rise to meet the increased costs.

approximately one-half of the amount an individual pays for health insurance is tax deductible. The "tax break" amounted to some $4 billion for individuals and $22 billion for business in 1980. This government subsidy of health insurance premiums averages 18 percent of the premiums and, in effect, offsets all of the charges associated with private insurance as well as part of the cost of service (Feldstein and Friedman, 1974; Feldstein, 1977).

Health insurance can also be viewed as a form of "precommitment" on the part of individuals who do not want monetary costs to influence their choice of medical care. By precommitting themselves through insurance, individuals do not have to make the choice between expensive, highly intensive care and cheaper, less intensive care (Fuchs, 1979). In addition, insurance is a form of self-control for individuals who feel they might spend all their money now, in the short term, and not have it in the long term when they need it for medical care; it therefore acts to relieve some of the tension in the conflict between long-term and short-term goals.

The Causes of Cost Inflation

The underlying causes of the inflation in overall expenditures on hospital care can be divided into four categories: (1) increased demand (demand-pull); (2) increases in the cost of producing care; (3) increases in the prices of inputs used to produce care; and (4) changes in the markets that supply inputs, particularly the labor market (supply-push).

When a product is demanded at a rate faster than it can be produced, the product is considered scarce and its price rises. At the same time, the demand rises for factors used in its production, and so the prices of the factors rise. This form of inflation has been labeled "demand-pull" and is considered a major cause of inflation in medical costs.

Although the explosion in health insurance during the past 25 years is the single most important factor in the increased demand for medical care, other factors have had an influence as well. Growth in population and increases in the average life span have contributed to the demand for medical care. The fastest growing age group is the 65-and-older category, whose per capita expenditures on health care are almost three times that of adults aged 19 to 64. In addition, many innovations in medical technology are extremely expensive and in-

crease the demand for medical care in a multipl
though the development of antibiotics and oth
cost-effective in saving lives, new developments
ogy, such as chemotherapy and organ transpl
pensive equipment and skilled personnel; by
of curing illness, such technology can be radically
The cost-increasing nature of medical technology will be discu
in Chapters 3, 4, and 9.

Several factors, aside from nationwide inflation and excess aggregate demand, have contributed to an increase in the cost of producing medical care. Malpractice insurance, a negligible problem 15
years ago, has increased an average of 29 percent a year from 1970 to
1978 (Freeland *et al.*, 1979). The threat of malpractice suits has
caused an increase in the number of tests ordered by physicians.
Complying with the numerous federal and state regulations and
reporting requirements also has contributed to the cost of medical
care. Lastly, cost-based reimbursement and the non-profit nature of
the industry leave little incentive for hospitals to try to reduce costs
and produce care in a more efficient manner.

In addition to demand-pull inflation and added costs, the hospital
industry has suffered from the nationwide inflation that affects all
industries. The price of fuel oil and coal for hospitals increased by 13
percent on an average annual basis and payroll expenses and employee benefits increased by 8.5 percent per year over the nine-year
period 1970–1978 (Freeland *et al.*, 1979). One infrequently publicized fact about the cost of inputs to the hospital industry is that the
cost of medical equipment and supplies has generally been 1 percent
to 3 percent below the consumer price index.

Fluctuations in the labor market may have contributed to a
"supply-push" inflation in the wages of hospital employees. During
periods of low unemployment, the wages of workers in low-wage
industries tend to increase, or "catch-up," relative to wages in
high-wage industries; but decrease when the level of unemployment
returns to normal. According to Salkever (1975), hospital wage rates
increased as unemployment fell from 6.7 percent in 1961 to 3.5
percent in 1969. In addition, to the extent that hospitals are considered to be a secondary market for unskilled workers, increasing
welfare payments and declining discrimination have contributed to a
narrowing of the wage differential (Salkever, 1975). The cost of labor
is an important consideration in hospitals, accounting for nearly 60
percent of total costs (Freeland *et al.*, 1979). In summary, conditions

he labor market have contributed to the overall increase in labor
xpense for hospitals, along with causes such as employee pressure
for higher wages, philanthropic wage setting, and a demand-pull
expansion of employment in hospitals. The demand-pull hypothesis
has most recently been supported by Furst and Markland (1980).
These authors have looked at the lead and lag relationship between
hospital capital investment and increases in operating cost between
1955 and 1977 and reject the hypothesis that plant assets lead to
changes in operating costs. The study concludes that hospital costs
rise in response to increased demand and changes in operating costs
lead to changes in plant assets—that is, in Figure 1.1, B stimulates E
and not the reverse.

Not to be overlooked is the role of the physician vis-à-vis the
supply of beds. Once a consumer enters a hospital, the cost of his
care becomes of secondary importance to him, because he is concerned only about getting well and he no longer controls the amount
of care provided. Taking responsibility for the consumer, the
physician-provider controls both supply and demand, acting as an
input broker for this patient. The physician demands the specialized
services of the hospital, while he supplies his personal services. The
consumer has little interest in the cost, because it is the insurance
carrier who pays the tab. In industries where consumers are unin-
sured and where technology improves slowly, efficiency and cost
containment are everyday commitments for managers. In the hospital industry,* however, the doctors hold power over the managers,
more than 90 percent of consumers are insured, and technology
changes rapidly; consequently, there is no incentive to economize.
The United States always ranks 11th behind Britain, Sweden, and a
number of socialist countries when evaluated by mortality statistics.
England and Sweden get better results and spend less of
their GNP on health care, because they put their money into ambulatory care and limit the growth in subspecialty technocrats by
fixing the supply of hospital beds (Battistella and Eastaugh, 1980). In
1946 these two countries and the United States had 240 acute hospital beds per 100,000 population. The American ratio has doubled

---

* In some sense, hospitals have grown "richer" than physicians, especially following
the passage of Medicare and Medicaid. Since 1950 the rate of physician price
inflation has been less than the rate of hospital price inflation (in Table 1.4, column
2-C is always less than column 3), although both the hospital industry and the
physician service industry are outperforming the general economy.

Table 1.4   Physician Services: Annual Rates of Increase in Expenditures, and Allocation of the Cost Inflation to Price, per Capita Use, and Population Shifts

| Time Period | (1)
Annual
Increase in
Total Expenses
for Physician
Services | Sources of Physician Cost Inflation | | | (3)
Annual
Increase
in Hospital
Price[1] |
		(2-A) Population	(2-B) Per Capita Use	(2-C) Price	
1950–1955	6.0%	1.7%	0.9%	3.5%	6.3%
1955–1960	9.1	1.7	4.1	3.3	6.5
1960–1965	9.0	1.5	4.9	2.6	6.6
1965–1968	9.8	1.1	2.5	6.2	11.3
1968–1971	10.9	0.9	2.9	7.1	14.6
1971–1974[2]	10.0	0.8	5.2	4.0	11.0
1974–1977	17.6	0.8	5.8	11.0	15.2
1977–1980	13.2	0.8	3.5	8.9	14.0

SOURCE: Health Care Financing Administration, Department of Health and Human Services, unpublished data.

[1] Charges per inpatient day.
[2] The Economic Stabilization Program was in effect 8/15/71 to 4/30/74.

since 1946 (Maxwell, 1975) whereas the other two countries have maintained the 1946 bed-per-population ratio (Department of Health and Social Security, 1978 and 1979).

The twin problems of inflation and oversupply of beds were largely caused by carte blanche government financing of Medicare, Medicaid, and the Hill-Burton program. The Hill-Burton program provided the seed money for doubling our bed-per-population ratio. Hill-Burton directly supplied hospital capital to the industry at zero price (see Chapter 9). The October 1976 policy statement of the Institute of Medicine pointed to curtailing the supply of hospital beds as the most important medicine for controlling costs.

Cost Containment

One may approach the problem of containing rising hospital costs from two directions. First, one may try to lower the cost of production of hospital care at any level of intensity by improving efficiency, by achieving greater economies of scale through building larger hospitals, or by redesigning the market to encourage competition. Second, one may try to curtail the current trend toward more intensive care through programs designed to limit supply expansion (for example, the Certificate of Need program), through preventive medicine, or through attempts to decrease the demand for medical care by encouraging greater cost-consciousness on the part of consumers.

Improving Efficiency

Essentially, any attempt to lower costs while not reducing the quality or intensity of care is an attempt to improve efficiency. Efficiency can be identified in three forms: technical, economic, and allocative. *Technical efficiency* refers to the relationship between input and output, irrespective of cost. If one cannot reduce the amount of input and still produce the same amount of output, then maximum technical efficiency has been achieved. In a hospital context, for example, inputs might be full-time equivalent employees and outputs would be days of care. *Economic efficiency* refers to the relationship between inputs and cost. When a day of care is provided at the minimum possible cost, there is economic efficiency. *Allocative efficiency* is achieved when one person, department, or service cannot be made better off without making another person, department, or service worse off.

An example of an improvement in economic efficiency that simultaneously decreases technical efficiency is the increased use of ancillary personnel. The substitution of nurse practitioners or physician assistants for physicians lowers the overall cost of care although it may result in the use of more employees. There are several reasons, however, why physicians may be reluctant to increase their use of ancillary personnel, including patient dissatisfaction, lower quality care, malpractice suits, costs of training, added managerial burden, and problems with licensure policies that restrict the activity of ancillary personnel (Human Resources Research Center, 1972).

One way to induce efficiency in the hospital industry is to encourage competition. To this end, the federal government has made an effort to foster competition and thereby decrease prices through new programs designed to alter the distribution of physicians geographically and across specialities. An increase in the concentration of physicians in an area seems to have a moderating effect on fees, at least with respect to general practitioners and surgeons (Sloan, 1976). HMOs and Surgicenters are competitive new entrants to medical markets whose growth has unfortunately been retarded by health planning. The merits of competitive health plans will be reviewed in Chapters 7 and 8.

The Merits of Prevention

One may consider the efficiency of medical care in a broader context by taking output as the overall health of the nation rather than simply as days of care. Victor Fuchs has stated that "when the state of medical science and other health-determining variables are held constant, the marginal contribution of medical care to health is very small in modern nations." In other words, one cannot simply add more doctors and hospitals and expect an equivalent improvement in health. Fuchs gives several reasons for this low marginal contribution. Patients and physicians use more discretion when physicians are scarce—that is to say, patients seek medical care less often when it is difficult to obtain, and physicians tend to concentrate on those patients who need care most. Many highly effective treatments such as vaccinations do not require the huge amounts of resources required by many generally less effective treatments such as heart transplants. As medical care proliferates, iatrogenic disease becomes a problem, exemplified by highly risky surgical interventions. Lastly, it is difficult to measure the output of medical care in terms of health, in that many factors other than medical care contribute to health—for example, nutrition and environment (Fuchs, 1979).

Studies that attempt to measure the health of the nation use indexes such as mortality rates, days of disability, effective life expectancy, or self-perceived health status. Some authors have gone a step further in evaluating the efficacy of the U.S. health care system by comparing these indexes with those of other modern nations. In 1970 the United States had the highest mortality rate of any OECD (Organization for Economic Cooperation and Development) nation for males 45 to 54 (Sorkin, 1975). In addition, the infant mortality rate for the United States was higher than for the majority of OECD nations.

As medical care consumes an increasing percentage of GNP with correspondingly little improvement in health, researchers have been led to consider the value of preventive medicine in cost containment. This can be viewed as a problem in allocative efficiency: At what point are resources better employed in the prevention of illness than in curing it? Charles E. Phelps (1978) states:

Studies cited from the literature show that many commonly accepted screening procedures have no observable payoff in health status or medical expenses saved. In stark contrast, personal behavioral decisions, such as smoking and dietary patterns, appear to have dramatic effects on health and mortality. Public policy appears to be better directed toward inducement of such health-producing behavior than inducement of further medical preventive procedures.

As evidence for the conclusions above, prepaid group practice plans (PGPP) have not been able to show that preventive measures such as physical examinations or multiphase screening are cost-saving. It would seem that private insurance companies would cover preventive care if it were cost-effective. Phelps suggests that the reason prevention is not covered by insurance companies is that it may not be effective, or, if effective, it may not be cost-saving. Even in the event that preventive services are cost-saving, the gains may be so far in the future or the elasticity of supply in the industry may be so high that insurance companies are unable to reap any benefits. One of the problems with preventive screening examinations is that the cost of treating false-positive results, along with adverse psychological effects, may outweigh the benefits of detecting a disease in its early stages (Phelps, 1978). In the same vein, Fuchs has suggested that if expensive cancer treatment programs did not exist, people might be more likely to follow their own prevention programs (Fuchs, 1979). In this case, it might be more important to encourage a change in behavioral patterns rather than to support research into expensive cancer treatments.

Economies of Scale

In considering what happens to the level of output as the level of input increases, we are addressing the issue of economies of scale. If output grows at the same rate as inputs are increased, then there are constant returns to scale (per unit costs are the same at any given level of output). If output increases at a rate greater than inputs are increased, then there are increasing returns to scale (per unit costs decrease at higher levels of output). If output grows at a rate less than the corresponding increase in inputs, then there are decreasing returns to scale (per unit costs increase as output rises).

Economies of scale are generally illustrated by the long run average cost curve (LRACC) in Figure 1.2. Hospital size is measured by either number of beds or average daily patient census. Output is typically measured by patient days, and in some cases patient dis-

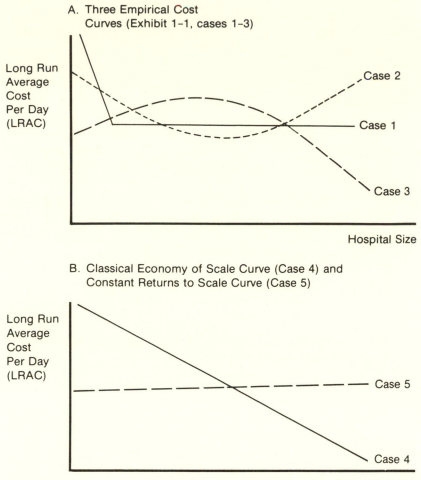

A. Three Empirical Cost Curves (Exhibit 1-1, cases 1-3)

Long Run Average Cost Per Day (LRAC)

Case 2

Case 1

Case 3

Hospital Size

B. Classical Economy of Scale Curve (Case 4) and Constant Returns to Scale Curve (Case 5)

Long Run Average Cost Per Day (LRAC)

Case 5

Case 4

Hospital Size

Figure 1.2 Relationships Between Hospital Size and Cost. (Case numbers are referred to in Exhibit 1.1).

charges or admissions. The classic configuration of the LRACC is the U-shape illustrated in Figure 1.2A, Case 2. Generally, average costs are expected to decrease as output increases up to a point of minimum average costs, after which diseconomies of scale may take over. This point of minimum average costs is the optimal size for a firm or hospital (or the optimal level of output). Diseconomies beyond a certain point may be the result of inefficient management in large-scale facilities, or they may reflect the costs of increased travel time for physicians and patients (Sorkin, 1975).

The central problem with applying the concept of economies of scale to hospital size is that hospitals do not produce a uniform product. Generally, the larger hospitals tend to treat more complex cases and to provide a much broader spectrum of care; thus a patient day in a small hospital is not equivalent to a patient day in a large hospital. Accordingly any study of economies of scale must take case mix into account.

Research studies on economies of scale in the hospital sector have found five different shapes of the LRACC (see Exhibit 1.1). Failure to account for case mix results in a U-shaped LRACC. When adjustment for case mix is made, the LRACC is found to be slightly

Exhibit 1.1   Survey of Studies Concerning Economies of Scale in the Hospital Sector

Case 1.   L-Shaped Average Cost Curve Found:

Feldstein, M. S., and J. Schuttinga. "Hospital Costs in Massachusetts: A Methodological Study," *Inquiry* 14:1 (March 1977), 22–31.

Francisco, E. W. "Analysis of Cost Variations Among Short-Term General Hospitals," in H. E. Klarman (ed.), *Empirical Studies in Health Economics*. Baltimore, Maryland: Johns Hopkins University Press, 1970, 321–332.

Lave, J. R., and L. B. Lave. "Hospital Cost Functions," *American Economic Review* 60 (June 1970), 379–395.

Case 2.   U-Shaped Average Cost Curve Found:

Carr, W. J., and P. J. Feldstein. "The Relationship of Cost to Hospital Size," *Inquiry* 4:2 (June 1967), 45–65.

Cohen, H. A. "Variations in Cost Among Hospitals of Different Sizes," *Southern Economic Journal* 33 (January 1967), 355–366.

Feldstein, M. S. *Economic Analysis for Health Service Efficiency*. Amsterdam: North-Holland Publishing Co., 1968.

Case 3.   Inverted U-Shaped Average Cost Curve Found:

Ingbar, M. L., and L. D. Taylor. *Hospital Costs in Massachusetts*. Cambridge, Massachusetts: Harvard University Press, 1968.

Case 4.   Downward Sloping Average Cost Curve Throughout:

Baron, D. P. "A Study of Hospital Cost Inflation," *Journal of Human Resources* 9 (Winter 1974), 33–49.

Berry, R. E., Jr. "Returns to Scale in the Production of Hospital Services," *Health Service Research* 2 (Summer 1967), 123–139.

Feldstein, P. J. *An Empirical Investigation of the Marginal Cost of Hospital Services*. Chicago, Illinois: University of Chicago, Center for Health Administration Studies, 1961.

Case 5.   Constant Returns to Scale:

Evans, R. G. "Behavioral Cost Functions for Hospitals," *Canadian Journal of Economics* 4 (May 1971), 198–215.

Lipscomb, J., I. E. Raskin, and J. Eichenholz. "The Use of Marginal Cost Estimates in Hospital Cost Containment Policy," in M. Zubkoff, I. E. Raskin, and R. S. Hanft (eds.), *Hospital Cost Containment: Selected Notes for Future Policy*. New York: Prodist Press, 1978, pp. 514–537.

downward sloping or flat for larger hospitals, indicating that economies of scale may exist although the economies may not be great
enough to justify much larger hospitals. An additional criticism of
studies of the LRACC is that highly aggregated cost data make it
impossible to separate the diseconomies due to size from those due
to inefficiency, thus potentially leading to wrong conclusions regarding the optimal hospital size (Finkler, 1979).

With regard to cost containment, achieving economies of scale
may not be our salvation, for throughout the series of studies the
LRACC was found to be very shallow. Economies of scale were
determined to be at most 16 percent between the largest and the
smallest hospitals in Figure 1.2 and Exhibit 1.1. The absence of
economies of scale hospital-wide may be puzzling to some analysts.
Much more significant economies of scale have been found on a
departmental basis, under conditions where the product is
homogeneous, by HAS (Hospital Administrative Services) researchers. Consequently, one would presuppose that if we could perform a perfect study adjusting for heterogeneous product mix of
patient cases, then economies of scale would be more significant than the 16 percent difference between the smallest and
largest hospitals in Figure 1.2B, Case 4. In summary, the data on
economies of scale is not persuasive enough to suggest that we close
all hospitals below a certain size. The increased travel time to consumers and staff associated with closing all below-average-size hospitals would probably outweigh the benefits accrued in increasing
returns to scale.

Limiting Supply

One attempt to bring under control the growing intensity of medical
care is through Certificate of Need programs which require formal
justification and review of proposed investment projects with costs
in excess of a specified dollar amount. All states receiving federal
funds are required to introduce Certificate of Need (CON) programs by 1980 (National Health Planning 1974). Previously, the
Social Security Act Amendments of 1972 required this type of control under Medicare, Medicaid, and Maternal and Child Health
reimbursement programs. There are two problems with CON programs. First, it is difficult to set specific, objective standards of need.
Second, CON programs have the adverse effect of limiting potential
competition by tangentially restricting the development of large
HMOs. An "improvement" to Certificate of Need programs was

suggested by the Carter Administration in 1977 and 1979: that a limit be placed on nationwide capital expenditures ("capital cap") and allocated among the states, thereby forcing local hospitals and planning agencies to more carefully evaluate trade-offs among various investment proposals.

Another potential approach to containing costs is state-sponsored prospective rate-setting programs. Prospective reimbursement in the context of the state rate regulatory process is generally regarded as the most effective present cost-containment approach. The seven regulated states had significantly lower inflation rates in the late 1970s (see Table 1.5). However, the lower inflation rate in total hospital expenses for these seven states may reflect factors in addition to the presence of state rate regulatory programs—for example, population growth in all seven states was below the national average.

Colorado might well have been counted as the eighth regulated state, because it had a rate program designed by Maryland state consultants for one year. The Colorado program was grossly understaffed and lacked the three-year start-up period that Maryland officials experienced. However, the anticipatory response to the Col-

Table 1.5 **Total Hospital Expenditure Inflation Rate for Regulated and Non-Regulated States, 1977–1980, for Non-Federal Short-Term General Hospitals**

Rate Regulatory Status	Annual Percentage Change in Total Hospital Expenses[1]			
	1977	1978	1979	1980
Highly Regulated States[2]: New York, Maryland, Massachusetts	10.5	8.7	8.8	12.3
Other Regulated States[3]: Connecticut, New Jersey, Washington, Wisconsin	12.7	11.0	10.9	14.2
43 Non-Regulated States[4]:	15.8	14.0	14.4	22.6
U.S. Total	14.2	12.6	13.0	19.7

SOURCE: American Hospital Association, *Annual Survey of Hospitals*, 1976–1980.

[1] Expressed as a weighted average, that is, the weight for each state is the amount of total expenses in the given year.
[2] Defined as mandatory rate setting programs implemented prior to 1976.
[3] Defined as mandatory rate setting programs implemented after 1976.
[4] The Behrens-Fisher statistic for comparing mean rates of increase in inflation of regulated and non-regulated states exhibits no statistically significant differences prior to 1976, that is, there is no support for suggesting that regulated states were predisposed to have low inflation rates.

orado program reduced the inflation rate from 3 percent above the national average in 1978 to 3 percent below the 1979 national average. Despite the impressive one-year performance, the Colorado legislature eliminated the program in 1980 in the spirit of deregulation and promoting competition. The annual cost of regulation was judged as prohibitively high ($1.6 million), but the benefits should justify the costs if the Colorado hospital inflation rate was to decrease by 0.5 percentage points. The net effect was to decrease the inflation rate by 6 percentage points; that is, the regulatory approach was cost-beneficial in the short term.

Because physicians are able to influence the demand for their services, the federal government has attempted recently to control the increasing use of medical services by curtailing the supply of physicians. This shift from the traditional policy of encouraging an increase in the supply of physicians involves restrictions on foreign medical school graduates and limitation of capitation payments to medical schools.

Limiting Demand

One strategy to curb the growing intensity of medical care is to reduce the demand for care by encouraging a greater level of cost-consciousness on the part of consumers rather than to decrease the supply. When consumers must pay for at least part of the cost of additional services, they choose to utilize fewer services than they would if fully insured. Thus the intention is to reduce the level of insurance by introducing more deductibles, coinsurance, and copayments. The trend is currently away from cost-sharing arrangements, however, both nationwide and in other countries, as unions and individuals seek the extensive "front-end" early dollar coverage. The public has lobbied for tax incentives to encourage insurance plans that excessively insure—that is, have lower coinsurance rates than are actuarially justified (Feldstein, 1977). In effect, public and individual decisions concerning health insurance could be considered as a form of precommitment, in that the potential patients have precommitted themselves to almost disregard price in medical resource consumption decisions. Our society probably will continue to dictate implicitly that no test or procedure be left undone to save a life, and we shall continue to experience a demand-pull inflation unique to medicine. But health care in general, and hospital care in particular, will feel increasing pressure from other sectors of the economy. For example, if medical care is "priceless," so is national defense and clean housing. Obviously, continued inflationary pursuit of the medical care goal will compromise other social goals, many of which are health-related.

The Agenda

In the following chapters we shall consider in some detail various aspects of social and institutional cost-containment issues. The problems of rising demand, consumer expectations, and the issue of unnecessary care are the subject of Chapter 2. Viewed in this light, no sensible analyst could conclude that medical technology *per se* is the cause of rising costs. However, curtailment of overcapitalization and inefficient physician ordering habits form an increasingly important set of issues. Economic techniques to perform technology assessment evaluations and change physician behavior, such as cost-benefit and cost-effectiveness analysis, will be reviewed in Chapters 3 and 4. To deal with the cost problem in the 1980s it will be necessary to restructure the financial incentive system. In order to understand the incentives structure, one must first survey the economic models of physician and hospital behavior (Chapter 5). The question of regulatory or competitive solutions will be the subject of Part Two in the text, Chapters 6–8. Part Three of the text, Chapters 9–12, will survey financial management issues relevant to hospital administrators, policymakers, corporate leasing and management chains, and medical schools. The concluding chapter will enable us to critically review and interrelate the disparate economic and financial management issues raised in the text. One final word of caution for those who believe that the unplanned medical economy is a "nonsystem" of scattered parts: Observe how systematically providers resist government attempts to institute change.

References

BATTISTELLA, R., and EASTAUGH, S. (1980). "Hospital Cost Containment." *Proceedings of the Academy of Political Science* 33:4 (Winter), 192–205.

Department of Health and Social Security (1978). *Digest of Health Statistics for England and Wales 1977.* London, England.

Department of Health and Social Security, Office of Health Economics (1979). "Scarce Resources in Health Care," *Milbank Memorial Fund Quarterly* 57:2 (Spring), 265–287.

FELDSTEIN, M. (1970). "The Rising Cost of Hospital Care." Discussion Paper No. 129, Harvard Institute of Economic Research.

FELDSTEIN, M. (1977). "The High Cost of Hospitals and What to Do About It," *The Public Interest* 12:48 (Summer), 40–54.

FELDSTEIN, M., and FRIEDMAN, B. (1974). "Tax Subsidies, the Rational Demand for Insurance and the Health Care Crisis." Discussion Paper No. 382, Harvard Institute of Economic Research.

FELDSTEIN, M., and TAYLOR, A. (1981). "The Rapid Rise of Hospital Costs," in M. Feldstein (ed.), *Hospital Costs and Health Insurance*, Chap. 1. Cambridge, Mass.: Harvard University Press.

FINKLER, S. (1979). "On the Shape of the Long Run Average Cost Curve," *Health Services Research* 14:4 (Winter), 281–289.

FREELAND, M., CALAT, G., and SCHENDLER, C. E. (1980). "Projections of National Health Expenditures, 1980, 1985, and 1990," *Health Care Financing Review* (Winter), 1–27.

FREELAND, M. S., ANDERSON, G., and SCHENDLER, C. E. (1979). "National Hospital Input Price Index," *Health Care Financing Review* (Summer), 37–52.

FUCHS, VICTOR (1979). "Economics, Health, and Post-Industrial Society," *Milbank Memorial Fund Quarterly/Health and Society* 57:2, 153–181.

FURST, R., and MARKLAND, R. (1980). "How Hospital Capital Investment and Operating Costs Relate," *Inquiry* 17:4 (Winter), 313–317.

GIBSON, R. (1980). "National Health Expenditures 1979," *Health Care Financing Review* 2:2 (Summer), 1–36.

Human Resources Research Center (1972). "Utilization of Ancillary Personnel by Physicians in Private Practice." Working Paper, University of Southern California.

JACOBS, P., BAUERSCHMIDT, A. D., and FURST, R. W. (1978). "Hospital Cost Inflation and Health Insurance: A Complex Market Model," *Inquiry* 15:3 (September), 217–224.

MAXWELL, R. (1975). "Health Care: The Growing Dilemma: Needs versus Resources in Western Europe, the U.S., and the U.S.S.R." A McKinsey Survey Report, McKinsey and Company, Inc.

NEWHOUSE, J. P., and TAYLOR, V. (1971). "How Shall We Pay For Hospital Care?" *The Public Interest* 6:23 (Spring), 78–92.

PHELPS, C. E. (1978). "Illness Prevention and Medical Insurance," *The Journal of Human Resources* 13 (Supplement), NBER Conference on the Economics of Physician and Patient Behavior, 183–207.

SALKEVER, D. S. (1975). "Hospital Wage Inflation: Supply-Push or Demand-Pull?" *Quarterly Review of Economics and Business* 15:33 (Autumn), 33–48.

SLOAN, F. (1976). "Physician Fee Inflation: Evidence from the Late 1960's," in R. Rosett (ed.), *The Role of Health Insurance in the Health Services Sector*. New York: Watson Academic, 321–354.

SORKIN, A. (1975). *Health Economics*. Lexington, Mass.: D. C. Heath.

Chapter 2

ECONOMIC MODELS OF PHYSICIAN AND HOSPITAL BEHAVIOR

> *The first step in the analysis of the medical-care market is a comparison between the actual market and the competitive model.*
>
> —KENNETH ARROW, 1963

> *An important general lesson in this example is that a theory can make "unrealistic" assumptions (in this case profit maximization) but still yield valid predictions. Thus a theory should not be rejected simply because its assumptions are unrealistic or even known to be wrong.*
>
> —JOSEPH NEWHOUSE, 1978

> *Arrow is misleading. . . . The competitive model is irrelevant to an analysis of the medical-care market; the relevant comparison is between the actual market and what equilibria could be achieved under alternative institutional arrangements.*
>
> —MARK PAULY, 1978

The literature on physician and hospital behavior has been characterized by two approaches: utility maximization models (Feldstein, 1970) or profit maximization models (Sloan, 1976). Supporters of the first approach view classical maxims concerning simple profit maximization as totally unrealistic. Supporters of the profit maximization approach view utility maximizers as unnecessarily fuzzy and complex. The situation is complicated because the hospital is an organizational anomaly. The principal input controlling the organization is a group of individuals—the physicians—who neither own nor work as employees of the firm. Rather than work with the unique aspects of the doctor-hospital interaction, most conservative economists have opted for standard competitive analysis of a two-element utility function (profit, and slack or leisure) as the best first approximation to physician and hospital behavior (Pauly and Redisch, 1973). Advocates of the profit maximization model maintain that if a multifaceted model and a simple model work almost equally well, one should prefer the simpler version. Models with "excessive" realism are viewed as a mixed blessing, because they complicate empirical implementation. In some cases, the simple and complex formulations perform equally well, but their explanatory power is too low to place any confidence in the models.

All economic models posit some degree of profit maximization in the physician's utility function, where profit is defined as net earnings above practice overhead costs and above an imputed basic wage for the profession. The specification of an imputed wage allows for formal consideration of the clinician's trade-off of leisure for income. The physician utility function (U) includes some of the following elements:

$$U = f \text{ (profit, leisure time, professional status, internal ethics, complexity of case-mix, study time to keep up-to-date, number of support staff under your supervision, etc.)}$$

Sometimes the utility function is stated in negative terms; for example, the disutility of working more or the disutility to the physician of coercing doctor-induced patient visits. In stark contrast to more traditional markets, the percentage of patient visits that is supplier-initiated is very high (39 percent, Wilensky and Rossiter, 1980). We can infer little about the medical necessity of these patient visits. Both groups of theorists, profit maximizers and utility maximizers, agree that physician behavior is too complicated to explain merely by profit motives, but the first group is adamant in asserting that, as in any other business, profit (net income plus perks) is the most important element.

Another element of the physician's utility function is the desire to treat an interesting complex of cases. Feldstein (1970) was the first to incorporate the need for interesting cases into a model. The inclusion of such provider taste variables in a model is often ridiculed by conservative economists, in spite of demonstrable physician mobility in pursuit of interesting cases. Many physicians are able to change their subspecialty, or mode of practice, or locus of practice (HMO, hospital-based, private office) every few years to ensure an interesting patient case-mix.

Supplier-Induced Demand

The conventional wisdom among health economists is that excess consumer demand grants physicians an unusually high degree of discretionary power to affect both the quantity and price of their services. Contrary to traditional competitive economic analysis, higher physician density per capita has been shown to correlate with higher (Dyckman, 1978; Institute of Medicine, 1976; Newhouse and Phelps, 1974) or unchanged (Holahan, 1978) physician fees. One should introduce the caveat that correlation does not prove causality; for example, the direction of causality might be reversed. Physician density increases where fees are currently higher and more easily inflated in the future. However, there are three main hypotheses for explaining the mechanism by which physicians might maintain income levels in response to increased physician density and presumably somewhat more active competition among physicians.

Feldstein (1971) suggests that when physician density increases physicians simply reduce the percentage of patient need that goes untreated in this market of permanent excess demand. Recent unpublished studies by the Canadian government support this theory and suggest that you could increase physician density five-fold above the national average and still have excess demand. Feldstein and others ignore the issue of whether this excess demand is medically necessary. Health marketing practitioners are attempting to grasp the prickly nettle of how physicians affect consumer taste and induce the consumption of unneccessary medical services. In this respect, the growing discipline of marketing that we will survey in Chapter 7 goes beyond the purview of traditional microeconomics; for example, one does not assume that preferences and taste are determined independently of the economic system. A second hypothesis advanced by a number of economists (Evans, 1974; Fuchs and Kramer, 1973) is that much of this new demand is physician-generated rather than permanently existing.

Both of these aforementioned hypotheses postulate a unique ability of physicians to affect consumer demand. If physicians are unable to maintain a target level of demand, they can still maintain a target income by increasing fees in response to declining demand for their services. This third hypothesis has been reported by Newhouse (1970b). These three hypotheses are not mutually exclusive. Physicians can maintain a target income by inflating prices, or treating more elective conditions, or doing some combination of the two. As we shall see in a later section, one group of physicians (general practitioners) has been found to be less capable of maintaining a target income because the market for their particular services is relatively competitive. Therefore, they must act as price-takers.

The question of the appropriate health manpower ratios per capita has been a subject for lively debate among public policy makers since 1960. As we shall see in Chapter 11, the federal government has played a large role in providing the funds to expand medical school output. If an increased per capita supply of a given type of physician appears to cause both slightly higher prices and higher utilization, then Congress might consider more substantial controls on medical school capacity and residency training programs. Checking the supply of physicians, including immigrating physicians, would go a long way toward containing the cost of medical care.

The benefits of a doctor oversupply (such as aggressive price competition) have currently not been flowing to the consumers because physicians band together in tight trade union groups (Feldstein, P., 1977). If the monopoly power of subspecialty unions is eroded in the future, and if the federal government selectively withdraws support from areas of specialization that are in oversupply, our society will explicitly be redistributing income to the physicians that provide primary care. This is the position taken by the Graduate Medical Education Advisory Committee Report (1980) to the Secretary of Health and Human Services. The report projects an oversupply of 60,000 to 70,000 physicians in 1990 and recommends a 17 percent reduction in medical school class size. The short-run effects of decreasing the supply of young doctors might be positive (reduced physician service expenditures), but the long-run effects of decreasing the stock of the most "hungry" competitive price-setters might be inflationary. An example of the postulated difference between the short-run and long-run economic effects of a change in the stock of suppliers is currently occurring in the case of deregulation of the natural gas industry. In order to avoid this long-run inflationary effect of a small number of suppliers, the natural gas market has recently been deregulated. In the market for natural gas, where in the short term deregulation appears inflationary, we see promising signs that after the current initial corrective bulge in prices, the policy may prove deflationary.

Fuchs (1978) has studied the surgeon manpower supply equilibrium and the problem of provider-induced demand. If surgeons do partially shift demand upward by 3–3.5 percent to compensate for a 10 percent expansion in surgeons per capita, and also increase price to minimize the potential reduction in income to a few percentage points, the current high number of surgical residency programs may be a major problem in cost containment. In the short term we could not reduce the supply of surgeon manhours, because the post-graduate training pipeline prevents surgical subspecialists from reaching their maximum productive level for 7–10 years. Surgeons have suggested from time to time that surgery should be done only by specialists, but they have not supported a policy that would discourage medical students from entering the field; rather, they minimize the effects of competition by finding new patients and new conditions on which to operate (Wennberg and Gittelsohn, 1973). It would be inappropriate to generalize too much from these two studies of surgeon behavior.

Supplier-induced demand as a function of an increased supply of hospital beds has frequently been held as an unquestionable tenet of health services research. In fact there is still a controversy among researchers as to whether hospital bed supply creates demand. For example, the estimated elasticity of bed supply on hospital utilization ranges from a low of 0.1 for Pauly (1980) to a high of 0.71 for Cullis *et al.* (1980). Are we to believe that a 10 percent increase in hospital beds per capita could produce anywhere from a 1–7.1 percent purely supplier-induced increase in hospital usage per capita? Empirical results concerning the price elasticity of demand for hospital care are more uniform (Table 2.1). Price elasticity refers to the responsiveness of the quantity of care demanded to changes in price, all other factors being held constant. For example, a −0.23 price elasticity with respect to hospital days translates into an expected 2.3 percent decline in hospital days resulting from a 10 percent increase in price. The price elasticity for minor or elective diagnoses is usually larger, but still inelastic (less than 1.0), whereas the price elasticity for life-threatening emergency care is very low; that is, price is of no consequence.

Pauly (1980) analyzed data from the DHEW Health Interview

Table 2.1   Summary of Seven Econometric Studies of the Price Elasticity for Hospital Care

Data Source	*Dependent Variable*	*Price Elasticity (computed at the mean)*
Newhouse and Marquis (1978)	Hospital Length of Stay	− .05
Feldstein (1977)	Hospital Days	
	(i) short run (1966–1973)	− .29
	(ii) long run (1959–1965)	− .13
Newhouse and Phelps (1976)	Hospital Days	− .23
Davis and Russell	(a) Admissions	− .5
(1972)	(b) Hospital Days	− .32 to −.46
Feldstein (1971)	(a) Admissions	− .43
	(b) Hospital Days	
	(i) short run (1963–1967)	− .26
	(ii) long run (1959–1967)	− .55
Rosenthal (1970)	(a) Length of stay	
	(depending on diagnosis)	0.0 to −.08
	(b) Patient Days	
	(depending on diagnosis)	− .01 to −.70
Rosett and Huong (1973), 1961 Expenditure Survey	Hospital and Physician expenditures (at 20% coinsurance)	− .35

survey and found little support for the hypothesis that there is any physician-induced demand in ambulatory care. One disturbing element in the Pauly regression results was the failure to find any influence of time cost on ambulatory demand. These results are in direct conflict with the findings of Acton (1975) concerning the importance of time cost in ambulatory demand functions: the longer the consumer waiting time or travel costs, the lower the demand. We will return to the question of provider-induced demand in a later section, physician pricing models, but first let us survey the literature concerning physician behavior.

Physicians' Supply Curves

Whether a physician works more or less as a result of an increase or decrease in physician wages is an important subject for public policy. Depending on the physicians' labor supply curve, they could decide to work harder and substitute more patient care for leisure (the substitution effect). Alternatively, physicians could decide that their income is sufficiently high to afford increased leisure time in preference to a higher workload. They would consequently work less (the income effect). An important point to remember is that even if the supply curve for a given individual physician is backward-bending (*SB* in Figure 2.1), the physicians' aggregate labor supply curve may instead be uniformly upward-sloping (*SF* in Figure 2.1) as is usually the case in most labor markets.

The research results on this issue are mixed. Feldstein (1970)

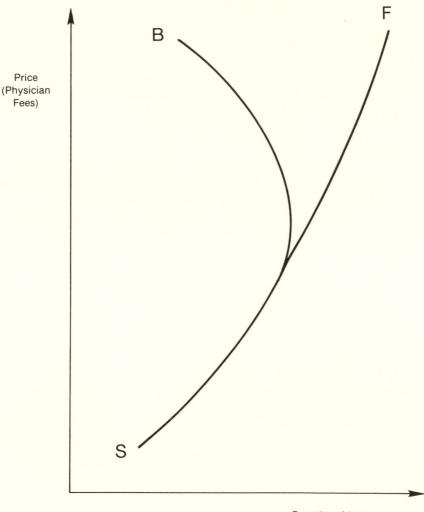

Figure 2.1   Physician Labor Supply Curve: Upward-Sloping Normality (SF) or Backward-Bending Response (SB).

finds strong support for the backward-bending supply curves. Sloan (1976) indicates no support for the position that physicians lie near the backward-bending portion of the labor supply curve, and reports very low elasticities of supply. Vahovich (1977) reports empirical results intermediate between Sloan and Feldstein; he finds slightly backward-bending supply curves and low elasticities of supply. In summary, physicians will not change their workload significantly in response to price controls or expanded health insurance coverage.

More recently, another study has corroborated the backward-bending labor supply hypothesis. Brown and Lapan (1979) also utilized aggregate time series data, but they operate under the hypothesis that physicians are price-taking utility maximizers rather than price-setters. Their findings support the view that physicians are on the backward-bending portion of their labor supply curve. A second interesting finding of this study is that nonphysician inputs (physician extenders, aides, etc.) substitute for declines in physician labor, so that the supply curve of physician-office services is always positively sloped (curve *SF* in Figure 2.1). These findings utilizing aggregate data corroborate the results of Reinhardt (1975) using data for individual physician practices. (We shall review the Reinhardt study in the context of federal manpower policy toward physician extenders in Chapter 5.) The inference to be drawn from the Brown and Lapan (1979) and Reinhardt (1975) findings is that the inflationary impact of physician price increases could be lessened if other inputs are substituted for physicians' time. Both studies call for increasing the number of trained physician extenders (physician assistants and nurse practitioners). The one dissenting opinion on this issue is the aforementioned study by Pauly (1980, Chapter 3). Pauly suggests that in the case of hospital care, hospitals provide too much hospital input and too small an input of physician time. The problem with this inference is that the sample under study was not representative of all hospitals. The author points out that the sample studied included only 165 small hospitals above 50 beds in size in predominantly rural counties containing just one hospital. On the other hand, if Pauly were correct it would solve another public policy problem: The anticipated doctor oversupply (GMENAC, 1980) of 60,000–70,000 could be eliminated if we somehow convinced physicians to work longer hours per diem in the hospital.

Physicians' Pricing Decisions

Physician behavior has been presumed to vary on three very basic dimensions: (1) whether physicians act as price-setters or price-takers, (2) whether prices are sufficient to clear the market of excess demand, and (3) whether demand can be shifted or induced. Six types of physician pricing models have been developed by economists. The first three models we shall survey assume that the physician is a price-setter; that is, third-party payers' reimbursement controls are not too constraining and lack of competition allows the professional considerable freedom to set fees. According to the longest standing physician pricing model, Monopoly Equilibrium (markets clear so that supply is brought into equilibrium with demand [see Glossary, "market clearing price"] and demand does not shift), physicians set prices as a discriminating monopolist (Kessel, 1958; Newhouse, 1970b). Price discrimination involves charging what the individual patient can bear, not as an altruistic method of charging the poor less, but rather as a method of reaping monopoly profits by capturing all the area under the demand curve.* The growth in insurance coverage has all but eliminated the physician's ability to price discriminate, except in the case of out-of-pocket subspecialty fees paid by the rich for "star" physicians to perform transplants or heart surgery. A number of court cases made it impossible for organized medicine to maintain the discriminating pricing policies of the 1950s (Havighurst, 1980).

The second model of physician pricing, Monopolist Demand Creation, also assumes that the market clears, but demand is shifted as a result of price-setting decisions. This model assumes the physician has the most power imaginable: like a simple monopolist he can set fees irrespective of what the other physicians are doing, and he can manipulate consumer wants and inflate demands if necessary. Evans (1974) supports this difficult-to-test theory with empirical evidence on supplier-induced demand in Canada. The author also defends the omnipotent pricing powers of physicians in an earlier work (Evans, 1973), which postulates that in markets with imperfect information on quality, the consumer is often lead to believe that higher price means higher quality. Solid evidence of consumers searching for

---

* A demand curve is the schedule of quantity sold at various prices if you offer one price to the entire marketplace. However, if a supplier could offer a spectrum of prices to the buyers so that each pays close to their maximum price, that would capture much more of the area under the demand curve, that is, the profits per unit of service would clearly be increased.

higher priced providers would be a revolutionary attack against economic normality in medical markets. Recently, this pricing model has been rejected by Pauly (1980).

A third physician pricing model involves Simple Monopolists Behavior in a Market of Chronic Excess Demand. This model is like model two in that physicians set prices irrespective of the market, but demand is not shifted and the market does not clear (excess demand is left unserved). This model is not manageable analytically; one can estimate neither a demand curve nor a supply curve. This model lacks advocates because it is largely untestable. It does have fleeting support from a number of different economists. Sloan (1976) advocates the idea of physicians acting as simple monopolists,* and Feldstein (1970) in rejecting static and dynamic competitive models suggests that physician services are in a state of permanent excess demand, subject to various modes of non-price rationing. Feldstein indicates that physicians benefit from a marketplace with permanent excess demand in which the profession can pick and choose among the most interesting case "material." In summary, none of these three models of physicians as price-setters is firmly established as empirical fact, but the first and third models do have some moderate level of support.

The last three models we shall survey are competitive models. Physicians are assumed to be such a small fraction of the marketplace that they must act as price-takers. With the exception of the market for general practitioners and family practitioners, comprising approximately 40 percent of all physicians, these competitive models are usually rejected by the econometric evidence of the authors. The fourth physician pricing model to consider is the classic Competitive Equilibrium Model. Under conditions of competitive equilibrium the market clears and demand is not shifted. This model has been tested on twenty years of time-series data by Feldstein (1970) and tested on cross-sectional data† by Newhouse (1970b), Fuchs and

---

* Another possibility is that physicians act in a monopolistically competitive manner (Masson and Wu, 1974): not as independent as the simple monopolist, but only slightly influenced by the pricing decisions of neighboring sources of care such as prepaid groups and practitioners in their own specialty.

† Time-series data can be indicative of short-run behavior because practice resources are relatively fixed in the short or middle run of 5–15 years. Cross-sectional analysis provides more information concerning long-run behavior, assuming the sample includes the range of various practice opportunities, in different stages of development. Analysis of a time series of cross-sections allows the researcher to construct a more complete set of structural equations for supply and demand relationships.

Kramer (1973), Kehrer and Knowles (1974), Newhouse and Phelps (1974), the Institute of Medicine (1976), and Dyckman (1978). All seven of these studies reject the competitive equilibrium hypothesis and report positive coefficients for physicians per capita or surgeons per capita in their price equations. The positive association between price and physician supply ratios is inconsistent with competitive models.*

Many health professionals are quick to claim that competition has been eliminated in medical markets. Some of the aforementioned studies do not include the obvious caveat that physicians are not a homogenous group. The possibility exists that some subgroups of physicians or surgeons do exhibit competitive pricing behavior. Four studies support this proposition. Steinwald and Sloan (1974) and Sloan (1976) report mostly negative association between general practitioner (GP) density and GP fees, and a lower negative association between general surgeons' density and their fees. Holahan *et al.* (1978) also found the same relationships for GPs, but rejected any correlation in the case of general surgeons or internists. More recently, McLean (1980) derived structural equations for both the supply of and demand for GP services utilizing the American Medical Association's eighth periodic survey of physicians. McLean rejects the hypothesis that the market for GPs is perfectly competitive, but the high net price elasticity (-1.75) indicates a considerable degree of competition in the market. This price elasticity is larger than the price elasticity reported in any of the studies summarized in Table 2.2. In summary, the competitive equilibrium model appears to have some validity in the case of general practitioners, and possibly general surgeons.

The fifth physician pricing model can best be summarized as the Oligopoly Target Income hypothesis. The target income theory of pricing suggests markups in prices as input costs inflate or demand declines. The model presumes that the market clears, demand will shift, and that demand can be manipulated by the physicians. The speed of adjustment depends on a number of factors including information collection costs. This model receives some support from Feldstein (1970), and relatively less support from Kehrer and Knowles (1974) and Vahovich (1977). The Feldstein study does not

---

* The observed low price elasticities in Table 2.2 are also not consistent with competition or simple profit maximization theories. The price elasticity of demand for certain individual physicians will be substantially larger than the market price elasticities reported in the table.

Table 2.2   Money-Price Elasticities and Time-Cost Elasticities of Eight Econometric Studies of the Demand for Physician Services

Data Source	Dependent Variable(s)	Elasticity with Respect to Price or Time
Newhouse and Marquis (1978)	Physician Visits	−1.00
Newhouse and Phelps (1976)	Physician Visits	− .15 to −.20
Phelps (1975)	Physician Visits (at 25% coinsurance)	− .20
Fuchs and Kramer (1973)	Physician Expenditures	− .15 to −.35
Acton (1975)	Demand Elasticity with Respect to:	(Time Elasticity)
	(a) Travel Time to MD's Office	− .25 to −.37
	(b) Waiting Time for Services	− .12
Phelps and Newhouse (1972)	Price Elasticity for:	
	(a) Physician Home Visits	− .35
	(b) Physician Visits	− .14
	(c) Lab, X-Ray, Ancillary Services	− .07
Davis and Russell (1972)	Outpatient Visits	−1.00
Feldstein and Severson (1964)	Physician Visits	− .19

provide very strong statistical support for this theory, reporting mixed results in his demand and price adjustment equations.*

Sloan (1976), and Steinwald and Sloan (1974) soundly reject the target income hypothesis. Green (1978) carries the argument one step further and reanalyzes the data from the Fuchs-Kramer (1973) study and fails to reject the hypothesis that physicians cannot induce demand. Unfortunately, it is almost impossible to distinguish demand shifts resulting from changes in consumer tastes from shifts caused by physician manipulation of information to the consumer, or from shifts that are simply responses to changes in time price faced by the consumer. In summary, we can at least infer that "physician supply creating demand" or the so-called "availability effect" is not uniform or pervasive in either model two or five.

---

* As the author (Feldstein, 1970) pointed out, reporting a low elasticity demand curve, finding a backward-bending supply curve, and inferring that price increases with excess demand seem very incompatible.

There is a sixth physician pricing model considered by Reinhardt (1975) and Pauly (1980). There is the possibility of Competitive Disequilibrium under Price Controls, that is, the market does not clear and demand is not shifted under private (insurance companies) or public (Economic Stabilization Program) price controls. Supply would consistently fall short of demand if the controls were too strict. This is the traditional case of excess demand under price ceilings: Physicians acting as price-takers only produce up to the point where marginal cost equals the price ceiling (typically less than what would be demanded of the physician at that "low" price, Ginsburg, 1978). There is no empirical support for assuming that physicians presently pursue this sixth pricing model (Newhouse and Phelps, 1976). There is some limited evidence that the subset of physicians serving Medicaid patients is unresponsive to price ceilings and to a 30 percent across-the-board reduction in Medicaid fees (Shwartz *et al.*, 1981). One might suggest that if a substantially lower level of reimbursement yields the same number of surgical and medical services thirty months later, then the initial fees were set arbitrarily high. It is heartening to learn that the only significant persistent drop in utilization occurred for the procedure most frequently labeled unnecessary, the tonsillectomy. One might question whether these results from Massachusetts would hold up over a longer time period or in other states that do not have such a high density of physicians per capita.

In summary, there may be types of physicians for which all six of these economic models fail to work, while other significant groups of physicians behave in a manner that is reasonably consistent with a number of these models. We shall now review some models of hospital behavior.

Physicians, Clubs, and the Agency Problem

Most of the early health economics literature contained simple utility maximization models of hospital behavior that ignored the influence of physicians. The first significant economic model that integrated the two groups of actors, physicians and hospitals, into a single theoretical framework was developed by Pauly and Redisch (1973). The authors model the hospital as a nonprofit physicians' cooperative. In one sense the Pauly and Redisch approach is a lineal descendent of the work by Buchanan (1966) on a theory of clubs.

Physicians are still agents looking out for their patient's best interests, but the physicians have a nonpassive* role in running the hospital like a doctor's club. Whether a physician joins the club (hospital) depends on the individual's net expected revenue, the expected service contribution to the club, and non-pecuniary factors. The hospital is run so as to maximize the net incomes of the physicians on the staff. Thus the club is a classic profit-making firm, except one input is held constant. The Pauly and Redisch (1973) seminal effort is a limited descriptive model of intrahospital dynamics, rather than a predictive model amenable to easy empirical testing.

Pauly (1974) found a positive relationship between physician income and hospital capital investment. This is certainly consistent with the view that the hospital is a producer cooperative operated to enhance doctors' incomes. The regression analysis was run on a cross-sectional sample of Internal Revenue Service and American Hospital Association data in thirty states. As with any statistical study, the results cannot prove a given model, but the results did not in any way reject the concept of the hospital as being operated to augment doctors' incomes. More recently, Shalit (1977) has suggested some indirect tests to discover whether the hospital is under the de facto control of a cartel-club of physicians. Membership in the cartel is not optimal for any individual member; they could do better in the short term on their own. His statistical support for the cartel theory from a cross-section of forty-six states in 1968 is rather weak, and all the relevant coefficients are insignificant if one redoes the two-stage least-squares equation with 1978 data.

The patient-physician-hospital relationship and the so-called "agency" problem (the physician acting as an agent for the patient with the hospital) has parallels in other sectors of the economy. The physician serves as an agent for the customer in much the same fashion as a gallery acts as an agent between the customer and the artist. In each case the agent claims to find and deliver the best quality care, but has a financial incentive to deliver the most costly style of care. Reder (1969) was one of the first economists to cast the doctor-patient relationship in light of the agency problem. One

---

* It might surprise some to realize that the earlier models of hospital behavior envisioned a rather passive role for physicians: Long (1964) and Rice (1966) Quantity Maximization models, Quantity and Output (Case-Mix) Prestige Joint Utility Maximization, or Simple Input Prestige Maximization (Lee, 1971; Feldstein, 1971; Newhouse, 1970b).

could speculate that new physicians in a market area act much like pure agents of the patient's interests, but when the physician has more than enough patients, patient utility can become a less important element of the physician's utility function. A dissatisfied customer is usually quickly replaced.

Currently there is no one "best" model for explaining physician and hospital behavior that adequately incorporates the characteristics of monopoly (e.g., supply restrictions, we shall review in Chapters 5 and 8) and competition (e.g., many hospitals and many physicians, subjects for Chapters 6 and 7). Many of the models require extensive utilization of proxy variables, provide a rather weak development of theoretical structure, and report *ad hoc* casual empirical tests.

Most of the published models or "think pieces" since publication of the Pauly and Redisch (1973) study have returned to the position that profit maximization of physicians is the most important element in any hospital's utility function. Granfield (1975), Cullis *et al.* (1980), Wilensky and Rossiter (1980), and Goldfarb *et al.* (1980) introduce a large number of distinct, competing goals into the hospital and physicians' utility functions. These goals include: quality maximization, case-mix complexity maximization, discretionary admission maximization, operating loss minimization, and prestige maximization. Some of the goals are incorporated into the model as part of the primal utility function, and other "goals" are introduced as slack or dual constraint variables.

Hospitals are not a homogenous group. Consequently, each of these models might be applicable to different types of hospitals. In this regard, Berry (1973) has provided a simple first-cut at grouping hospitals for economic analysis. Berry identified four basic hospital types, listed in order of increasing average cost per diem: basic service hospitals (33 percent of AHA members), quality-enhancing service hospitals (31 percent), complex service hospitals (23.5 percent), and total community service hospitals (12.5 percent). The Pauly and Redisch model might be most applicable to the first two types of hospitals: small facilities, with almost no residents or student nurses, comprising 64 percent of hospitals but less than 27 percent of the hospital days.*

---

* The productivity chapter in the Pauly (1980) text analyzes a sample of 165 small rural counties. Each county had just one short-term general hospital with at minimum 50 beds. As stated earlier, this sample was not intended to be representative of American hospitals. It is unclear whether these hospitals contribute much to the hospital costs escalation problem.

Better models will need to be constructed to explain the behavior of large University Medical Centers, representing one third of the total community service hospital cluster. These hospitals are more likely to impose explicit rents on physicians with admitting privileges, in the form of obligations to perform charity service in clinics, low pay service in emergency rooms, and low pay service on utilization review committees. Other elements in the physician's utility function—such as prestige among peers—obviously benefit from affiliation with the large teaching hospital. There are many complexities that we shall introduce in this regard in characterizing teaching hospitals (Chapter 12) as a four-headed firm: hospital administration, physicians that are medical school loyalists, independent physicians, and totally hospital-based hospital-reimbursed physicians.

Physician-Induced Investment

Overcapitalization is the most frequently mentioned problem of the hospital industry. Granfield (1975) was the first to suggest that the hospital industry is subject to the Averch-Johnson (1962) hypothesis; hospitals are regulated, protected from competition, and consequently overcapitalized. In Chapter 8 we shall test an econometric model for positive or negative effects of regulation on hospital capital investment.* The entire network of health planning and Certificate-of-Need regulations has been designed in theory to give nonphysicians the wherewithal to reject physician requests for excessive capital investment. From the standpoint of physician utility preferences, overcapitalization in the hospital sector is helpful if it increases slack capacity (and thus the certainty that physicians can get their patients admitted) and increases technology availability. Having an excess capacity of diagnostic and therapeutic equipment is "efficient" for physician utility maximization in a number of ways: It increases income from interpretation of test results, decreases waiting time for information to be acquired, potentially improves care quality, etc.

---

* To place the issue in a broader context, Bower (1966) reviewed the Averch-Johnson hypothesis for the electric utility industry and found a professional agent of the public interest, the engineer, whose power over the investment structure is at least as impressive as the physician community's influence over hospital trustee boards.

Hospital overcapitalization may be optimal for the physician staff, but the investment pattern is seldom socially optimal. One ramification of the Averch-Johnson hypothesis is that we would expect that firms would be regulated or constrained from maximizing profit. This hypothesis will be considered in Chapter 5. One corollary of the Averch-Johnson hypothesis is that the cost of capital to the hospital is less than the cost of capital in less regulated private markets. That hypothesis will be confirmed in Chapter 9, and the policy implications of tax-free hospital bonds and "free" fully reimbursed interest charges will be discussed. In this era of fluctuating interest rates, one is surprised that third-party payers have not created reimbursement incentives that encourage hospitals to await lower interest rates in the short term, that is, that the payers would pay only a capital allowance (nonprofit firm's return on equity) equivalent to a fixed fraction of gross plant assets (from which the institution would have to meet all capital costs).

Another aspect of the Averch-Johnson effect suggested by Kahn (1971) is a tendency to bargain less rigorously with outside suppliers. One recent study supports this hypothesis. The General Accounting Office (1980) has recently provided dramatic evidence of hospitals paying 200–300 percent more than necessary for certain supply items (oxygen, recording paper, and irrigating solution). The study concluded that hospitals in the same cities were paying excessive prices for the same supplies for one-fourth of the supply items where cost comparisons were made available by the hospitals. The supply companies benefit from the present cost reimbursement system that does not penalize one Pittsburgh hospital for paying $4.20 per roll of recording paper, while the neighboring facility pays only $1.12 per roll.

One might question whether current regulations or public utility style regulations are appropriate for American hospitals. Dewey (1979) argues that in the case where one industry receives an exemption from an otherwise universally enforced law against collusion, the exempted industry can expand output and attract resources from other industries. The hospital industry, fueled by a demand-pull inflation and protected from potential competitors like HMOs (Chapters 6 and 8), might be a dramatic example of the "Dewey" phenomenon. Hospitals' share of Gross National Product has increased four-fold in thirty years, and that does not include the prolific growth in physician resources devoted to the hospital care process.

We can make one quick test as to whether the Averch-Johnson (A-J) effect might be operating in the hospital sector. If the A-J effect is operating in the hospital industry, those physicians that are most frequent users of the hospital as their workshop should find their incomes improved the most. This hypothesis is supported by national average increases in physician income, where the most hospital-based specialties had the highest growth in income (Table 2.3). This result is certainly consistent with the Averch-Johnson effect, but it does not prove the A-J hypothesis. In summary, the probable allocative distortions produced by the combined effect of increased health insurance coverage and the A-J effect has yielded hospital overcapitalization and physician overspecialization. There are too many specialists and too few generalists. We will discuss health manpower issues in a broader context at the end of Chapter 5, but it seems plausible to suggest that a reduction in hospital over-capitalization might yield a reduction in returns for hospital-based specialists, and thus reduce the incentive to enter subspecialty training programs.

Marketing and Physician Behavior

Health marketing concepts and applications will be the subject of Chapter 7. The intent of this section is to indicate the potential influence of physicians on hospitals and vice versa. Physicians have an incentive to keep their retailer—the local hospital—afloat and well equipped. Many physicians view their relationship with the hospital as analogous to the relationship of a free-lance mechanic to a garage, except that the clinical setting must be substantially cleaner. The medical staff, like the mechanic, is not required to pay rent for user privileges. In this context, we shall review three basic models for describing the patient service production process.

If one assumes that the physicians control the medical-hospital producer-retailer channel, the clinician can achieve maximum profits by forcing the retailer (hospital) to purchase inputs and produce services that just cover the hospital's costs. The physician as the producer (manufacturer) controls the supply in the distribution channel and can largely dictate the price for nonphysician providers in the channel. It is in the physicians' interest to have the retailers (hospitals) provide a very expensive, technologically intensive style of service. The professional fees of the physicians are proportionally higher when interpreting and performing the more technologically

Table 2.3   Trends in Net Income by Specialty, Indexed to Pediatrician Income, 1968–1980

Specialty	1968	1971	1974[1]	1978	1980 est.	Percentage of Patient Visits at a Hospital 1978[2]
Anesthesiology						
(a) Average Net Income (ANI)[3]	$35,954	47,293	54,365	67,000	77,900	
(b) ANI as a % of Pediatricians' ANI	114.0	122.8	129.1	132.9	135.9	90
(c) Growth in ANI Since 1968 (%)	—	31.5	51.2	86.3	116.7	
Surgery						
(a) Average Net Income	$43,907	54,045	60,510	75,800	89,210	
(b) ANI as a % of Pediatricians'ANI	139.3	140.4	143.7	150.4	155.6	53
(c) Growth in ANI Since 1968 (%)	—	23.1	37.8	72.6	103.2	
Internal Medicine						
(a) Average Net Income	$35,552	42,869	51,390	64,300	75,600	
(b) ANI as a % of Pediatricians' ANI	112.8	111.3	122.0	127.6	131.8	41
(c) Growth in ANI Since 1968 (%)	—	20.6	44.5	80.9	112.6	
Obstetrics and Gynecology						
(a) Average Net Income	$40,572	51,062	61,693	70,600	77,740	
(b) ANI as a % of Pediatricians' ANI	128.7	132.6	146.5	140.1	135.6	26
(c) Growth in ANI Since 1968 (%)	—	25.9	52.1	74.0	91.6	
General Practice						
(a) Average Net Income	$33,671	39,823	44,727	52,400	58,700	
(b) ANI as a % of Pediatricians' ANI	106.8	103.4	106.2	104.0	102.4	22
(c) Growth in ANI Since 1968 (%)	—	18.3	32.8	55.6	74.3	
Pediatrics						
(a) Average Net Income	$31,527	38,503	42,112	50,400	57,340	
(c) Growth in ANI Since 1968 (%)	—	22.1	33.6	59.9	81.9	16
Average American Worker[4]						
(c) Growth in Family Income Since 1968 (%)	—	23.2	66.3	126.7	179.4	
(d) Growth in the Consumer Price Index, All Items, Since 1968 (%)	—	16.4	41.7	87.5	141.8	

[1] The Economic Stabilization Program was in effect from 8/15/71 to 4/30/74.
[2] Held, P. J., and Reinhardt, U. (1979). *Analysis of Economic Performance in Medical Group Practices*, Final Report to DHEW, Contract HRA-106-740119. Princeton, N.J.: Mathematica Policy Research, Inc.
[3] *Profile of Medical Practice* (1980), annual source book, Center for Health Services Research and Development. Chicago, Illinois: American Medical Association.
[4] U.S. Department of Commerce, Bureau of the Census (1980). *Statistical Abstract of the United States 1980*. Washington, D.C.: U.S. Government Printing Office.

sts and procedures. Prevailing fee-for-service medical a one-level distribution channel (where the number of s determines the length of the channel) consisting of ....cian (manufacturer) and the hospital (retailer) providing care to the consumer.* Medical care provided in the inner city is typically a two-level channel of physician (manufacturer), teaching hospital (wholesaler intermediary), and satellite clinic (retailer) providing the product to the consumer. The physician must set prices in reference to the demand function for professional plus hospital services combined, since physician and hospital services are complements. Consequently, making maximum use of hospital resources, collecting maximum possible fees for test interpretation, and supporting profit minimization in the hospital supports profit maximization for individual physicians.

Alternatively, if one assumes that the retailer controls the production channel, as in the case of a Health Maintenance Organization (HMO), the plan can achieve maximum profits by hiring physician services at below market prices. A third alternative is to assume that the physicians and hospitals or HMO plans pursue profit maximization while allowing a "necessary" profit margin to the other party. Such a compromise may result in an inefficient equilibrium at a price between P' and P'' producing a quantity of service ranging between Q' and Q'' in Figure 2.2. To maximize profits physicians set marginal physician revenue equal to their marginal costs, implying a transaction with the hospital involving Q' units of care at price P'. To maximize hospital revenues in excess of costs, hospitals would prefer a transaction with the physicians involving fewer units of service (Q'') at a higher level of reimbursement (P'').

Prepaid group health plans are one of the few markets where health facility managers and physicians are on a relatively equivalent bargaining basis. The management of new HMOs must frequently report to the private risk bearers who supplied the venture capital. As we shall see in Chapter 6, these managers must also report to the public risk bearers who provide the necessary financing for the operation from the federal treasury, but their true employer is the private risk bearers. In contrast to the tradition-burdened hospital

---

* An alternative perspective is to view the hospital as the manufacturer producing a product to be delivered to both the patient and the physician. In Chapter 7 the hospital is viewed as the dominant manufacturer; in Chapter 12 both the physician and the hospital are taken as equally dominant manufacturers of health care services.

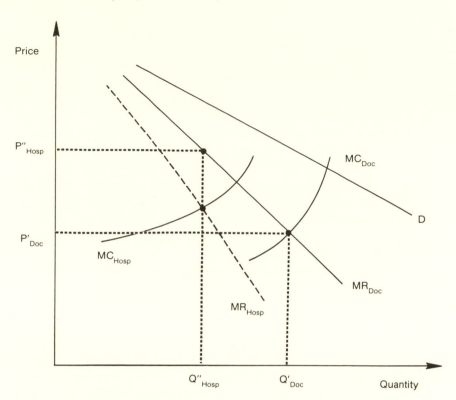

Figure 2.2 Potential Equilibrium in the Doctor-Hospital Producer-Retailer Production Channel for Hospital Services.

industry, HMO sponsors are always putting on the pressure and searching the market for better managers. The market for HMOs is less stable than the hospital industry, in that there is a much higher chance of exit (going out of business). Consequently, the owner-sponsors of the HMO search for the best quality managers to deal with the potential growth opportunities in the market for prepaid group health care.

Hospital Regulation and Financial Health

The aim of any prospective reimbursement system, be it as simple as the Western Pennsyvania budget projection or as complex as New Jersey Diagnostic Related Group projections, is to give hospitals a target unit cost. Among cluster groupings of similar hospitals, the target is intended as a second-best alternative to perfect competition. Target setting becomes an exercise in futility if special interests are allowed to exclude everything beyond the administrator's clear control: ancillary utilization, union wages, energy costs, interest rates, malpractice premiums, etc.

The cardinal sin of hospital oligopolists is to be too profitable. The hospital sector has been highly successful in convincing the media that they are not excessively capitalized or profitable. Among administrators one hears frequent laments that physician-induced overcapitalization has substantially reduced hospital operating margins. Administrators talk of "managing for survival" and increasingly being forced to trade wealth derived from charge payers and profit centers (lab, radiology, etc.) for the subsidization of loss leaders (for example, maternity care) and cost payers. Increasingly, hospital managers must cut new "frills" such as health education programs. In the 1980s hospital administrators may have to cut the slack even more to maintain a reasonable operating margin. Hospital administrators have successfully utilized their oligopoly power in many states to force Blue Cross and state government to reduce contractual allowances for cost payers to below the 5–7 percent level. For example, the Maryland Hospital Association forced the state rate review commission to cost out the real economies of scale in paperwork that should accrue to bulk payers. As a result of this unpublished study, the discount allowance was reduced to below 4 percent in 1981.

Hospital Collusion

The amount of collusion among hospitals is seldom mentioned in the literature. There are many reports of dramatic increases in shared services across hospitals and a large increase in the number of multi-hospital systems.* Hospitals must have an individual incentive to join or there must be compulsion, such as health planning. The members and potential members of informal or explicit multi-hospital contracts face a number of strategic problems. It is beyond the scope of this chapter to analyze these strategic problems in the

---

* According to the American Hospital Association, 90.2 percent of hospitals share services and departments with neighboring hospitals, and 26 percent are members of multi-hospital systems (Johnson, 1980). Multi-hospital systems account for more than 31 percent of the acute care community hospital beds in the nation. Non-profit multi-hospital systems are popular in Indiana, Illinois, Michigan, Missouri, Kansas, and Wisconsin. Investor-owned proprietary multi-hospital arrangements are flourishing in California, Texas, and most southern states.

context of multi-attribute utility functions and the theory of games. Instead, we shall suggest a taxonomy of three extensive forms of multi-hospital integration that go beyond simply having a shared laundry or computer services contract.

The newest and most comprehensive mode of sharing is the vertical integration of unlike institutions in a given area. Patients are moved through a referral or feeder system from primary care centers to secondary care hospitals to tertiary care University Medical Centers. Each hospital offers a limited scope of services and knows its position in the hierarchy. Vertical shared oligopoly arrangements among hospitals rarely exist for long periods of time because the system requires such a high degree of cooperation and coordination. Hospitals will only participate in the vertical arrangement if the cost of supporting the centralized system is less than the perceived benefits of keeping the oligopoly operating. An example of this type of vertical integration is the uncontracted arrangement between ten secondary care hospitals and one big tertiary care hospital in Chicago. Whenever the big hospital needs a Certificate-of-Need or rate increase from planners and regulators, the smaller hospitals go as a group to lobby on behalf of the big hospital. The ten smaller hospitals benefit from the assured referral network and the improved physician retention rates that followed formal affiliation with the large teaching hospital. Such collaborative activities among hospitals, even concerning price-output decisions, are not subject to the Sherman Antitrust Act. The Federal Trade Commission does not have jurisdiction over nonprofit firms unless the FTC can demonstrate that the organized acts of collusion are directed for the "profit" of the group members. The FTC currently pursues a limited antimonopoly procompetition strategy, which directly contradicts the approach of health planners in other branches of government who "bless" the "right" hospitals and blanket the nation with monopoly-creating health plans.

The other two types of multi-hospital integration involve different modes of horizontal integration: cooperation and coordination among like institutions. The first mode of horizontal integration could be labeled Horizontal Segmented Oligopoly, typically in the face of significant competition from HMOs, IPAs, or federal hospitals. In the face of competition, hospitals are more likely to share clinical services and administrative services. Physicians typically are more risk-averse about sharing clinical services, because they might lose their patients to other hospitals. But in the face of external pressure from the large prepaid group competitor, physicians are more likely to support the sharing of clinical services in order to contain costs and make fee-for-service medicine more competitive (see Chapter 6 for a more detailed discussion of competition).

The third type of multi-hospital integration will be labeled Horizontal Shared Oligopoly. This is the most prevalent mode of sharing and simply involves: (1) dividing up the service market among like institutions and (2) emphasizing the sharing of administrative services. In the case of a Horizontal Shared Oligopoly, the combination of the risk-averse increasing utility function of the local physicians with the risk-averse utility function of the hospitals results in a net risk-averse behavior pattern (Eastaugh, 1978), that is, sharing of clinical services is not prevalent.*

The Horizontal Shared Oligopoly members often express an ambivalent attitude toward rate regulation and planning regulations. For example, the eight burn centers in one state extensively lobbied state government not to deregulate their industry. The group members wanted continued strict rate regulation to protect the group from the potential ravages of a price war. The members also wanted continued strict Certificate-of-Need regulation to protect them from price or quality competition from any new entrant to their market. Further research is needed to determine which models are most appropriate for various hospital market and physician market situations.

Conclusion

In this chapter we have briefly surveyed a number of empirical and theoretical models of physician and hospital behavior. The six physician pricing models reviewed are summarized in Figure 2.3. Prominent among the possible ways of containing medical costs is providing the physicians and managers with better information concerning the benefits and effectiveness of various tests, techniques, and procedures. The studies detailed in Chapters 1 and 2 are best described

---

* In the case of increasing utility functions, as attribute P increases in value (patient referrals to another neighboring provider), the group risk-aversion function converges to the upper limit; behavior tends to be risk-averse. Consequently, for increasing utility functions, as P increases, $U(P)$ increases and for higher values of $U(P)$ we predict the providers should behave in an increasingly conservative fashion. Conversely, administrative services have a low potential for creating strategic difficulties between the hospital and the physicians, so no one will care if they are shared extensively with other hospitals.

1.	2.	3.	4.
Demand Shifts	Market Clearing Prices Achieved	Physicians Are Price-Setters	Physicians Are Price-Takers
NO	YES	**Model 1—** Monopoly Equilibrium	**Model 4—** Competitive Equilibrium
YES	YES	**Model 2—** Dynamic Demand Shifts	**Model 5—** Oligopolistic Target Income Levels
NO	NO	**Model 3—** Chronic Excess Demand Disequilibrium	**Model 6—** Exogeneous Price Ceilings

Figure 2.3 Taxonomy of Six Economic Models for Physician Behavior.

as positive economics. These studies are descriptive in nature and sometimes are intended to predict the dynamics and inner workings of the health services delivery sector. In the following two chapters we shall survey a number of normative economic models. The techniques, such as cost-benefit and cost-effectiveness analysis, are decision-making models designed to guide resource decisions, from building a facility to deciding what technique should be the standard operating procedure. The truth is, of course, that normative techniques are typically used to help provide better informed decisions at the margin, rather than dictate cook-book decision-making. In our pluralistic society, the decision makers are wise to keep the experts on tap, rather than on top (Price, 1965).

References

ACTON, J. (1975). "Nonmonetary Factors in the Demand for Medical Services: Some Empirical Evidence," *Journal of Political Economy* 83:3 (May), 595–614.

ARROW, K. (1963). "Uncertainty and the Welfare Economics of Medical Care." *American Economic Review* 53:4 (December), 941–973.

AVERCH, H., and JOHNSON, L. (1962). "The Firm under Regulatory Constraint," *American Economic Review* 52:4 (December), 1052–1069.

BERRY, R., (1973). "On Grouping Hospitals for Economic Analysis," *Inquiry* 10:4 (December), 5–12.

BOWER, R. (1965). "Rising Capital Cost versus Regulatory Restraint," *Public Utilities Fortnightly* 65:5 (March 4), 31–33.

BOWER, R., and R. ROHR (1975). "Utility Rate Structure Design: Theory in Practice," *Eastern Economic Journal* 2:3 (July), 189–204.

BROWN, D., and LAPAN, H. (1979). "The Supply of Physicians' Services," *Economic Inquiry* 17:2 (April), 269–279.

BUCHANAN, J. (1966). "An Economic Theory of Clubs," *Economica* 32:1 (January), 1–14.

CULLIS, J., FORSTER, D., and FROST, C. (1980). "The Demand for Inpatient Treatment: Some Recent Evidence," *Applied Economics* 12:1 (March), 43–60.

DAVIS, K., and RUSSELL, L. (1972). "The Substitution of Hospital Outpatient Care for Inpatient Care," *Review of Economics and Statistics* 54:2 (May), 109–120.

DEWEY, D. (1979). "Information, Entry, and Welfare: The Case for Collusion," *American Economic Review* 69:4 (September), 587–594.

DYCKMAN, Z. (1978). *A Study of Physician Fees*, Staff Report (March), Council on Wage and Price Stability, Executive Office of the President, Washington, D.C.

EASTAUGH, S. (1978). "Determinants of Overutilization," unpublished dissertation, School of Hygiene and Public Health, Johns Hopkins University.

EVANS, R. (1973). *Price Formation in the Market for Physician Services in Canada, 1957–1969.* Ottawa: Queen's Printer.

EVANS, R. (1974). "Supplier-Induced Demand: Some Empirical Evidence and Implications," in M. Perlman (ed.), *The Economics of Health and Medical Care.* New York: Wiley, 162–173.

FELDSTEIN, M. (1970). "The Rising Price of Physicians' Services," *Review of Economics and Statistics* 52:2 (May), 121–133.

FELDSTEIN, M. (1971). "Hospital Cost Inflation: A Study in Nonprofit Price Dynamics," *American Economic Review* 61:5 (December), 853–872.

FELDSTEIN, M. (1977). "Quality Change and the Demand for Hospital Care," *Econometrica* 45:7 (October), 1681–1689.

FELDSTEIN, P., and SEVERSON, R. (1964). "The Demand for Medical Care," in *Report of the Commission on the Cost of Medical Care.* Chicago: American Medical Association, 56–76.

FELDSTEIN, P. (1977). *Health Associations and the Demand for Legislation: the Political Economy of Health.* Cambridge, Mass.: Ballinger.

FUCHS, V. (1978). "The Supply of Surgeons and the Demand for Surgical Operations," *Journal of Human Resources* 13 (Supplement), 35–56.

FUCHS, V., and KRAMER, M. (1973). "Determinants of Expenditures for Physicians Services in the United States, 1948–1968," Paper Series, National Bureau of Economic Research.

General Accounting Office (1980). "Hospitals in the Same Area Often Pay Widely Different Prices for Comparable Supply Items," Report HRD-80-35 (January 21). Washington, D.C.: U.S. Government Printing Office.

GINSBURG, P. (1978). "Impact of the Economic Stabilization Program on Hospitals: An Analysis with Aggregate Data," in M. Zubkoff *et al.* (eds.), *Hospital Cost Containment: Selected Notes for Future Policy.* New York: Prodist, 293–323.

GMENAC (1980). *Graduate Medical Education National Advisory Committee Re-*

port to the Secretary, *DHHS* 1:1 (September), 1–123.

GOLDFARB, M., HORNBROOK, M., and RAFFERTY, J. (1980). "Behavior of the Multiproduct Firm: A Model of the Nonprofit Hospital System," *Medical Care* 18:2 (February), 185–201.

GRANFIELD, M. (1975). "Resource Allocation Within Hospitals: An Unambiguous Analytical Test of the A-J Hypothesis," *Applied Economics* 7:4 (December), 241–249.

GREEN, J. (1978). "Physician-Induced Demand for Medical Care," *Journal of Human Resources* 13 (Supplement), 21–34.

HAVIGHURST, C. (1980). "Antitrust Enforcement in the Medical Services Industry: What Does It All Mean?" *Milbank Memorial Fund Quarterly* 58:1 (Winter), 89–124.

HOLAHAN, J., HADLEY, J., SCANLON, W., and LEE, R. (1978). *Physician Pricing in California*, Urban Institute working paper, report 998–10.

Institute of Medicine (1976). *Medicare-Medicaid Reimbursement Policies: Part III*, Volume 3. Washington, D.C.: National Academy of Sciences.

JOHNSON, D. (1980). "Multihospital System Survey." *Modern Healthcare* 15:4 (April), 57–64.

KAHN, A. (1971). *The Economics of Regulation: Principles and Institutions*, Volume 2, Institutional Issues. New York: Wiley, 53–59.

KEHRER, B., and KNOWLES, J. (1974). "Economics of Scale and the Pricing of Physicians' Services," in D. Yett. (ed.), *An Original Comparative Economic Analysis of Group Practice and Solo Fee-for-Service Practice* (DHEW Report). Springfield, Virginia: National Technical Information Service.

KESSEL, R. (1958). "Price Discrimination in Medicine," *Journal of Law and Economics* 1:1 (October), 20–53.

LEE, M. (1971). "A Conspicuous Production Theory of Hospital Behavior," *Southern Economic Journal* 38:7 (July), 48–59.

LONG, M. (1964). *The Economics of Health and Medical Care*. Ann Arbor: University of Michigan, 211–226.

MASSON, R., and WU, S. (1974). "Price Discrimination for Physician's Services," *Journal of Human Resources* 9:1 (Winter), 63–79.

McLEAN, R. (1980). "The Structure of the Market for Physicians' Services," *Health Services Research* 15:3 (Fall), 271–280.

NEWHOUSE, J. (1970a). "Toward a Theory of Nonprofit Institutions: An Economic Model of the Hospital," *American Economic Review* 60:1 (March), 64–71.

NEWHOUSE, J. (1970b). "A Model of Physician Pricing," *Southern Economic Journal* 37:2 (October), 174–183.

NEWHOUSE, J., and PHELPS, C. (1974). "Price and Income Elasticities for Medical Care Services," in M. Perlman (ed.), *The Economics of Health and Medical Care*. New York: Wiley, 139–161.

NEWHOUSE, J., and PHELPS, C. (1976). "New Estimates of Price and Income Elasticities of Medical Care Services," in R. Rosett (ed.), *The Role of Health Insurance in the Health Services Sector*. New York: Watson Academic, 261–312.

NEWHOUSE, J., and MARQUIS, M. (1978). "The Norms Hypothesis and the Demand for Medical Care," *Journal of Human Resources* 13 (Supplement), 159–182.

PAULY, M., and REDISCH, M. (1973). "The Not-For-Profit Hospital as a Physicians Cooperative," *American Economic Review* 63:1 (March), 87–99.

PAULY, M. (1974). "Hospital Capital Investment: The Roles of Demand, Profits and Physicians," *Journal of Human Resources* 9:1 (Winter), 7–20.

PAULY, M. (1978). "Is Medical Care Different?" in W. Greenberg (ed.), *Competition in the Health Care Sector*. Germantown, Md.: Aspen Systems, 11–35.

PAULY, M. (1980). *Doctors and Their Workshops: Economic Models of Physician Behavior*. Chicago: University of Chicago Press.

PHELPS, C. (1975). "The Effects of Insurance on the Demand for Medical Care," in R. V. Anderson *et al.* (eds.), *Equity in Health Services: Empirical Analysis in Social Policy*. Cambridge, Mass.: Ballinger.

PHELPS, C., and NEWHOUSE, J. (1972). "The Effect of Coinsurance: A Multivariance Analysis," *Social Security Bulletin* 35:6 (June), 20–29.

PRICE, D. (1965). *The Scientific Estate*. Cambridge, Mass.: Harvard University Press.

PRIEST, C. (1970). "Possible Adoption of Public Utility Concepts in the Health Care Field," *Law and Contemporary Problems* 35:4 (Autumn), 839–848.

REDER, M. (1969). "Some Problems in the Measurement of Productivity in the Medical Care Industry," in V. Fuchs (ed.), *Production and Productivity in the Service Industries*. New York: Columbia University Press.

REINHARDT, U. (1975). *Physician Productivity and the Demand for Health Manpower*. Cambridge, Mass.: Ballinger.

RICE, R. (1966). "Analysis of the Hospital as an Economic Organism," *Modern Hospitals* 106:4 (April), 87–91.

ROSENTHAL, G. (1970). "Price Elasticity of Demand for Short-term General Hospital Services," in H. Klarman (ed.), *Empirical Studies in Health Economics*. Baltimore: Johns Hopkins University Press, 104–124.

ROSETT, R., and HUANG, L. (1973). "The Effect of Health Insurance on the Demand for Medical Care," *Journal of Political Economy* 81:2 (March-April), 281–305.

SHALIT, S. (1977). "A Doctor-Hospital Cartel Theory," *Journal of Business* 50:1, 1–20.

SHARELL, S. (1979). "Risk Sharing and Incentives in the Principal and Agent Relationship," *Bell Journal of Economics* 10:1 (Spring), 55–73.

SHWARTZ, M., MARTIN, S., COOPER, D., LJUNG, G., and WHALEN, B. (1981). The Effect of a 30 Percent Reduction in Physicians' Fees on Medicaid in Massachusetts," *American Journal of Public Health* 71:4 (April), 370–375.

SLOAN, F. (1976). "A Microanalysis of Physicians' Hours of Work Decisions," in M. Perlman (ed.), *Economics of Health and Medical Care*. New York: Wiley, 302–325.

SLOAN, F. (1976). "Physician Fee Inflation: Evidence from the Late 1960's," in R. Rosett (ed.), *The Role of Health Insurance in the Health Services Sector*. New York: Watson Academic, 321–354.

STEINWALD, B., and SLOAN, F. (1974). "Determinants of Physicians' Fees," *Journal of Business* 47:3 (October), 493–511.

VAHOVICH, S. (1977). "Physicians' Supply Decisions by Specialty: TSLS Model" *Industrial Relations* 16:1 (February), 51–60.

WENNBERG, J., and GITTELSOHN, A. (1973). "Small Area Variations in Health Care Delivery," *Science* 182:4008 (December 14), 1102–1108.

WILENSKY, G., and ROSSITER, L. (1980). "The Magnitude and Determinants of Physician-Initiated Visits in the United States." Proceedings of the World Congress on Health Economics, September 8–11, Leiden University, the Netherlands.

Chapter 3

COST-EFFECTIVENESS
AND COST-BENEFIT ANALYSIS

Nothing is pure and entire. All advantages are attended with disadvantages.

—David Hume

One cool judgment is worth a thousand hasty councils. The thing to do is to supply light and not heat.

—Woodrow Wilson

Cost-effectiveness and cost-benefit analysis have been applied in many preventative, diagnostic, and treatment contexts. Over the past decade methods have improved for prospectively collecting better data sets and incorporating intangible quality-of-life valuations into the calculus for weighing benefits against costs. Further cooperation between clinicians, economists, and epidemiologists is a healthy trend. Political scientists are prone to argue over valuation in dollars, reflecting a basic misunderstanding of the trade-off concept and a need to combine and compare benefits and costs in comparable units. The purpose of this chapter is to review the state of the art of cost-effectiveness and cost-benefit analysis in evaluation of medical technologies. Economic evaluation of new or expensive technologies has become a central issue in the public debate about rising medical care costs. Historically, the growth in technology has stimulated a concomitant increase in the numbers and salaries of health care employees. Warner (1978) and Fuchs and Kramer (1973) characterize the new health technologies prior to 1955 as being cost-saving (physician time-saving and usually quality-enhancing), whereas the technologies introduced since 1955 have tended to be

55

cost-increasing. Physicians and economists frequently express their hope that these expensive and/or physician-using technologies are partially justified by their quality-enhancing properties.

Basic Concepts

The objective of cost-benefit analysis is to maximize net benefits (benefits minus costs, appropriately discounted over time). The objective of cost-effectiveness analysis is to rank order the preferred alternatives for achieving a single goal or specified basket of benefits. Cost-effectiveness analysis is not any easier to perform than cost-benefit analysis if multiple varieties of benefit are specified (man-years, work-loss days, reduced angina), except that in doing cost-benefit one must value the intangible benefits in commensurate dollar terms. Operationally, ethical questions can be raised if the benefits and costs accrue to different social groups. For example, a clinic scheduling system that minimizes wasted time for the physician through multiple overlapping appointments may be a net benefit of a few hundred dollars per doctor at the expense of many more dollars of patient time.

In economic sectors where competitive markets fail to exist, such as the health care or water resource sectors, cost-benefit analysis aims to do what supply and demand forces accomplish in competitive markets. The price system will not equalize marginal benefits and marginal costs if market failure exists, that is, price disequilibrium occurs in highly insured consumer markets (Fuchs, 1972). Another criterion of choice is to maximize the ratio of benefits to costs, discounting the numerator and denominator to present value dollars. Alternative programs (or procedures or services) are then ranked by benefit-cost ratios, and the programs with the highest payoff ratios are selected until resources are exhausted or until the ratio equals one. This approach is equivalent to maximizing net present value within a budget constraint. A third, outmoded decision criterion is to support a project if the internal rate of return exceeds the predetermined discount rate. The internal rate of return criterion can lead to different resource decisions from the net present value criteria if programs are of different sizes or have varying time horizons.

If a technology is found to be the most cost-effective alternative, then the next question is whether it is cost-beneficial. For example, Acton (1973) first evaluates which of five program alternatives is most efficacious and which is most cost-effective in reducing deaths from heart attacks, which he follows by a valuation of life and intangible benefits to assess whether the benefits make the program worth the costs for society. One obvious advantage of cost-benefit analysis is that it leads to a positive (go) or negative (no go) net present value for the procedure being evaluated, and does not require a cost-effectiveness cutoff level to decide whether a project can be done within the resource constraints. However, many more complete cost-effectiveness analyses are performed than cost-benefit analyses, because intangible benefits pose difficulties with valuation and the choice of a discount rate is simpler in cost-effectiveness evaluations (Feldstein, 1970).

If a technology is found to be cost-beneficial, the only question left is whether the risk is socially acceptable for public financing of the service. Society may have some preference for the social classes that are to face an unacceptable risk, even if it is known in advance that the total risk is insufficient to make the benefit-to-cost ratio less than one. Safety, as measured by risk analysis, is a relative concept. No test or therapy that provides any benefit has ever been completely safe. Physicians, like all professionals, have learned to live comfortably with the reasonable notion that we must forego some safety to achieve any net benefit.

The critical point to convey to the reader is that cost-effectiveness and cost-benefit analysis are increasingly taking their appropriate position in the evaluation (pre-diffusion) stage prior to the marketing decision. The rationale of this emerging public policy is that the costs (in lives and in dollars) of foregoing economic and efficacy evaluation may often be much greater than the costs of a well-designed evaluation. One "consumerist" benefit of increasing reliance on economic evaluation is that it must force those in power to be explicit about (1) valuation of life biases (across social class) in cost-benefit calculations and (2) the resource cut-off level utilized in cost-effectiveness analysis.

It is certainly not necessary to conduct economic analysis and randomized clinical trials on every new technology, and certainly not on most existing ones. However, the uncontrollable economic pressures for efficiency are apt to result in more federal funding of cost-benefit and cost-effectiveness studies through the National Center for Health Care Technology. More evaluations will be funded and utilized in decision making if government continues to pay a large fraction of the medical bills.

The traditional basis of clinical medicine suggests that the physician should make every effort to provide all possible avenues of care to the patient. The idea of scarcity of resources has no role in this code of ethics, except during wartime. The medical ethic is increasingly being criticized relative to the public health ethic which suggests that every clinician has an obligation to inquire about underserved potential patients and foregone man-years of life that go untreated because physicians serve a technological imperative and a profit imperative (that is, serve the patients who are technically interesting or profitable, then attend to the other cases).

Methods of Analysis

There has been a high degree of public and political disenchantment with model builders that provide narrow definitions of direct benefits and ignore the limitations of their very crude data bases. The typical accounting costs of billed charges or incurred expenses are too narrow a definition of cost for the economic analyst. Confusion frequently exists when members of the medical profession attempt to do a cost analysis. For example, the cost to society of not having airbags must not exclude accident victims that are DOAs (dead on arrival). In the arena of cost-effectiveness analysis between medical treatment versus surgery, surgeons frequently omit DOTs (dead on table) from the analysis in order to make surgery look better relative to medical treatment. The tendency is to go far afield in counting benefits and to neglect some costs, such as the pain of surgery or the overhead costs of the operating room. Cash expenditures are too limited a definition of cost. True cost to society can only be measured in opportunity cost terms. In the parlance of economics, the cost of any item or service is the foregone benefit that you sacrificed in order to obtain it.

Estimating the economic burden of a disease involves the measurement of prevalence, the assessment of impact on the individual's health status and other people's well-being, and the eventual quantification of direct and indirect costs associated with these impacts. For example, Berry and Bolond (1977) estimated the cost of alcohol abuse at $31.4 billion in 1971. Half of the alcohol abuse burden on the economy results from lost economic production ($14.9 billion), $8.3 billion is generated in direct health care service costs, and the residual $8.2 billion results from motor vehicle accidents, fires, crime, and other less tangible impacts. In many cases indirect costs can be the largest component of the analysis. Klarman estimated the present value of eradicating syphilis at $3.1 billion, with 42 percent of this total benefit accounted for by erasure of the "stigma" associated with the discovery of the disease. The study assumed that people were willing to forego 1.5 percent of their earnings to avoid the stigma associated with the disease (Klarman, 1965).

Measurement of Indirect Benefits

Direct benefits of health services or public health programs are measured by the foregone medical care costs. Often the direct benefits of eliminating a disease are a fraction of the indirect benefits. For example, in 1979 HEW estimated the direct benefits of eliminating medical expenditures on smokers at $5 billion annually, and the indirect benefits were estimated at $12 billion in terms of foregone worker productivity. Mushkin (1962) separates indirect benefits of health programs into three categories: reduction of premature death, avoiding lost working time (morbidity), and avoiding lost capacity to be productive after returning to work (debility). The first and second measures, mortality and morbidity, have been well researched. However, our ability to quantify debility remains a topic for future research. Expected earnings replaced income as the relevant measure of indirect benefits in the 1960s (Rice, 1966). Cooper and Rice (1976) produce annual tabulations of the present value of lost earnings due to mortality under alternative discount rates and annual estimates of the foregone earnings due to disability. In some cases potential morbidity reduction represents 90 percent of indirect benefits (skin diseases), and in other cases potential mortality reduction represents 90 percent of indirect benefits (neoplasms).

The value of housewives' services has also recently entered the benefit picture, although their services are still omitted from the gross national product. Klarman (1967) measured housewives' services by the wages they could earn (using alternative wages they could earn as an opportunity cost measure), while Weisbrod (1968) measures their replacement value by the cost of employing a housekeeper. The only strength of the Weisbrod approach is that it estimates housewives' worth as an increasing function of family size: A housewife is more expensive to replace in larger families. The opportunity cost concept is more persuasive, since housewife value is a function of education attainment and occupation. Foregone earnings as an estimate of indirect benefits is relatively easy to estimate, although some radical economists might question the assumption that earnings are a suitable measure of social benefit. The resultant biases implicit in measuring benefits in terms of earnings reflect imperfections in the labor market such as racism and sexism.

Most economists became disenchanted during the 1970s with the gross output approach of valuing a person's life as discounted expected future earnings. For example, concluding that visits to a rheumatology clinic were cost-beneficial only for males merely reflects an artifact of the sex bias in earnings data; women earn less (Glass, 1973). A variant of this approach, subtracting out consumption to yield net output, was considered ill advised, because killing elderly or handicapped individuals would be "valued" as an act that confers a net benefit to society. Fromm (1965) suggested a third approach, valuing life on the basis of the life insurance premiums one is willing to pay. However, the life insurance approach only measures a person's willingness to compensate others following death, rather than the value set on one's own life.

The most prevalent assessment approach in the 1970s has been the "willingness to pay" approach suggested by Schelling (1968) and measured initially by Acton (1973). Both authors realized that quantity multiplied by price was at best equal to a minimum benefit of health services to the society, since it does not account for the many consumers who would be willing to pay more than the price.

Consumer's surplus of benefit involves estimating a measurable proxy, the area under the entire demand curve. Figure 3.1 illustrates the concept of measuring benefit by the amount of money that each person is willing to pay rather than go without the service. For a hypothetical example of selling bone marrow transplants to people with aplastic anemia, in the figure some 48 individuals are willing to pay $10,000 to receive the treatment.

All individuals are not willing to pay the same amount under hypothetical conditions of equal wealth across all individuals. Individuals face different risks; for example, the treatment is painful and often causes potentially fatal side-effects under which the new transplanted marrow cells attack the liver, skin, and other organs. The *ABC* shaded area above the price line *AB* is the sum of money equal to the consumer's surplus. The surplus represents a dollar measure of the excess of satisfaction over consumer dissatisfaction. Individuals 1–6 are willing to pay an extra $10,000 above the price ($10,000),

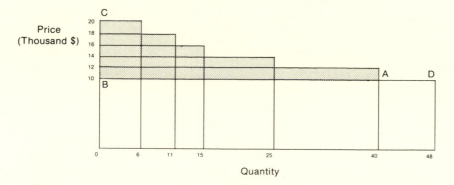

Figure 3.1 Hypothetical Demand Curve for Bone-Marrow Transplant Therapy (Aplastic Anemia Patients). (The shaded regions represent the consumer's surplus.)

individuals 7–11 are willing to pay an extra $8,000 each, individuals 12–15 are willing to pay an extra $6,000, individuals 16–25 are willing to pay an extra $4,000, and individuals 26–40 are willing to pay an additional $2,000 each. Consequently, the net benefits are $480,000 (price times quantity) plus $199,000 consumer's surplus.

This analysis assumes that the consumer is well informed and that the social value of transplants for anemia patients is the sum of the individual values. One might argue for adding on a psychic benefit for expressing the value that all members of society place on the assurance that if they have this rare type of anemia, the bone marrow transplant will be available.

In contrast to this life-or-death approach, Acton (1973) questioned the willingness to pay to reduce the probability of death from 0.002 to zero ($56), and linearly extrapolated this finding to conclude that the imputed value of human life was 500-fold larger ($28,000). This explicit linear relationship between risk and reduction and willingness to pay is not justified by that author. The willingness-to-pay approach can also be criticized on the grounds that life is probably valued much higher for identified individuals than for members of a hypothetical population. Consumers and physicians tend to value identified individual lives more than statistical anonymous foregone lives, yet physicians are often criticized for placing a substantially higher value on identified individuals than society, with its limited resources, can afford to place on the average citizen.

The willingness-to-pay approach is an improvement relative to the economic theory of human capital developed by Becker (1964) and others. In contrast to the human capital approach for measuring foregone expected earnings, the willingness-to-pay approach provides a consumer measure of the sum total of indirect benefits and intangible benefits. For example, Acton's experimental subjects were provided with an ex-ante problem of deciding how much to spend in reducing various kinds of risk of death from heart attack. Klarman (1974) and Acton (1973) have each criticized the study based on the small sample size and the apparent underestimation biases. Recently, Thaler and Rosen (1976) estimated marginal valuations of safety for select hazardous occupations from the 1967 Survey of Economic Opportunity earnings data to impute the value of a life saved at $176,000. Utilizing actuarial data, the authors estimated that workers in certain high-risk occupations demanded $176 a year to accept an extra death risk of 0.001 per year. Thaler and Rosen concluded that a society of workers would together be willing to pay $176,000 (in 1967 dollars) per life saved. More recently, Bailey (1980) adjusted the Thaler and Rosen estimate to allow for inflation, indirect taxes, and special benefit programs (OASI and worker compensation), and concluded that $303,000 (in 1978 dollars) was a more reasonable estimate of the value of a life saved. A range of estimates of $28,000 to $303,000 may strike some as being erratic, but our ability to design questionnaires and estimate benefits is constantly improving. Members of "humanitarian" professions often provide outrageous reactions to what they describe as utilitarian econometric pyrotechnics for valuing life. However, benefits are measured in dollars not for dollars' sake, but to symbolize foregone social programs or sacrificed lives.

Measurement of Intangible Benefits

Valuation is not a consideration in competitive markets, because marginal benefit is assumed to be equal to price. However, when prices fail to exist (water resources) or price is deemed a defective measure of value (health services), an attempt is made to impute value or "shadow price." Shadow price values can be imputed by asking individuals what they would be willing to pay for relief from pain, grief, discomfort, and disfigurement. For example, if a year of life is valued by a willingness-to-pay measure of $28,000, and a woman would sacrifice a year of life to avoid losing her breast(s) (Abt, 1977), this suggests a shadow price of $28,000 for a mastectomy. In this situation, Abt suggests that the additional costs for a few more drugs and drinks would bring the annual average shadow price of grief and worry to about $3,000. Often times the analyst can only identify the need to shadow price an intangible benefit. For example one intangible that is difficult to shadow price is the benefit of restored fertility capacity that follows a successful kidney transplant.

The shadow price concept can also be applied to arrive at quality weights for adjusting the value of additional years of existence. Klarman (1965) utilized an analogous disease approach to measure the willingness-to-pay value of escape from early manifestations of syphilis by the proxy disease psoriasis, and the late manifestations of syphilis by the proxy of terminal cancer cases. Direct data acquisition for "unstigmatized" medical conditions like cancer and psoriasis was more easily accomplished than directly working with syphilis victims. Economists must work with physicians to develop proxies and weighting schemes for capturing the multiplicity of dimensions of health care outputs. Inappropriate priorities might be set if survival probabilities are not integrated with quality-of-life factors.

The consumer utility literature has benefited from the recent development of more sophisticated scales for measuring preference functions and indifference curves. Stewart *et al.* (1975) and Grogono and Woodgate (1971) developed refined, but unvalidated, scales for measuring physical, social, psychiatric, and mobility limitations. The psychometric approach provided only marginal improvements over the 1948 Visick scales. Recently, multi-attribute utility theory has been applied to evaluate the benefits of treating sore throats (Giaugue and Peebles, 1976) and cleft lips in children (Krischer, 1976). Indifference curve analysis has been suggested as another approach to quantifying benefits. Newhouse (1979) has described an indifference curve along which combined sickness, pain, and restricted activity day composite measures of suffering are weighted equally undesirable. The best practical application of these concepts is provided by Weinstein *et al.* (1977) in their assessment of quality-of-life considerations after coronary artery bypass surgery. Quality-of-life outcome measures include pain at rest, pain with minimal activity, pain with mild activity, pain with strenuous activity, and no pain. Quite predictably, a potential surgical patient places a higher utility value on no pain if he avoids exercise. A utility function to value outcomes was specified as a function of life style and life expectancy. The data are highly subjective, but reliance on imperfect analysis provides more insights than analytical nihilism.

Cost-effectiveness analysis is more frequently completed because intangible benefits need only be estimated, not valued. Cost-effectiveness analysis requires only that all benefits be expressed in commensurate units so that the cost of achieving a specified level of benefits might be minimized. Cost-effectiveness is not any simpler than cost-benefit analysis if multiple varieties of benefit are specified (lives, years, pain), except that in doing cost-benefit analysis one must also value intangible benefits.

Net Present Value Analysis: Discounting

The uneven distribution of costs and benefits over time poses little conceptual difficulty for the analyst. One simply reduces the stream of future costs and benefits to net present value by discounting. The most common rationale for discounting social programs to present value reflects the uncertainty of the future: A benefit in hand is worth two in the future. In contrast, health economists' have downplayed the business sector rationale for discounting which is the time value of money. In the business sector uncertainty is always incorporated through the use of decision trees. A form of discounting, Net Present Cost Analysis, will be used in Chapter 10 to evaluate buy/lease decisions for new equipment.

The discount rate is designed to reflect the opportunity cost of postponing benefits or expenditures for an uncertain future. Arrow and Lind (1970) posit that the yield on private investment can be properly regarded as the appropriate opportunity yield for public investment only if the subjective cost of risk-bearing is the same for the average taxpayer as it is for the private investor. Musgrave (1969) indicates that the benchmarks should be a function of the source of financing; private consumption has a higher discount rate than public investment. What is most frequently misunderstood by non-economists is that inflation is only one part of the rationale for discounting. Even if all benefits were adjusted for the projected rate of inflation, discounting would still be necessary to account for the social rate of time preference. Discounting future years of life implies no utilitarian value judgment. It only presumes that benefits and costs must be juxtaposed and measured in commensurable dollar units at a single given discount rate. Choice of a discount rate is of no consequence for a short-lived program with benefits and costs concentrated within one to two years.

Selection of the rate of discount is a crucial parameter in most net present value calculations. For example, Jackson *et al.* (1978) reported that elective hysterectomy is only justified on tangible cost grounds if the discount rate were under 4 percent. Waaler and Piot (1970) reported in a recent cost-effectiveness analysis of tuberculosis control measures that discount rates greater than 6 percent favor case-finding and treatment, whereas a lower discount rate would favor a vaccination program. Discount rate selection is crucial for evaluating screening programs that yield benefits 20–60 years in the future. A prediction that technology will become more cost-increasing in the future argues for a lower discount rate selection in order to make lifesaving more valuable in future years. This viewpoint is supported by the suggestion that technology is reaching a state of diminishing returns where even an optimistic 50 percent reduction in the three leading causes of death (cardiovascular disease, cancer, and motor vehicle accidents) would add less than one year of life for people aged 15–65 (Tsai *et al.*, 1978). There are three basic varieties of discount rates: (1) The corporate discount rate if the private sector borrowed the funds, (2) the government borrowing rate on bond issues in the marketplace, and (3) the social discount rate to enable programs and procedures with benefits far in the future to prove more acceptable.

The social discount rate is probably the most often used because of the strength of the intergenerational equity argument. For example, a $25 million one-shot project in 1980 with a payoff of $75 million in the year 2000 only has a positive net present value if the discount rate is 6 percent or less. The typical social discount rate is on the order of 4–6 percent. However, a bias against the value of future generations might still remain apparent to some futurists if they realized that at a 5 percent discount rate, 30 deaths in 2050 are exactly equivalent to 1 death in 1980. To those political scientists and welfare economists concerned with ethical issues, any discount rate will have some slight bias in favor of present generations (a counterargument might be Keynes' rejoinder that "in the long run we are all dead").

Opportunity cost principles argue for a high discount rate. The true cost of a health care investment is the return that could have been achieved if the resources had gone elsewhere in the private sector. For Mishan (1976) and Fisher (1973) the relevant comparison is not the expected rate of return, but the expected rate of return net of the subjective costs of risk-bearing. The first option, the corporate discount rate, is obviously overinflated since it includes both a risk premium and a markup for corporate taxes. In order to achieve equivalent after-tax investor earnings, a corporation must offer stockholders a 13.5 percent return (that is, a 27 percent before-tax gross return) to compete with a riskless municipal bond returning 9.5 percent and allowing a 4 percent risk premium. Operationally, the second choice, government borrowing rates, serves as the upper bound in most analyses. Given the implicit assumption that the discount rate is not changing over time, the most prudent course of action is to perform a sensitivity analysis of the net present value under a range of discount rates. If a sensitivity analysis can demonstrate that selection of a discount rate does not affect the recommendations, then the tenuousness of the assumption will not be a source for concern.

The last discounting issue that must be considered is the selection of an appropriate downward adjustment to reflect the degree to which the medical price index exceeds the consumer price index (CPI). Klarman *et al.* (1968) were the first to incorporate a net discount rate adjusted downward by 1–2 percent to reflect the extent that growth in medical prices exceeded the growth in the CPI. More recently, Jackson *et al.* (1978) utilized a downward adjustment of 5 percent to reflect the excess of medical inflation relative to inflation in the general economy. This net discount rate factor reflects the value of direct health service foregone costs (benefits) that would also have increased by the excess of the medical price index over the CPI. If cost containment programs were to bring the medical inflation rate to parity with the CPI, as was almost done in 1979, then this adjustment would be unnecessary.

Applications of Cost-Benefit Analysis to Therapeutic Treatment

There is a lack of consensus among both analysts and decision makers regarding how to value the intangible benefits of health programs. Most decision makers find the valuation process in cost-benefit analysis difficult, and do not trust analyses that depend on gross approximations, small samples, and a poor data base. These decision makers are willing to violate the efficiency criteria and invest more in hospitals and physicians than society receives as a return on the dollar. Society might profit from having a more healthy skepticism concerning therapeutic treatments. Many therapies will exhibit dramatic benefits on introduction and require no cost-benefit analyses. For example, the dramatic 90 percent decline in the fatality rate from heart block exhibited after introduction of cardiac pacemakers in 1968 is a classic example of a clearly cost-beneficial new treatment mode. However, as Lewis Thomas (1977) has observed, modern medicine increasingly creates "half-way" technologies like bypass surgery or heart transplants and "complex" technologies like hemodialysis. Thomas reserves the label of a truly "sophisticated" technology for therapeutic treatments that eliminate the disease and restore the patient to prior health status. Consequently, a therapy like coronary artery bypass surgery is not sophisticated because it does nothing for the disease (arteriosclerosis). It has been assessed as having a low cost-effectiveness ratio because it does little to prolong life, but it almost always reduces chest pain for the 95–98 percent of patients surviving the operation (Weinstein *et al.*, 1977).

Somewhere between 2 and 20 percent of new treatments might be prime candidates for cost-benefit studies to decide whether the benefits are worth the costs to society. A smaller percentage of established therapies might also deserve the same cost-benefit analysis. The policy issue is seldom one of cost-beneficial yes or no, but rather an issue of frequency. Obviously, if clinicians start treating more non-serious cases, the frequency of treatment skyrockets. For example, prophylactically treating slightly symptomatic conditions of appendectomy (Neutra, 1977), or completely asymptomatic conditions of disease without consequence (for example, cholecystectomy, Ingelfinger, 1968) will dramatically decrease the benefit-to-cost ratio. It has been estimated that a program to treat asymptomatic silent gallstone carriers (15 million) would cost at least $45 billion (Fitzpatrick *et al.*, 1977). One of the intangible benefits of doing an economic evaluation is that it may suggest to the medical community that they decrease overutilization by increasing the degree of discrimination through improved clinical interpretation skills. This policy is good medicine and good economics. For example, Neutra (1977) has suggested that decreasing the removal rate of normal appendices will lead to slightly lower rates of perforation and other complications. One study in China (1974) has reported a mere 0.2 percent mortality rate from non-surgical treatment of appendicitis.

Very few complete cost-beneficial studies have been published. Many times a limited cost-benefit analysis will lead to the most socially cost-effective clinical decision rules. For example, Schoenbaum *et al.* (1976) suggests that a single rubella vaccination at 12 years or at two ages would be better than the typical norm of a single vaccination for all children at an early age. Berwick *et al.* (1975) suggest that hypercholesterolemia screening and treatment for children is more cost-beneficial than treatment and/or screening in adult years. This later study considers the issue of whether childhood screening is best done on the umbilical cord, all school age children, or high-risk school age children. The study suggests that selection of the discount rate determines whether the screen should be as liberal as 238 mgm for normal nonfamilial children or as conservative as 252 mgm for 10-year-old high-risk familial hypercholesterolemics. Sometimes the selection of a decision rule depends on how many intangible benefits are loaded onto the analysis. For example, prevention of Down's syndrome (mongolism) is a cost-beneficial screening venture for women over 40, but the screening for women age 35–39 is justified only if more disastrous pyschological sequelae for the parents are postulated following the birth of an abnormal child.

Cost-benefit analysis can provide the justification for new or mandatory screening and treatment programs. Layde *et al.* (1979) report a benefit-to-cost ratio of two ($4 billion/$2 billion) for a new multitiered alpha-fetoprotein screening program for detecting neural defects for a theoretical cohort of 100,000 American women. The mock analysis was necessary because the only existing data came from a small sample in Scotland. The study neglects many ethical issues and intangible benefit problems with a test that has only a 64 percent sensitivity, that is, the failure to identify an abnormality in a screened woman may result in more costly psychological sequelae than if the child had not been tested and declared healthy *in utero*.

Cost-benefit analysis can also be used to support expansion of an existing treatment program. Ward (1977) reports that an $8 billion hypertension control program would return a benefit to society of $10 billion. The suggestion that 6.1 million Americans with diastolic blood pressure above 105 mm undergo drug therapy was the byproduct of a 1967–1969 controlled clinical trial on treatment effectiveness of males visiting Veterans Administration facilities. The two problems with hypertension control center around the side effects of the drugs (dizziness, impotence, and malaise) and the problem of maintaining a high degree of patient compliance in nonexperimental situations. Finnerty *et al.* (1971) report that patient compliance was 84 percent in the experimental situation, but only 16 percent if the patient did not receive the "red carpet treatment." Before the nation spends $6 or $8 billion on hypertension, it seems reasonable to require that we make sure that the technology is effective (will not fail under normal conditions).

Frequently, the economic analyst is asked to perform a cost-benefit evaluation on a questionable treatment or mandatory screening program. For example, the Farber and Finkelstein (1979) cost-benefit study of mandatory premarital rubella-antibody screening dampened the initial enthusiasm for the program. In some cases, the evaluators need only look at the touted benefits in a more scientific fashion, with a randomized controlled trial, to conclude that the treatment has zero benefits. For example, the New York University 1973 study group, finding that hyperbaric oxygen provided no benefits for the elderly, eliminated enthusiasm for the treatment that had been stimulated by an unscientific study published in a nationally acclaimed journal in 1969 (Jacobs *et al.*, 1969). The oxygen "treatment" cost $2500 per week in 1970. The easy acceptance of a faulty, but profitable, treatment seems to be rather unprofessional if one views medicine as a science. For example, the time lag between general acceptance and proof of zero benefits was seven years in the case of gastric freezing as a cure for ulcers (1962–1969) and five years for internal mammary artery ligation surgery (1956–1961). The duration of the acceptance of faulty treatments was much longer in the early 1900s. For more than a quarter of a century, physicians tried to cure constipation with surgery (1906–1933) and treat menopausal symptoms with ptosis surgery (1890–1928) (Barnes, 1977).

Health education, which has been assailed by skeptics, is a popular current example of a new approach to improving the effectiveness of medical care. Table 3.1 represents the results of a limited benefit-cost comparison of four approaches to increasing patient compliance to anti-hypertensive medications. The study sample included 402 patients randomly assigned to experimental and control groups. The emphasis of the study concerned the efficacy of utilizing a triage process, whereby patients are subdivided into groups more predisposed to benefit from a given health education approach. The benefits of the triage method for achieving medication compliance clearly outweigh the cost only in the case of the highly depressed patients (24.3 percent of the sample), as defined by responses to five of the seven items used in the depression scale questionnaire. The benefit-to-cost ratio for the group (2.2) compares favorably with the

Table 3.1 Simple Benefit-to-Cost Comparisons of Triage Options Versus the Option Not to Triage in Achieving Improved Medication Compliance Among Hypertensives

Option	Triage	Type of Patients	IHC[1]	Health Education Intervention(s)	Benefit-Cost Ratio
1	Yes	High Level of Depression	65–26	Family Reinforcement (FR)	2.20[2]
2	Yes	Medium Level of Depression	58–33	FR + Message Clarification	1.15
3	Yes	No Depression	65–35	FR + Message Clarification	1.33
4	No	All Patients	60–32	FR + Message Clarification	1.24

[1] IHC = Increase in number of high compliers with treatment versus control per hundred patients.

[2] Only option 1 has a significantly better ratio for triaging in comparison to not triaging.

average benefit-to-cost ratio of 1.24 for hypertension control for persons in the age range of 35–65 (Option 4). In other words, triaging only the 24 percent highly depressed subpopulation and providing family member reinforcement is more cost beneficial than giving everyone the special health education intervention. Previous studies demonstrating a cost-benefit ratio in the 1.1–1.3 range may not stand the test of time in claiming a statistically significant ratio above the 1.0 level when applied to a larger population or applied to a non-experimental population that will be less susceptible to the Hawthorne effect. Individuals are known to change their behavior more dramatically under experimental conditions due to the mere fact of being under concerned observation.

Applications of Cost-Effectiveness Analysis

The purpose of cost-effectiveness analysis in the therapeutic arena is to identify the preferred alternatives. Physician preoccupation with survival probabilities must not preclude measurement of quality-of-life factors in performing a cost-effectiveness analysis. Cost-effectiveness analysis still requires that intangible factors be measured; however, they do not have to be valued. Typically the search for preferred alternatives involves comparisons of less invasive treatment versus radical surgery, for example, simple versus radical mastectomies, medical treatment versus bypass surgery, medical treatment versus doing a vagotomy for common duodenal ulcers, pyloroplasty versus antrectomy surgery for intractable duodenal ulcers, and internal urethrotomy versus uteral reimplantation for vesicoureteral reflux. In some cases the preferred alternative depends on treatment location, for example, home dialysis versus facility-based dialysis. Ten percent of American dialysis visits are done at home, compared with 6 percent in the Japanese proprietary system and 60–70 percent in the non-profit British system. The stimulation of a less profitable, but more cost-effective delivery point (home) may produce a $50 million net savings (Sparer and McKeon, 1979).

Cost-effectiveness analyses usually report either costs per unit of desired benefit achieved, or units of tangible benefits per dollar expended. For example, Schweitzer and Keating (1978) report a cost-effectiveness ratio for bone-marrow transplants of $433,000 per leukemia patient saved ($22,000 per man-year saved) and $125,000 per aplastic anemia patient saved ($8,000 per man-year saved).

Romm and McKeon (1979) report a cost-effectiveness measure of 81 visits per $1000 for a solo doctor and physician extender compared to 57 visits per $1000 for a physician operating in solo practice.

However, in some analyses, the need for computing any ratio is obviated by the lack of any differential in effectiveness between treatment modes. In such cases, the lower cost mode is preferable. One randomized study (Hill *et al.*, 1978) of the cost-effectiveness of home versus hospital (CCU) care for heart attack victims (mild cases, originally seen at their homes) found no statistically significant difference in the six-week mortality between the two groups (13 percent). Another controlled trial (Hampton and Nicholas, 1978) that randomly allocated mobile coronary care unit (MCCU) and routine ambulances to answer emergency calls found no differential in prehospital coronary mortality rates (47 percent). Despite the comments on high costs of CCUs and MCCUs, and in view of the concern for lack of substantially improved outcomes following the public expenditure of more resources for such technologies, groups of cardiologists continue to support the more institutionalized modes of therapy. Coincidentally, the cardiologists derive higher fees from hospital utilization. The prudent decision maker might suggest that CCUs and MCCUs should continue to be utilized in carefully controlled pilot study settings until effectiveness can be clearly established. One does not want to impede innovation if a period of trial and improvement can produce a more cost-effective alternative.

Many physician-directed cost-effectiveness analyses ignore larger social issues in considering questions of whether a given procedure during an operation is worth the effort. For example, Skillings *et al.* (1979) reject the concept of routine operative cholangiography since the technique detected only two unsuspected cases of "silent" gallstones at an average cost of $6612. The authors reject operative cholangiography if performed either routinely or for isolated silent small stones in the gallbladder. The Skillings study ignores the issues of false-positives (reported diseased when in fact healthy) yielding unnecessary surgery and mortality associated with increased time under anesthesia. However, including these negative benefits would only reinforce the case against operative cholangiography. Recently, Alon *et al.* (1979) performed a randomized trial and cost-effectiveness analysis of bypass patients treated under bubble oxygenators and membrane oxygenators. The more expensive membrane oxygenator brings no lasting benefits beyond the second postoperative day and is therefore only recommended for extended open heart procedures on high-risk patients. In some cases the analysis is touted as a cost-benefit analysis, when in fact it does not technically even qualify as a cost-effectiveness analysis. For example, a myringotomy with tube insertion is labeled cost-beneficial compared to the possibility of a foregone tympanoplasty simply because the relative fees are $75 and $925, respectively (Armstrong and Armstrong, 1979).

An example of a complete and technically competent cost-effectiveness analysis is the comparison by Piachaud and Weddell (1972) of medical versus surgical removal of varicose veins. Fifty men and two hundred women were allocated at random to either surgery or injection-compression sclerotherapy. Direct costs were four-fold higher for the surgical group. The treatment in the medical group involved seven clinic visits, in comparison to the surgical treatment that required three to four days of hospitalization and two clinic visits. The time cost to the patient was 100 hours for surgery and 30 hours for medical treatment. The opportunity cost to the economy was 31 workless days for surgery and 7.5 days for medical therapy. After three years of follow-up, there existed no clinical basis for selecting either mode of therapy. There may be many treatments or procedures in medicine that, like varicose vein surgery, are effective, but less cost-effective than a recently developed alternative. The widespread disdain for randomized experimentation and the general acceptance of existing techniques among the physician community might retard the research and development of more efficient and equally effective alternatives.

Policy Considerations and Conclusions

Cost-benefit analysis should increasingly assist government and third-party insurance carriers in inhibiting the financing of half-way technologies that provide palliative relief but not a definitive treatment. If it is politically difficult to underfinance therapies that are not cost-beneficial, then government can intervene on the development side to limit technological diffusion to a few well-evaluated pilot studies. If the evaluation suggests that the treatment mode is definitive and worth the price tag, then the new technology should diffuse through the medical sector.

It would take a high degree of naive optimism to suggest that economic analysis can produce a matrix of relative benefits, measured in terms of quality adjusted years of life saved, for the multitude of health services from which government or Blue Cross could read off our best buys. However, economic evaluation and decision analysis do not merit the unmitigated pessimism of Ransohoff and Feinstein (1976), who characterized it as a "computerized Ouija board." As Albert (1978) has recently pointed out, the true role of evaluation in medicine will lie between the pessimism of the Ouija board and the naive optimism of a "new Rosetta stone." The direct value of economic evaluation is that it can erode some of the areas of the unknown that surround the benefit-to-cost assumptions implicit in the behavior of physicians and administrators. Evaluation should be viewed as a consumerist cause if it forces those in power to be explicit about valuation assumptions in cost-benefit calculations and the resource cut-off level required in cost-effectiveness ranking decisions. The indirect benefit of economic evaluation is that it might teach health professionals to apply their craft only to the point where the marginal benefits equal the marginal costs. Economists' and regulators' credulity has been taxed by the disorderly diffusion of every new unproven technology. A possible intangible benefit of the evaluation process lies in the hope that cost-effective clinical decision-making principles will seep into the subconscious cognitive process of American physicians and result in a less costly style of medical care.

Cost-benefit principles will increasingly influence program evaluation and basic decisions about whether certain modes of regulation are worthwhile or are in need of dramatic change, such as a reduction in scope or better targeting of the effort. While speculation abounds as to whether PSROs are on balance desirable or cost-beneficial, little has been reported prior to 1980 as to the benefits and cost of utilization review activities. The 1980 Congressional Budget Office (CBO) study found a disappointing benefit to cost ratio of 0.4, indicating that PSRO review of Medicare patients, representing 46 percent of hospital patient days, had reduced Medicare stays by only 1.5 percent. Previous crude cost estimates by the PSRO program had assumed that the days of care foregone (saved) would be equivalent to an average hospital day of ancillary services consumed. The CBO study pointed to the ratio of marginal cost to average cost as an appropriate multiplier, because those days of stay saved do in fact reside in the latter part of the patient's hospitalization episode—days in which few tests or procedures are performed. Cost and effectiveness issues related to PSRO performance evaluation will be discussed in Chapter 12.

It is impossible to do a cost-benefit analysis of a hospital. Rather, hospitals should be viewed as flexible collections of medical technologies, where the benefit-cost possibilities of each technology need to be assessed separately. From the foregoing discussion it is clear that economists should be encouraged to address themselves to clinical applications of normative economic techniques (cost-benefit, cost-effectiveness, decision analysis). Aside from public health applications of cost-benefit analysis to polio and syphilis, few complete studies have been conducted to date. Many studies avoid the issue of valuation and perform limited cost-effectiveness analyses, and in the other cases the retreat is to provide only societal cost estimates of the impact of a disease or condition. The possible candidates for cost-benefit analysis in the 1980s range from the mundane to the exotic. Included on the HEW National Center for Health Care Technologies list of candidates are dental x-rays, soft tissue x-rays, diagnostic ultrasound, fetal monitoring, barium enemas, renal disease treatments, cell cytology reliability, radio-isotope scanning, and computerized axial tomography (CAT) scanning. Since the measurement of intangible benefits may pose some difficulty, cost-effectiveness analysis will often provide the more practical tool for evaluation.

In view of the uncertainties implicit in any technological assessment effort, one might question whether medicine should lock itself into an expensive and unproven therapy, such as bone marrow transplants, as a type of standard treatment. A sliding fee schedule could be employed to make the utilization of expensive marginal technologies less profitable for the physicians. In order to create a positive incentive for physicians to evaluate and get experience with a new test or treatment, the fee could increase as the service is proven to be more valuable. This concept of a technology evaluation-sensitive fee schedule has already been suggested by Gaus and Cooper (1978). Another possible positive planning solution to stimulate less costly behavior may be the allowance of replacement cost reimbursement for depreciation at projected (higher) market prices if the hospital introduces cost-reducing technologies or tests, and/or phases out cost-increasing equipment and services of unproved efficacy. Negative planning solutions such as Certificate-of-Need program sanctions are another possible solution that will be reviewed in Chapter 8. However, the coercion implicit in an effective negative planning approach inevitably adds to bureaucracy and creates barriers to innovation. Society should fear also any movement toward technology prohibition that creates disincentives for scientific inquiry merely because the economy cannot afford the implementation costs of every resulting procedure. The nation must strike some sort of balance between the relative risks of disorderly-promiscuous-diffusion versus orderly-slow-diffusion of new technologies, treatments, and tests.

References

ABT, C. (1977). "The Issue of Social Cost in Cost-Benefit Analysis of Surgery," in J. Bunker, B. Barnes, and F. Mosteller (eds.), *Costs, Risks, and Benefits of Surgery*. New York: Oxford University Press.

ACTON, J. (1973). "Evaluating Public Programs to Save Lives: The Case of Heart Attacks," Rand Corporation Report R-950-RC. Santa Monica: Rand Corporation.

ALBERT, D. (1978). "Decision Theory in Medicine: A Review and Critique," *Milbank Memorial Fund Quarterly* 56:3 (Summer), 362–400.

ALON, L., TURINA, M., and GATTIKER, R. (1979). "Membrane and Bubble Oxygenator: A Clinical Comparison in Patients Undergoing Bypass Procedures," *Herz* (German) 4, 56–62.

ARMSTRONG, B., and ARMSTRONG, R. (1979). "Tympanostomy Tubes: Their Use, Abuse, and Cost-Benefit Ratio," *Laryngoscope* 89:3 (March) 443–449.

ARROW, K., and LIND, R. (1970). "Uncertainty and the Evaluation of Public Investment Decisions," *American Economic Review* 60:3 (June), 364–378.

BAILEY, M. (1980). *Reducing Risks to Life: Measurement of the Benefits*. Washington, D.C.: American Enterprise Institute.

BARNES, B. (1977). "Discarded Operations: Surgical Innovation by Trial and Error," in *Costs, Risks, and Benefits of Surgery, op. cit.*, 109–123.

BARTEL, A., and TAUBMAN, P. (1979). "Health and Labor Market Success: The Role of Various Diseases," *Review of Economics and Statistics* 61:1 (February), 1–8.

BECKER, G. (1964). *Human Capital*. New York: National Bureau of Economic Research.

BERRY, R., and BOLAND, J. (1977). *The Economic Cost of Alcohol Abuse*. New York: The Free Press.

BERWICK, D., KEELER, E., and CRETIN, S. (1975). "Screening for Cholesterol: Costs and Benefits." Report from The Center for the Analysis of Health Practices, Harvard School of Public Health.

China Medical Group (1974). Report of The Acute Abdominal Conditions Research Group, "Some Problems in Nonoperative Treatment of Acute Appendicitis," *China Medical Journal* 2, 21–40.

COCHRANE, A, (1972). *Effectiveness and Efficiency*. London: Nuffield Provincial Hospitals Trust.

COOPER, B., and RICE, D. (1976). "The Economic Cost of Illness Revisited," *Social Security Bulletin* 39:1 (February), 21–36.

FARBER, M., and FINKELSTEIN, S. (1979). "A Cost-Benefit Analysis of a Mandatory Premarital Rubella-Antibody Screening Program," *New England Journal of Medicine* 300:15 (April 12), 856–859.

FEINSTEIN, A. (1977). "Clinical Biostatistics: The Haze of Bayes, The Aerial Palaces of Decision Analysis, and The Computerized Ouija Board," *Clinical Pharmacology and Therapeutics* 21:4 (April), 482–496.

FELDSTEIN, M. (1970). "Choice of Technique in the Public Sector," *Economic Journal* 80:320 (December) 985–990.

FINNERTY, F., *et al.*, (1971). "Reasons for Poor Clinic Attendance," *Clinical Research* 19:10 (October), 500–510.

FISHER, A. (1973). "Environmental Externalities and the Arrow-Lind Public Investment Theorem," *American Economic Review* 63:4 (September), 722–726.

FITZPATRICK, G., NEUTRA, R., and GILBERT, J. (1977). "Cost-Effectiveness of Cholecystectomy for Silent Gallstones," in *Costs, Risks, and Benefits of Surgery, op. cit.*, 246–261.

FROMM, G. (1965). "Civil Aviation Expenditures," in R. Dorfman (ed.), *Measuring the Benefits of Government Investment*, 172–230. Washington, D.C.: The Brookings Institution.

FUCHS, V. (1972). "Health Care and the U.S. Economic System," *Milbank Memorial Fund Quarterly* 50:2 (April) 211–237.

FUCHS, V., and KRAMER, M. (1973). *Determinants of Expenditures for Physicians' Services in the United States.* Rockville, Md.: U.S. Government Printing Office.

GAUS, C., and COOPER, B. (1978). "Technology and Medicare: Alternatives for Change," in R. Egdahl and P. Grertman (eds.), *Technology and the Quality of Health Care.* Germantown, Md.: Aspen, 225–236.

GIAQUE, W., and PEEBLES, T. (1976). "Application of Multidimensional Utility Theory in Determining Optimal Test-Treatment Strategies for Streptococcal Sore Throat and Rheumatic Fever," *Operations Research* 24:5 (September-October), 933–950.

GIBSON, G. (1976). "Regionalization and Emergency Medical Services: The Dance of the Lemmings," in E. Ginzburg (ed.), *Regionalization and Health Care.* DHEW, Washington, D.C.: U.S. Government Printing Office.

GLASS, N. (1973). "Cost Benefit Analysis and Health Services," *Health Trends* 5:1 (January), 51–60.

GROGONO, A., and WOODGATE, D. (1971). "Index for Measuring Health," *Lancet* 2:7738 (November 1) 1024–1029.

HAMPTON, J., and NICHOLAS, C. (1978). "Randomized Trial of Mobile Coronary Care Unit for Emergency Calls," *British Medical Journal* 10:6120 (April 29), 1118–1122.

HILL, J., HAMPTON, J., and MITCHELL, J. (1978). "A Randomized Trial of Home-versus-Hospital Management for Patients with Suspected Myocardial Infarction," *Lancet* 1:8069 (April 22), 837–844.

INGELFINGER, F. (1968). "Digestive Disease as a National Problem-Case V—Gallstones," *Gastroenterology* 55, 102–110.

JACKSON, M., LOGERFO, J., DIEHR, P., WATTS, C., and RICHARDSON, W. (1978). "Elective Hysterectomy: A Cost-Benefit Analysis," *Inquiry* 15:3 (September), 275–280.

JACOBS, E., WINTER, P., and ALVIS, H. (1969). "Hyperoxygenation Effects of Cognitive Functioning in the Aged," *New England Journal of Medicine* 281:13 (October 2), 753–757.

KLARMAN, H. (1965). "Syphilis Control Programs," in R. Dorfman (ed.), *Measuring Benefits of Government Investments.* Washington, D.C.: The Brookings Institution, 367–410.

KLARMAN, H. (1967). "Present Status of Cost-Benefit Analysis in the Health Field," *American Journal of Public Health* 57:11 (November) 1948–1953.

KLARMAN, H. (1974). "Application of Cost-Benefit Analysis to the Health Services and the Special Case of the Technologic Innovation," *International Journal of Health Services* 4:3 (Fall), 325–352.

KLARMAN, H., FRANCIS, J., and ROSENTHAL, G. (1968). "Cost Effectiveness Analysis Applied to the Treatment of Chronic Renal Disease," *Medical Care* 6:1 (January-February), 48–54.

KRISCHER, J. (1976). "The Mathematics of Cleft Lip and Palate Treatment Evaluation: Measuring the Desirability of Treatment Outcomes," *The Cleft Palate Journal* 13:4 (April), 165–180.

LAYDE, P., ALLMEN, S., and OAKLEY, G. (1979). "Maternal Serum Alpha-Fetoprotein Screening: A Cost-Benefit Analysis," *American Journal of Public Health* 69:6 (June) 566–573.

MISHAN, E. (1976). *Cost-Benefit Analysis*. New York: Praeger.

MUSGRAVE, R. (1969). "Cost-Benefit Analysis and the Theory of Public Finance," *Journal of Economic Literature* 7:3 (September), 797–806.

MUSHKIN, S. (1962). "Health as an Investment," *Journal of Political Economy* 70:5 (October), 129–157.

NEUTRA, R. (1977). "Indications for the Surgical Treatment of Suspected Acute Appendicitis: A Cost-Effectiveness Approach," in *Costs, Risks, and Benefits of Surgery, op. cit.*, 277–307.

NEWHOUSE, J. (1979). *The Economics of Medical Care*. New York: Addison-Wesley.

PIACHAUD, D., and WEDDELL, J. (1972). "The Economics of Treating Varicose Veins," *International Journal of Epidemiology* 1:3 (Autumn), 287–299.

RANSOHOFF, D., and FEINSTEIN, A. (1976). "Is Decision Analysis Useful in Clinical Medicine?" *Yale Journal of Biology and Medicine* 49:2 (May), 165–179.

RICE, D. (1966). "Estimating the Cost of Illness," Health Economics Series No. 6. Washington, D.C.: U.S. Government Printing Office.

ROMM, J., and MCKEON, M. (1979). "Survey and Evaluation of the Physician Extender Reimbursement Study: Cost-Effectiveness." System Sciences Inc. Consultants Report to DHEW, Health Care Financing Administration.

SCHELLING, T. (1968). "The Life You Save May Be Your Own," in S. Chase (ed.), *Problems in Public Expenditure Analysis*. Washington, D.C.: The Brookings Institution, 127–162.

SCHOENBAUM, S., HYDE, J., BARTOSHESKY, L., and CRAMPTON, K. (1976). "Benefit-Cost Analysis of Rubella Vaccination Policy," *New England Journal of Medicine* 294:6 (February 5) 306–310.

SCHWEITZER, S., and KEATING, M. (1978). "The Cost-Effectiveness of Bone-Marrow Transplant Therapy." Paper given at The American Public Health Association Annual Meeting, Los Angeles, October 17.

SKILLINGS, J., WILLIAMS, J., and HINSHAW, J. (1979). "Cost-Effectiveness of Operative Cholangiography," *American Journal of Surgery* 137:1 (January), 26–30.

SPARER, G., and MCKEON, M. (1979). "Renal Dialysis—A Case Study Useful for Assessing Approaches to Catastrophic Health Insurance." System Sciences Inc. Consultants Report to DHEW, Health Care Financing Administration.

STEWART, A., WARE, J., and JOHNSTON, S. (1975). "Construction of Scales Measuring Health and Health-Related Concepts from The Dayton Medical History Questionnaire," in *The Conceptualization and Measurement of Health in the Health Insurance Study*. Santa Monica: Rand Corporation.

THALER, R., and ROSEN, S. (1976). "The Value of Saving a Life: Evidence from the Labor Market," *National Bureau of Economic Research* 40, 265–298.

THOMAS, L. (1977). "On the Science and Technology of Medicine," *Daedalus* 106:1 (Winter), 35–46.

TSAI, S., LEE, E., and HARDY, R. (1978). "The Effect of a Reduction in Leading Causes of Death: Potential Gains in Life Expectancy," *American Journal of Public Health* 68:10 (October), 966–971.

VISICK, A. (1948). "A Study of the Failures After Gasterectomy," *Annals of the Royal College of Surgeons* 3, 266–281.

WAALER, H., and PIOT, M. (1970). "Use of an Epidemiological Model for Estimating the Effectiveness of Tuberculosis Control Measures," *Bulletin of the World Health Organization* 43, 1–16.

WARD, G. (1977). "National High Blood Pressure Program." Report from The National Institutes of Health to the Congressional Office of Technological Assessment.

WARNER, K. (1978). "Effects of Hospital Cost Containment on the Development and Use of Medical Technology," *Milbank Memorial Fund Quarterly* 56:2 (Spring) 187–211.

WEINSTEIN, M., PLISKIN, J., and STASON, W. (1977). "Coronary Artery Bypass Surgery: Decision and Policy Analysis," in *Costs, Risks, and Benefits of Surgery*, *op. cit.*, 342–371.

WEISBROD, B. (1968). "Income Redistribution Effects and Benefit-Cost Analysis," in S. Chase (ed.), *Problems in Public Expenditure Analysis*. Washington, D.C.: Brookings Institution, 177–209.

Chapter 4

THE ROLE OF TECHNOLOGY ASSESSMENT

*Beware of little expenses; a small leak will sink a great
ship.*

—Benjamin Franklin

*The interests of the federal programs are not well
served by a declining access to data or by ambiguous
distinctions between research and policy analysis.*

—Herbert Klarman

Medical technology assessment is becoming an increasingly important topic for physicians and health policy makers. Formal training in
cost-effective clinical decision making for residents and medical students is a potential alternative to further coercive federal cost containment efforts. If further regulatory ventures are to be avoided,
and the dual goals of cost containment and quality achieved, physicians should be taught in their formative clinical years to apply
parsimony and efficiency principles in ordering tests and treatments.
This chapter will examine the question of whether exposure to such
instruction changes attitudes among medical students electing to
take a course on decision analysis and health economics. Further
research is needed as to the timing and content of the most cost-
effective means of promoting cost-effective clinical decisions. Ethical
and social issues raised by cost-benefit and cost-effectiveness applications will also be discussed.

Economics and Medicine

Future physicians must realize that cost-benefit analysis and cost-effectiveness analysis are tools that can produce better informed decisions. However, as we have seen in Chapter 3, these two analytical techniques have occasionally been oversold in the health sector because of the multiplicity of dimensions of health service output and the difficulty of comparing disparate types of health benefits. Economic techniques should not be sold as value-free mathematics. However, without such analysis, decision making will remain *ad hoc*, with the assumptions hidden and the value judgments implicit. Some decision makers may want their values and assumptions to be kept secret and free from refutation, rather than to be made public and explicit.

The Congressional Office of Technology Assessment (U.S. Congress, 1980) evaluation of cost-effectiveness and cost-benefit applications in the health field concluded that the conceptual and practical limitations of the techniques are such that they should not be considered definitive tools that produce "correct" decisions. For example, construction of a hospice may not be justified merely by the projected medical cost savings, but the humanitarian intangible benefits (bereavement support, etc.) might more than justify the investment. According to the Office of Technology Assessment report, the analyst's role is one of information-generation and decision-assistance, because limited resources typically preclude valuation of intangible benefits.*

American society has been predisposed to rationing the availability of a new hospital technology through planning legislation. Traditionally once the supply is in place we deal ineffectively with rationing decisions. For example, Rettig (1978) documents a classic case of the physician community's inability to cope with ethical issues in the rationing of renal dialysis care after Shana Alexander published the November 1962 *Life* magazine article, "They Decide Who Lives, Who Dies." The American tradition has been to make

---

* The Office for Medical Applications of Research at The National Institutes of Health also works in the area of technology assessment, for example, funding consensus development sessions to study the safety and appropriate conditions for use of drugs, devices, and procedures (Perry and Kalberer, 1980). The Reagan Administration is currently considering merging a third technology assessment study group (National Center for Health Care Technology) with the aforementioned NIH group. Organized medicine has supported this attempt to merge centers and substantially reduce their total budgets. The American Medical Association has always argued that technology assessment is the responsibility of the private medical community.

local selective choices through critical care committees rather than to implement an "all or none" rationing decision; that is, everyone is allowed access or no one is allowed access as with most European countries. Recently, a lawyer has written a hypothetical Supreme Court Decision for the year 2000 that upholds the concept of a national lottery for distribution of artificial hearts (Annas, 1977). The author points out that American society cannot accept "all or none" rationing.

Frequently, economic evaluations consider questions of whether a procedure or treatment should be done more or less frequently. For example, Cole (1976) reports that performing one million prophylactic hysterectomies would save $1.4 billion (mostly in the form of 35,000 prevented cases of cancer), but cost $2.9 billion. The Congressional study on unnecessary surgery estimated the cost of excess and inappropriate elective surgery at $4 billion in 1976 (U.S. Congress, 1976).

Since the reader may not have conceptualized excess utilization in graphic terms, Figure 4.1 illustrates three possible scenarios for

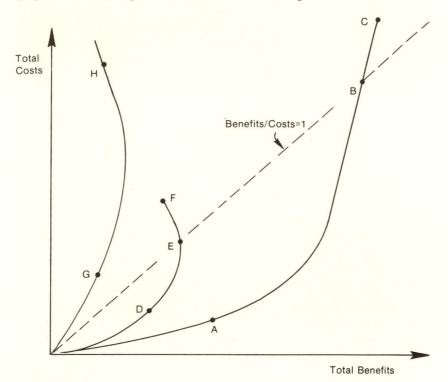

Figure 4.1 Three Hypothetical Production Functions of Total Treatment Benefits as a Function of Total Costs.

medical treatment production functions. Curve *AB* represents a cost-beneficial treatment mode such as heart pacemakers. If the technology were inappropriately utilized or prophylactically pre-scribed for an indiscriminately large fraction of the population, the assessed technology could move along the curve into the region *BC* where benefits do not justify costs. Hypothetical curve *DE* might represent the benefit-cost range when surgeons perform only 50,000 coronary artery bypass operations annually, but the treatment may appear unjustified (region *EF*) if the operative incidence increases to 90,000 annual bypass cases. The third hypothetical curve *GH* is an example of a treatment mode that is never cost-beneficial (for example, gastric freezing for ulcers, Miao, 1977). Unfortunately the public had to endure the fad from the introductory usage stage at point *G* (1962) to peak popularity at point *H* (1968), before the faulty treatment mode (gastric freezing) was finally discredited (1969).

Ethical and Social Issues

In the United States we allow any individual who can afford it to buy any technology, and we selectively finance transplants and less effec-tive technologies from the public treasury. Questions of cost-benefit and resource limitations do disturb some American physicians and prompt the medical community to ask how we can afford dialysis and transplants during a resurgence of polio and other childhood dis-eases. In contrast to England, America has said that a citizen should not be barred from the opportunity to receive tertiary care services if he or she can afford them. Whereas England has made the slogan "health care as a right" operational by funding all primary and sec-ondary care service activities, frequently individuals are not allowed to buy even proven technologies that are judged too expensive for the society. One of the demands during the British hospital strikes in the mid-1970s was that private pay patients not be allowed to have medically unnecessary services performed. For the 94 percent of the British population utilizing the British National Health Service as their primary provider, publicly funded bypass surgery and heart and renal transplants are now available for those willing to wait two to four months. In America, obtaining most basic medical services is done through a process similar to the search for any other consumer good (that is, the family plans and budgets for the purchase), but obtaining very expensive new services is very often a matter of chance. It is possible that this situation reflects consumer preferences, in that the American consumer may value the assurance that comes with knowing that his nation can provide the utmost care for a given individual following the onset of a catastrophic disease.

Economic evaluation of common diseases will probably continue to receive more critical assessment than innovations for rare diseases that pose a less significant net financial burden in spite of the higher unit costs. An innovation like coronary bypass surgery has attracted the attention of the health services research community in the United States because expenditures have rocketed from zero to $2 billion per year within a single decade. Economic impact considerations should be a critical determinant in selecting the procedures for randomized clinical trials (RCT). Neuhauser (1979) has pointed out the dangerous limitations that short-sighted ethical considerations impose if they become the sole determinant of RCT experimentation. He argues that in some cases proposed sham operations (for example, telling the patient the operation was performed when in actuality it was not) should not be stopped by the local human subject committee of the hospital. For example, internal mammary artery ligation therapy was exposed by eight pairs of sham operations as an ineffective multi-million dollar mode of treatment. Neuhauser suggests an appropriate reward for the eight patients who saved our economy and the public chest: "Each should receive $1 million tax-free and be flown to the White House to shake hands with the President." The economy may be wasting tens of billions of dollars on unnecessary care because of the failure to perform RCTs.

The less tangible quality-of-life benefits comprise an increasing proportion of medical care benefits. For example, elective surgical expenditures are properly intended to achieve less tangible goals than mortality or morbidity rate reduction, such as relief of disability, pain, and disfigurement. Such quality-of-life factors are to be identified, then quantified in terms of their equivalent social costs by shadow pricing, and finally balanced against commensurate shadow prices for quantity of life. Advocates of the "willingness-to-pay" approach suggest the maximization of lives saved (Zeckhauser, 1975) as the social objective function. Mishan (1971) has pointed out that while our enlightened society can hardly avoid making these analytical efforts, shadow pricing and value weighting present a multitude of difficulties for research. Because consumers are provided with imperfect information, individuals' "willingness-to-pay" will sometimes be underestimated (e.g., vaccinations) and other times overestimated (e.g., laetrile).

Valuation problems still tend to plague most analyses. Subjective

questions concerning valuation and effectiveness are largely a product of the values and occupation of the respondent. For example,
CAT scanner effectiveness to a radiologist is measured by whether
the pictures are clearer and the information is more detailed. The
economist must represent the public interest and ask whether there
is a connection between CAT scanning yielding better diagnosis,
resulting in better treatment, and ultimately improving patient outcome. The radiologist's definition of effectiveness might argue for
7000 CAT scanners, but a more economical viewpoint might suggest
that we need 800 or 400. Another dilemma that the economic analyst
faces is the unsubstantiated thesis of ever-improving technology,
that is, the assumption that any evaluation will be obsolete when
completed since medical science is improving so fast. Yet another
problem faced by the analyst attempting to do a prospective study is
refusal by the physicians to pursue randomized controlled trials if
any hint of inferiority among the alternatives can be raised as a "red
herring" to prevent the experiment. However, difficult decisions
will increasingly need to be made concerning the allocation of scarce
resources. Contrary to the conventional wisdom, the majority of
Americans would like to place a dollar value on human life. According to a 1981 national Harris Poll, 52 percent of the American public
believe that government and the courts must attempt to place an
economic value on human life. Only 34 percent of the national
sample of the population disagreed with the need to put a dollar
value on life, and 14 percent responded "not sure" or "it depends"
(APHA, 1981).

The multiplicity of quality-of-life dimensions for weighting health
benefits will always require the use of consensus decision making
and value judgments. How else can our society weigh the value of a
55-year-old's life saved against a 5-year-old's case of blindness prevented? Encapsulated in that classic quip that economists "know the
price of everything and the value of nothing" comes the realization
that there are theoretical limitations to either market prices or
willingness-to-pay prices in valuing benefits. Prices do not reflect
the value of externalities and other assurances (of capacity if needed)
enjoyed by nonusers of the service, and the imperfectly informed
user of the service may fail to appreciate all the direct or indirect
benefits accrued. Another ethical and measurement problem unique
to health services involves the issue of irreversibility of death, that
is, the ability of the marketplace to proxy value through the price
system is applicable to television sets but not to human life (Cook

and Graham, 1977). Purchase of a television is reversible, but loss of a life is not. The most obvious "problem" assumption in applying cost-benefit or cost-effectiveness analysis is that the tools disregard all equity considerations of redistribution of income. These highly reductionist and normative techniques presume the distribution of purchasing power in the society is efficient.

One cannot simply assume that cost-benefit analysis is a mere extension of an efficient price system that enables us to select or finance medical services that yield an excess of social value over resource cost. The price system and labor markets are imperfect, and equity considerations must be involved. However, one should not underestimate the value of cost-benefit or cost-effectiveness calculus, because the process of analysis asks explicit questions of valuation that politicians might want to blur, such as why do we spend $25,000 to give one executive a bone marrow transplant or bypass operation while foregoing five years of life for twenty-five ghetto dwellers suffering from rheumatic fever or hypertension. The popular dislike for quantifying value judgments prevents the exposure of unconsciously inaccurate or insidious assumptions. Public disclosure of economic analysis and the assumptions that were dictated to the analyst has the potential for maximizing compassionate concern for non-discriminatory "Who Shall Live?" decisions. As recently as 1979, physicians have taken the elitist view that cost-benefit analysis is a less satisfactory alternative to hospital committee *ad hoc* decisions (Turnbull *et al.*, 1979).

Value judgments increasingly will have to be made by the courts. For example, should patient X be provided with chloromycetin if the drug is known to correlate weakly with fatal anemia. Taking the drug increases the risk of dying from aplastic anemia from 1 in 500,000 to 1 in 40,000. How shall we decide when changing a probability distribution constitutes "causing" an event? This question has been raised in a wide range of circumstances, from auto safety to the case of swine flu vaccination side effects.

Consumer Cost Issues

The growth in third-party financing of medical care has frequently been criticized for funding excessive and/or inappropriate therapies. One postulated negative effect of health insurance is the increased financing of useless technologies like gastric freezing for ulcers. An-

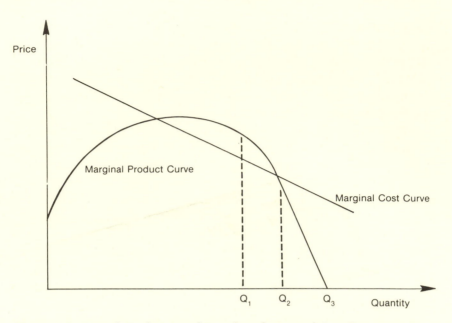

Figure 4.2   Hypothetical Marginal Benefit and Marginal Cost Curves.

other postulated negative byproduct of the growth in health insurance is the utilization of treatments to an excess (see points *C, F, H* in Figure 4.2). The growth in health insurance coverage provided health care institutions with the wherewithal to expand service capability and produce service at the point where the cost exceeds the benefit. As health insurance becomes more comprehensive and the consumer's out-of-pocket cost falls to zero, health service institutions continue to provide care beyond the point where marginal cost is equal to marginal benefit (Q_2) up to point Q_3 (see Figure 4.2). The situation is somewhat analogous to that of the consumer who visits an automobile showroom and asks the dealer to select a car for him, price being no object. Because the dealer's profit margin is higher if he provides a Mercedes rather than a Mustang, the customer will never see the Mustang.

The present American economy cannot afford a Mercedes for every consumer (point Q_3). In defense of production at point Q_3 is the argument by American medicine that they must do the utmost for each patient irrespective of cost. Many economists argue that society can barely afford the Mustang unless we decrease utilization rates by increasing the co-insurance paid by patients. Future physicians should realize that relaxing the degree of clinical discrimination and increasing the quantity of care provided per illness episode (intensity) can only bankrupt our health economy. Moreover, doing the utmost for everybody will save a few lives but at an ever diminishing rate. Production of Q_3 minus Q_1 additional units of medical service ignores the opportunity cost of spending that money on housing or pollution control. Some analysts would hope that every dollar wasted in the medical economy is a dollar not utilized on defense or nuclear power. However, it is the broader health economy of prevention and public health that is being squeezed by the growth in the medical economy.

Economic and Decision Theory Tools for Reducing "Little Ticket" Expenditures

A consideration to be dealt with in technology assessment is that there is more to cost containment than simply preventing the purchase of $500,000 machines. Many health planners assume that the cost problem will disappear if only society can control the purchase of "big ticket" items and so reduce the availability of expensive therapeutic treatment approaches. However, a number of recent studies (Maloney and Rogers, 1979) have suggested that "little ticket" items, such as laboratory tests and diagnostic procedures, comprise the bulk of the cost crisis iceberg. Diagnostic charges account for over 25 percent of total hospital expenditures, and diagnostic testing costs have been increasing at almost double the rate of total hospital costs (see Chapter 12). The efficiency and increased costs of performing more diagnostic tests are central issues in the public debate about rising medical costs. Twenty-fold variations in the number of diagnostic tests utilized by groups of interns did not measurably affect the outcome following care for a cohort of patients with ambulatory hypertensive disease (Daniels and Schroeder, 1977). The surgery study presented in Chapter 12 suggests that physician characteristics, such as degree of medical school affiliation and percentage of foreign medical graduates, are the best predictors of the number of elective tests ordered. John Knowles (1969) was one of the first physicians to link the cost and efficiency issues:

> One should ask how many renal arteriograms in patients with hypertension have resulted in the surgical or medical cure of the patients' hypertension. . . . Increasingly we shall be asked to answer such questions, for our resources are not infinite nor is our share of the Gross National Product.

In considering the cost effectiveness value of diagnostic tests, clinicians and medical students should be encouraged to consider three issues: the reliability of test interpretation among physicians, the specificity of the test, and the marginal costs and benefits of additional testing. With respect to the reliability issue, there is wide disagreement among physicians upon what constitutes a significant change in diagnostic test results for the same patient (Skendzel, 1978). The previously cited study by Daniels and Schroeder (1977) indicated a strong but not statistically significant correlation between poor clinical outcome and laboratory costs, suggesting that physicians who tend to be less competent use the laboratory more. There is a growing body of evidence indicating physician confusion in the interpretation and application of information contained in diagnostic tests. This confusion tends to result in suboptimal patient care and high medical costs.

Obviously diagnostic tests do not disclose the presence or absence of disease. They are merely tools to detect the presence or absence of particular signs or symptoms from which the presence or absence of a specific disease may be predicted. The following diagram illustrates the two-step sequence from testing to diagnosis.

$$\text{Diagnostic test} \xrightarrow{(1)} \text{The sign or symptom} \xrightarrow{(2)} \text{Disease}$$
$$\text{is + or } - \qquad\qquad \text{is present}$$
$$\text{or absent}$$

There are two points of potential slippage, each with its own implications, in the diagnostic testing procedure. Type one (1) breakdowns are often due to inadequate technology which is translated into an inability to detect the target sign or symptom with adequate accuracy. It follows that these breakdowns often can be remedied by improving technology. Type two (2) breakdowns occur when the presence or absence of the target sign or symptom has a low predictive value for the presence or absence of disease. These breakdowns are inherent in the test and usually cannot be remedied.

Sensitivity and specificity analysis have traditionally been used to measure the efficacy of diagnostic tests. These values are determined by performing the test on two selected groups of subjects, those with disease and those without disease. They answer the questions: Given that the patient has the disease, how likely is he to have a positive test? Conversely, given that the patient doesn't have the disease, how likely is he to have a negative test? Sensitivity and specificity are rarely both 100 percent because diagnostic tests measure biologic variations that are then used to predict disease. These variations are usually distributed over a range of values roughly conforming to a normal curve. The curves representing the range of laboratory values of the diseased and the non-diseased population overlap. The more overlap, the greater the trade-off between sensitivity and specificity.

Diagnostic tests are used for at least three purposes: discovery, confirmation, and exclusion. Discovery tests must have high sensitivity and are used to detect disease in patients who seem healthy. Confirmation tests must have high specificity and are used to verify disease in situations of strong suspicion.* Exclusion tests must have high sensitivity and are used to rule out disease in situations of suspicion, but are too expensive to use for discovery purposes. A test can be used for one, two, or all three purposes. Physicians and medical students should be encouraged to develop strategies utilizing combinations of tests that allow the achievement of both high sensitivity and high specificity.

The importance of the specificity or false-positive issue has been raised recently in the context of fetal monitoring and renovascular disease screening among hypertensives. Banta and Thacker (1979) report that the direct annual costs of electronic fetal monitoring in 1977 were $80 million, but that the indirect costs to both mother and child could exceed $300 million annually. The benefits of fetal monitoring are to be found in the degree to which early detection of fetal distress prevents mental retardation or death. The poor specificity of this diagnostic tool gives rise to many false-positive indications of fetal distress, contributing to 100,000 additional unnecessary Caesarian sections in 1977 (costing $222 million). Future controlled clinical trials are necessary to determine whether there is a "best" mode of monitoring among the five (internal electronic monitoring, external electronic monitoring, diagnostic amniocentesis, scalp sampling, and ultrasonography). Banta and Thacker point to the need to acknowledge increased risk to the mother associated with pelvic infections or death from unnecessary operations, estimated at $58 million for 1977. In addition, there is another $50

---

* Sometimes it is better to avoid the confirmation test (e.g., a biopsy) and treat all highly suspect cases with the therapy [e.g., the anti-viral drug adenine arabinoside for herpes virus encephalitis (HVE)]. Braum (1980) has demonstrated that it is better on the average to avoid the risk of brain biopsy and directly administer the drug on the basis of other tests.

million of estimated costs associated with the risk of infant hemorrhaging, respiratory distress, and infection at the site of the electrode.

A potential explanation for why fetal monitoring became so popular in a matter of months might center around what Foltz and Kelsey (1978) call "the nation's ideology to support the maximum utilization of new technologies." Two clinical trials by Haverkamp *et al.* (1976, 1979) of the effectiveness of electronic fetal monitoring versus basic nurse monitoring found no significant differences. Our medical technology is all too quick to accept new diagnostic techniques that have been founded on faulty evaluations or have poor specificity in the average hospital. Two examples are the CEA (carcinoembryonic antigen) test for colonic cancer and the NBT (nitro-blue tetrazolium) test in the diagnosis of bacterial infection. Both tests were promoted to medical students in 1973, then found to be substantially less effective by 1975–1976 (Ransohoff and Feinstein, 1978).

A fourth case of the importance of considering the costs associated with poor test specificity has been provided by McNeil and Adelstein (1975). The effect of high sensitivity but poor specificity in the primary screening modality for detecting renovascular disease among hypertensives ($83 intraveneous pyelogram plus $100 renography) can be improved by subsequent arteriography at a cost of $375 (1975 prices). This subsequent angiogram increases the specificity to a perfect 100 percent, but the new information is hardly worthwhile since case finding is not associated with improved survival figures and surgical treatment following the angiogram was found to be no more efficacious than medical treatment prior to testing (McNeil, 1977). However, improved specificity and case finding through pulmonary angiography ($300) and perfusion lung scanning ($125) have been demonstrated to be worth the 40 percent increased costs for diagnosis of pulmonary embolism in young patients.

Having addressed the reliability and specificity issues in cost-effectiveness analysis, the third issue left for discussion is marginal costs. Neuhauser and Lewicki (1975) performed a marginal cost analysis on the value of doing a fifth or sixth sequential stool guaiac, in reaction to the recommendation by Gregor (1969) and the American Cancer Society (Leffall, 1974) that six guaiacs be done on all persons over 40 years of age to detect asymptomatic colon cancer. Even with a diagnostic test of high sensitivity (92.67 percent), the marginal cost of the sixth test ($47.1 million per cancer case detected) was 20,000 times the average cost per case discovered. Although six sequential stool guaiacs, followed by barium enemas for all positive guaiacs, will identify virtually all "silent" colon cancers, is it worth $47.1 million to detect that one rare case when the resources could be used elsewhere? Physicians are too oriented toward citing simple average costs ($4 for the first stool guaiac, and $1 for each subsequent guaiac) to recognize the devastating implications that the recommendation of up to six guaiacs could have on medical costs. For example, physicians would neglect the 41 percent of total diagnostic costs devoted to incorrectly diagnosing (false-positive) colon cancer and then ruling out presence of the disease with a $100 barium enema. Maximization of specificity (the minimization of false-positives) has the added benefit of reducing needless patient anxiety, in addition to the tangible benefits of reducing unnecessary care, iatrogenic morbidity, and mortality.

One final problem in assessing new tests or techniques concerns the issue of substitutability. New diagnostic procedures can seldom be judged 100 percent accurate, perfect substitutes for the old methods. For example, computerized axial tomography scanning (CAT) may be considered by physicians to be cost-effective simply because it replaces other costly, painful, and invasive diagnostic procedures. However, some radiologists have suggested that head scans cannot be considered merely a substitute for pneumo-encephalography, arteriography, and other techniques. For example, many more CAT head scans are being performed than would be necessitated by replacement of all the prior techniques. The Office of Technological Assessment (U.S. Congress, 1978a) study suggests that hospitals with high percentages of negative scans are using the machine as a less than cost-beneficial blind screening tool. If we do eventually conclude that head scanning is safe, reliable, and cost-effective if used judiciously, a question still remains as to whether body scanners are necessary. The paucity of evidence supporting CAT technology does not seem to justify $388 million of expenditures in 1976. Abrams and McNeil (1978) suggest that body scanning should not be the primary diagnostic echelon. This disclaimer ignores the fact that CAT scanning can have efficacy at the best quality hospitals, but lacks cost-effectiveness at the average or below-average hospital if utilized too frequently. Some of the best hospitals are adding to the cost containment problem by developing "replacement" equipment for the CAT scanner (Ritman *et al.*, 1980). This new machine, the Dynamic Spatial Reconstructor or DSR, costs $5 million and has not been subjected to any form of cost-benefit or cost-effectiveness analysis.

Physician Involvement or Increased Federal Intervention?

The existence of growing federal regulation in the health field is a byproduct of the observation that the imperfect private sector has been little help in selecting the programs and services that are to be available as a reimbursable expense in the clinical armada. Consequently, as a matter of public policy, the Congressional Office of Technological Assessment (U.S. Congress, 1978b) has suggested a sequence for evaluating medical technology: Consider efficacy, cost-effectiveness, cost-benefit, and then safety. Efficacy is concerned with measuring the benefit of a technology under ideal conditions of use, for example, the Mayo Clinic and Johns Hopkins Hospital. Cost-effectiveness is a measure of the relative benefits and costs, to society, of various technologies applied to the same problem area under average conditions of use. Consequently, a technology can have efficacy in the best hospitals, but be cost-ineffective for general use. Cost-effectiveness is measured by the ratio of costs to tangible benefits, expressed as cost per man-year saved or cost per quality adjusted man-year saved or cost per disability-year prevented.

The estimation of direct benefits is usually a simple process of measuring what costs are foregone as a result of the consumption of the service under evaluation. One frequently mentioned caveat to the problem of benefit estimation is double-counting or overestimating the benefit of eliminating one disease if there is a simultaneous presence of multiple diseases. Weisbrod (1961) was one of the first to recognize that patients who avoid one cause of death (cancer) may have a higher susceptibility to another competing cause of death (heart disease). The bias in the benefit estimation process is to overstate the benefits projected from reducing the prevalence or incidence of any single disease category, that is, the whole is smaller than the sum of the individual parts. The estimation of intangible benefits is also a major problem in most studies. One of the most overlooked intangible benefits is the patient reassurance factor. However, if the false-positive rate is too high, the intangible negative benefit of unnecessary patient distress could outweigh the net amount of patient assurance.

Physician involvement in the process of doing cost-benefit or cost-effectiveness research is crucial. Construction of a decision tree is the first step in most cost-effectiveness analyses designed to assist in the selection of alternative approaches to patient care. It allows the practitioner to incorporate the predictive values obtained from appropriate therapeutic procedures into a wider framework. This analysis is not purely mechanical and requires input from a group of experienced clinicians. The twin problems of "dirty" data and unreasonable assumptions could be eliminated if heavy handed regulators allowed clinicians to have more input in the design phase, funded better epidemiological studies, and sponsored more randomized controlled clinical trials. For example, we should begin funding clinical trials to assess the relative cost-effectiveness of zeugmatography (with magnetic, rather than radiation "images" of the patient) versus the more established CAT scanning technique.

Teaching Medical Students

The purpose of this section is to outline one approach to teaching cost-effective clinical decision making and to measure the degree of attitudinal change produced by a brief course in this area. The elective course was offered to third-year medical students at Cornell Medical College. As medicine has grown more technological, the decision process has also become more statistically complex. Unfortunately, the recent medical school graduate's statistical knowledge has not kept pace with the growth in medical science. In a recent study at four Harvard teaching hospitals only 20 percent of fourth-year medical students, 15 percent of internal medicine residents, and 20 percent of attending physicians correctly responded to a question that required the application of elementary statistical analysis to diagnostic test results (Cassells *et al.*, 1978).

A potential benefit of injecting economic content into the medical school curriculum is that the new clinicians might informally utilize cost-effective clinical decision making principles to provide equivalent quality of care at less cost. The Association of American Medical Colleges, the American Hospital Association, and the American Medical Association House of Delegates have endorsed cost education for physicians during the undergraduate and postgraduate educational process. If we are to make intelligent decisions on how to improve the quality of care and contain the cost of services, it is our responsibility to discover the most effective means of training physicians to make economical decisions. The hope is that formal training in decision analysis and economics can yield more rational decisions, and perhaps better patient outcomes, or at least more informed choice if economy happens to conflict with the pursuit of the "highest possible" quality of care. The norm for the 1980s may have to be the provision of the best possible patient outcomes within the constraint of a given amount of available resources, for example, 10 percent of Gross National Product for health care.

If some of the principles of cost-effective clinical decision making would permeate into the subconscious cognitive processes of American physicians, a less costly style of medical care might result. Continuing education programs may affect practicing physicians' behavior, but it might be more cost-beneficial to bring formal discussion of these issues to medical students and help them reflect upon their future role as clinicians. Most of the previous effort in this area has concentrated on house staff (AMA, 1978). The approaches include identifying those individuals with out-of-line utilization profiles, testing residents with a price list of hospital charges, and asking the young clinician if the marginal information gain of the test justified the cost (Lyle *et al.*, 1979).

The next section will review the results of the pre-course and post-course attitude survey of the students. The course had three major themes. The first basic theme is that physicians must understand the role of cost-benefit analysis in "big ticket" resource priority decisions and other policy determinations. The second course theme is that physicians should increasingly utilize and participate in cost-effectiveness evaluations to constrain the proliferation of "little ticket" expenses for tests and procedures. Thirdly, clinicians should be interested in preserving professional autonomy by cooperating with the health policy decision makers rather than being co-opted by the growth in federal intervention. If further regulation is to be avoided and the dual goals of cost containment and improved patient care achieved, health practitioners must be taught to utilize diagnostic tests more appropriately and treatment modes more effectively.

Student Attitude Survey

There is inevitably an imperfect link between attitudes and behavior. Nevertheless, attitude shifts are taken as a proxy estimate of program effectiveness because researchers seldom have the option to wait five years and do a prospective field survey to measure shifts in post-graduate clinical behavior. The self-report attitudinal instrument utilized in this study did not rely on a single question to detect the depth or presence of an attitude. Instead, the four basic constructs (interest in reducing costs, concern with decision science techniques, concern with economics and biostatistics, and advocating maximum consumer information) were measured by a number of questions. Providing four-to-seven ordinal attitudinal (agree strongly, mildly, disagree mildly, strongly) items for each construct aids in minimizing the error that could result from student misinterpretation of single items.

The instrument was constructed so that the responses were anonymous, while allowing for the recognition of individuals before and after the course. The anonymity of the survey response was intended to minimize the potential bias that could occur if respondents were to hide their true attitudes and bend their answers to conform to the attitudes of the instructor. Of the 80 third-year Cornell Medical students based in New York City during the month in which the Cost-Effective Clinical Decision Making Course was offered, 56 filled out a pre-course questionnaire. Of these 56, 29 elected to take the course and completed a post-course questionnaire. The two basic research questions involved how the course affected the attitudes of the 29 course takers, and how the 27 respondents who elected not to take the course differed from the 29 course participants.

A number of nonparametric statistical tests demonstrated the significant impact of the course on attitudes and the selection bias between course takers and nontakers. The Kolmogorov-Smirnov Test* demonstrated that the sample of course takers was more predisposed to cost-effective clinical decision making ideas compared to those electing not to take the course for six of the twenty items. Course takers were significantly predisposed to being pro-consumerists (two items significant at the 0.01 level), mindful of the need for medical cost containment (three items significant at the 0.05 level), and conscious of the necessity for decision analysis applications to medicine (one item significant at the 0.05 level).

In the case of the 29 students who completed questionnaires before and after the course, the Wilcoxon matched-pairs test provided

---

* Siegel, S. (1956). *Nonparametric Statistics*. New York: McGraw-Hill.

a measure of the significance of attitudinal change. Those completing the course had not significantly shifted their ideas on consumerism and the need for cost containment. However, there was a significant shift with respect to applications of decision analysis to medicine (two items were significant at the 0.02 level, two additional items at the 0.05 level). Completion of the course also affected positively their respect for health economics (one item was significant at the 0.01 level, two additional items were significant at the 0.05 level).

The students most in need of a course in this subject area appeared to be the least likely to take the course. Multivariate discriminant analysis provided an accurate prediction of participation (yes, no) in the course. Of the 56 respondents, 78.6 percent were correctly classified, and the two groups were statistically different (Chi squared $= 4.09$, $p < 0.05$, d.f. $= 1$). In order to investigate further the question concerning the dichotomous variable of course selection, a probit model was tested for the twenty agree/disagree items. One of the early applications of this maximum likelihood technique in the health field was provided by Finney (1972). In our situation, the model was statistically significant in explaining the course selection (Chi squared $= 51.78$, $p < 0.05$). The two items significant at the 0.01 level were: "Patients should have convenient access to their medical record," and "Physicians should answer the patient in a quantitative probabilistic fashion if the patient asks for such specific information." The only other statement responses significant at the 0.05 level were: "Appropriate applications of statistical tools in differential diagnosis can significantly lower medical costs," and "Understanding of statistical tools is necessary to properly interpret diagnostic test results." The results seem to argue for making the course a requirement since the students most in need of decision science materials are the least likely to voluntarily select such a course.

Conclusions

Health practitioners, especially physicians, must be taught more economics and biostatistics in order to use diagnostic information appropriately and effectively and arrive at the best treatment mode.* Formal training in decision analysis can be applied to im-

---

* Duncan Neuhauser has suggested that the Hippocratic oath be rewritten in the 1980s as follows: "I swear by Apollo, the physician, and Aesculapius, and health and all heal and all the Gods and Goddesses that, according to my ability and judgment, *and cost considerations*, I will keep this oath and stipulation."

prove patient care in a therapeutic setting as well as to assist medical practitioners in understanding the priority setting and policy determinations that society will make regarding the future medical practice. Criticism of statistical tools usually is based upon the subjective estimates included in the formulas, alleging that what appears to be objective analysis is really no better than the examiner's best guess. This criticism will become less justified as decision makers begin to realize that (1) all decisions incorporate subjective estimations and (2) only through disciplined analysis can this subjectivity be evaluated. The recent proliferation of courses in the area of cost education or cost-effective clinical decision making is a healthy trend for those interested in evaluative research and medical cost containment. If we are to contain costs and maintain patient service quality, it is our responsibility to discover the most effective approaches to making economical clinical decisions.

References

ABRAMS, H., and MCNEIL, B. (1978). "Medical Innovations of Computed Tomography—Part II," *New England Journal of Medicine* 298:6 (February 7), 310–318.

American Medical Association (1978). *Cost-Effective Medical Care.* Chicago: Resident Physicians Section, American Medical Association.

American Public Health Association (1981). "Poll Shows Americans Would Put Dollar Value on Life," *Nation's Health* 20:2 (February), 3.

ANNAS, G. (1977). "Allocation of Artificial Hearts in the Year 2002: Minerva v. National Health Agency," *American Journal of Law and Medicine* 3 (Spring), 59–76.

ARTHUR, W. (1981). "The Economics of Risks to Life," *American Economic Review* 71:1(March), 54–64.

BANTA, D., and THACKER, S. (1979). "The Premature Delivery of Medical Technology: A Case Report—Electronic Fetal Monitoring," DHEW, National Center for Health Services Report. Rockville, Md.: U.S. Government Printing Office.

BODEN, L. (1979). "Cost-Benefit Analysis: Caveat Emptor," *American Journal of Public Health* 69:12 (December), 1210–1211.

BRAUN, P. (1980). "The Clinical Management of Suspected Herpes Virus Encephalitis," *American Journal of Medicine* 69, 895–899.

CARELS, E., NEUHAUSER, D., and STASON, W. (eds.) (1980). *The Physician and Cost Control.* Cambridge, Mass.: Oelgeschlager, Gunn and Hain, Inc.

CASSELLS, W., SCHOENBERGER, A., and GRABOYS, T. (1978). "Interpretation by Physicians of Clinical Laboratory Results," *New England Journal of Medicine* 299:17 (October 26), 999–1001.

COLE, P. (1976). "Elective Hysterectomy: Pro and Con," *New England Journal of Medicine* 295:5 (July 29), 264–265.

COOK, P., and GRAHAM, D. (1977). "The Demand for Insurance and Protection:

The Case of the Irreplaceable Commodities," *Quarterly Journal of Economics* 91:1 (February), 143–156.

DANIELS, M., and SCHROEDER, S. (1977). "Variations Among Physicians in Use of Laboratory Tests: Relation to Clinical Productivity and Outcomes of Care," *Medical Care* 15:6 (June), 482–487.

EASTAUGH, S. (1981). "Teaching the Principles of Cost-Effective Clinical Decision Making to Medical Students," *Inquiry* 18:1 (Spring), 28–36.

FEIN, R. (1971). "On Measuring Economic Benefits of Health Programs," in *Medical History and Medical Care*. London: Nuffield Provincial Hospitals Trust, 181–217.

FINNEY, D. (1972). *Probit Analysis*, third edition. Cambridge, Engl.: Cambridge University Press.

FOLTZ, A., and KELSEY, J. (1978). "The Annual Pap Test: A Dubious Policy Success," *Milbank Memorial Fund Quarterly* 56:4 (Fall), 426–462.

GREGOR, D. (1969). "Detection of Silent Colon Cancer in Routine Examinations," *CA: Cancer Journal for Clinicians* 19:6 (November-December), 330–337.

HAVERKAMP, A., THOMPSON, H., McFEE, J., and CETRULO, C. (1976). "The Evaluation of Continuous Fetal Heart Rate Monitoring in High-Risk Pregnancy," *American Journal of Obstetrics and Gynecology* 125:3 (June 1), 310–318.

HAVERKAMP, A., ORLEANS, M., LANGENDOERFER, S., McFEE, J., MURPHY, J., and THOMPSON, H. (1979). "A Controlled Clinical Trial on the Differential Effects of Fetal Monitoring," *American Journal of Obstetrics and Gynecology* 134:4(June 14), 399–408.

KNOWLES, J. (1969). "Radiology: A Case Study in Technology and Manpower," *New England Journal of Medicine* 280:24 (June 12), 1323–1329.

LEFFALL, I. (1974). "Early Diagnosis of Colorectal Cancer," *CA: Cancer Journal for Clinicians* 24:3 (May-June), 152–159.

LYLE, C., BIANCHI, R., HARRIS, J., and WOOD, Z. (1979). "Teaching Cost Containment to House Officers," *Journal of Medical Education* 54:11 (November), 856–862.

MALONEY, T., and ROGERS, D. (1979). "Medical Technology—A Different View of the Contentious Debate Over Costs," *New England Journal of Medicine* 301:26 (December 27), 1413–1419.

McNEIL, B., and ADELSTEIN, S. (1975). "Measures of Clinical Efficiency: The Value of Case Finding in Hypertensive Renovascular Disease," *New England Journal of Medicine* 293:5 (July 31), 221–226.

McNEIL, B. (1977). "The Value of Diagnostic Aids in Patients with Potential Surgical Problems," in J. Bunker, B. Barnes and F. Mosteller (eds.), *Costs, Risks, and Benefits of Surgery*. New York: Oxford, 77–90.

MIAO, L. (1977). "Gastric Freezing: An Example of the Evaluation of Medical Therapy by Randomized Clinical Trials," in *Costs, Risks, and Benefits of Surgery*, *op. cit.*, 198–211.

MISHAN, E. (1971). "Evaluation of Life and Limb: A Theoretical Approach," *Journal of Political Economy* 79:4 (July-August), 687–705.

MUSHKIN, S. (1979). *Biomedical Research: Costs and Benefits*. Cambridge, Mass.: Ballinger.

NEUHAUSER, D., and LEWICKI, A. (1975). "What Do We Gain from the Sixth Stool Guaiac?" *New England Journal of Medicine* 293:5 (July 31), 226–228.

NEUHAUSER, D. (1979). "The Public Voice and the Nation's Health," *Milbank Memorial Fund Quarterly* 57:1 (Winter), 60–69.

PERRY, S., and KALBERER, J. (1980). "The NIH Consensus-Development Program and the Assessment of Health Care Technologies," *New England Journal of Medicine* 303:3 (July 17), 169–172.

RANSOHOFF, D., and FEINSTEIN, A. (1978). "Problems of Spectrum and Bias in Evaluating the Efficacy of Diagnostic Tests," *New England Journal of Medicine* 299:17 (October 26), 926–930.

RETTIG, R. (1978). "Lessons Learned from the End-Stage Renal Disease Experience," in R. Egdahl, and P. Gertman (eds.), *Technology and the Quality of Health Care.* 153–173. Germantown, Md.: Aspen Systems.

RITMAN, E., KINSEY, J., ROBB, R., GILBERT, B., HARRIS, L., and WOOD, E. (1980). "Three-Dimensional Imaging of Heart, Lungs, and Circulation," *Science* 210:4467 (October 17), 273–280.

SCHETTLER, R., and PARINGER, L. (1980). "A Review of the Economic Evidence on Prevention," *Medical Care* 18:5 (May), 473–484.

SKENDZEL, L. (1978). "How Physicians Use Laboratory Tests," *Journal of the American Medical Association* 239:11 (March 13), 1077–1080.

TURNBULL, A., GRAZIANO, C., BARON, R., SICHEL, W., YOUNG, C., and HOWLAND, W. (1979). "The Inverse Relationship Between Cost and Survival in the Critically Ill Cancer Patient," *Critical Care Medicine* 7:1 (January), 20–23.

United States Congress (1976). 94th Congress, 2nd Session, Subcommittee on Oversight and Investigations of the Committee on Interstate and Foreign Commerce. *Report on the Cost and Quality of Health Care: Unnecessary Surgery.* Washington, D.C.: U.S. Government Printing Office.

United States Congress, Office of Technology Assessment (1978a). "Policy Implications of the Computed Tomography Scanner," Report to the U.S. Congress, F. Robbins, Study Chairman. Washington, D.C.: U.S. Government Printing Office.

United States Congress, Office of Technology Assessment (1978b). *Assessing the Efficacy and Safety of Medical Technologies.* Washington, D.C.: U.S. Government Printing Office.

United States Congress, Office of Technology Assessment (1980). *Cost-Effectiveness and Cost-Benefit Analysis in Health Care: Methodology and Literature Review,* Volume II. Washington, D.C.: U.S. Government Printing Office.

WEISBROD, B. (1961). *Economics of Public Health.* Philadelphia: University of Pennsylvania Press.

ZECKHAUSER, R. (1975). "Procedures for Valuing Lives," *Public Policy* 23:4 (Fall), 419–464.

Part Two

WHICH ROAD: REGULATION OR COMPETITION?

Chapter 5

CONSUMERISM, RATE REGULATION, AND ALTERNATIVE MANPOWER PROGRAMS

The informational inequality between physician and patient also means that the patient's freedom of choice must in practice be delegated in great part to the physician. He must determine the treatment and the referral to specialists or to hospital. But this responsibility imposes rigidities upon the physician; there is an obligation to engage in "best practice." . . . The patient should be provided with more information.

—KENNETH ARROW

Discourse between provider and patient is one of the most healing of resources, and is also the least expensive. The proper ethical relationship is to have a full exchange of information.

—MORRIS ABRAM

A physician may want to hire a new health practitioner for a number of reasons. This could involve either the provision of additional types of medical services, such as preventive care or patient education, or more careful and systematic diagnosis for those medical problems that require it. The ability to give more thorough examinations may result in lower hospitalization rates.

—ALAN SORKIN

Consumerism will be defined in this chapter as the promotion of citizens' interests through the provision of information concerning the quality, cost, and availability of services. Whether one advocates the free flow of information or competing health plans, all of the recent consumerism reform strategies are designed to give patients more power. If the debate between "competition" and "regulation" is to be the cornerstone question for public policy, it must be cast in a light that reflects the fact that government is the dominant purchaser of medical care. The most dramatic example is in hospital care, where government finances 43 percent of hospital expenses (Chapter 1). The government share of patient days is higher than its share of expenses (approximately 50 percent) due to the fact that government supports more longer staying, older patients with chronic conditions. Medicare and Medicaid patients over the age of 65 represent 36 percent of the patient days in non-federal short-term community hospitals. The government has a responsibility to the taxpayers to be a prudent purchaser of medical care. Consequently, the government will ask for some degree of regulatory control.

The critical policy question for the 1980s is what degree of regulation will be required and what degree of competition will be encouraged. Those who have an unfailing faith in competition advocate major changes in the tax laws and the health insurance industry. In Chapter 6 we shall survey the national health industry reform proposals for injecting competition into the system. The purpose of this chapter is to suggest two small scale strategies for promoting the competitive ideal. The first strategy to be advanced is the provision of more consumer information concerning hospitals and physicians. We will then review the issue of regulatory "style" in the context of state hospital rate regulation programs. The intent of this section is to explore the possibility of exporting successful and less interventionist rate regulatory approaches to overregulated or nonregulated states. Lastly, the strategy of promoting physician extenders as a means to improve consumer satisfaction, and perhaps decrease costs, is advanced.

Regulatory Proposals to Contain Costs

The double-digit annual inflation rate in hospital costs continues to be the most substantial problem facing health administrators and policy makers at both micro and macro levels. Since 1950, the percentage of gross national product devoted to hospital care has increased from 1.0 to 3.8 percent. State officials interested in containing local contributions to Medicaid are the primary advocates of cost control in the Congress. In fact, it was a misnomer to refer to the 1979 administration bill H.R. 2626 as a cost containment bill. The bill was a revenue containment proposal that presumed hospital administrators would prefer to contain costs rather than run deficits. The purpose of the following three sections is to outline the nature and limitations of revenue caps before proposing a link between the reimbursement process and public disclosure of relevant quality of care information.

The legislative history of hospital cost containment dates back to 1971 and the initiation of the Economic Stabilization Program (ESP). Between 1971 and 1974, the Congress and the administration learned two important lessons about hospital behavior under price controls. First, phases I–III of ESP suffered under the conventional assumption that price per diem should be monitored. The regulators learned that per diems are manipulable by increasing average length of stay, so phase IV controls initiated in June of 1973 emphasized cost per admission. By 1976, the regulators had learned that admission rates are also manipulable, so the subsequent 1977 and 1979 administration bills (H.R. 6575 and H.R. 2626) provided disincentives to increasing admissions (only half the average revenue per admission would be allowed) and incentives for decreasing admissions (declines of less than 6 percent would not diminish revenues). The second lesson of the ESP program is that all inpatient revenues, not just federal and state funds, received by a hospital need to be controlled. Consequently, both Carter Administration bills requested a cap on all revenues of 9.0 percent in the 1977 version and 9.7 percent in the 1979 version. The 1979 Kennedy version of the hospital cost containment bill (S. 570) had a more liberal revenue cap of 10.9 percent per annum. In November 1979, the much amended hospital "cost control" bill containing an 11.6 percent cap was defeated by Congress.

The private sector was quick to prepare a response to the original 1977 administration proposal. After H.R. 6575 stalled in committee, Congressman Rostenkowski challenged the hospital industry to provide voluntary action or face tough controls in the future. Reacting to six years of Congressional discussion of hospital cost containment, the American Hospital Association, American Medical Association, and Federation of American Hospitals formed a National Steering

Committee in November of 1977 to support a "Voluntary Effort" to reduce hospital cost inflation to 11.6 percent by 1979. The voluntary effort was successful in being below its 13.6 percent target for a 2 percent decline during 1978. The 1978 inflation rate as measured by the American Hospital Association's monthly panel survey of 1760 hospitals was 12.8 percent. Few spokesmen for the hospital industry denied the need for more regulation if their Voluntary Effort failed to halt the rapid increases in hospital expenditures. However, industry spokesmen were quick to redefine their measure of success when the 1979 hospital inflation rate increased to a dismal 13.4 percent. Advocates of the Voluntary Effort argued that adjustments for the unanticipated upwards climb in the inflation rate from 6.6 percent in November 1977 to 13.3 percent for 1979 made the Voluntary Effort a categorical success. Federal officials counterargued that the general inflation rate for a market basket of consumer goods was irrelevant, and the more appropriate hospital price index escalated at a rate of only 9.9 percent in 1979. Although the entire economy was plagued with single-digit inflation for much of the 1970s, hospital industry groups have always defended double-digit inflation rates (Table 5.1) as necessary for meeting their "special" need to provide a constantly expanding vista of new technologies. The rate at which hospitals increased intensity of services in 1979 equaled 3.8 percent. However, this 3.8 percent growth rate was significantly lower than the rate of 4–4.5 percent in the 1970s. One of the explicit goals in the Carter Administration hospital cost containment proposal was to limit increases in intensity of services to 1 percent per year.

Most economists argue that although hospital services represent a classic example of market failure, regulation cannot be relied on as the panacea to the cost problem. For example, Salkever (1978) suggests fostering institutional changes and better provider incentives to deliver less costly care as the medical economy enters a growth period where the physician–population ratio will increase 35 percent from 1976 to 1995. Granting that regulation has failed in other sectors of the economy, such as the railroad industry, economists can be found who nevertheless argue that further regulation holds some promise for containing costs in the hospital sector. States with mandatory hospital rate regulation had a rate of inflation that was 3–4 percent lower per patient day and per hospital admission in 1977 and 1978 when compared to the 44 states without mandatory rate regulation (Biles *et al.*, 1980). A more recent regression study by Coelen and Sullivan (1981) suggests that the states

Table 5.1   1968–1980 Inflation Rates in Hospital Costs, Costs per Patient Day, Revenues per Patient Day, Hospital Revenues, and the Consumer Price Index (CPI)

Year	(A-1) Total Hospital Cost (percent)	(A-2) Hospital Costs per Diem (percent)	(B-1) Hospital Revenues per Diem (percent)	(B-2) Total Hospital Revenues[1] (percent)	(C) CPI[2] General Economy (percent)
1968	17.6	11.5	12.3	17.4	4.9
1969	16.6	15.5	14.5	16.1	5.4
1970	17.2	13.9	13.6	17.1	5.9
1971	11.0	12.3	12.5	11.2	4.3
1972	12.1	10.4	9.9	11.6	3.3
1973	12.0	9.2	8.5	11.3	6.2
1974	16.0	12.2	13.2	17.0	11.0
1975	17.5	16.2	16.4	17.8	9.1
1976	19.1	15.0	15.9	20.1	5.8
1977	15.6	14.4	14.9	16.2	6.5
1978	12.8	12.1	12.1	12.8	7.7
1979	13.4	11.5	11.7	13.4	11.3
1980	16.7	13.0	13.5	17.3	12.4

SOURCE: Office of Public Policy Analysis, American Hospital Association, panel survey of 1,300–1,700 hospitals selected as a random stratified 20 percent sample of AHA member hospitals.

[1] Gross patient revenue, not gross net charges.

[2] Consumer Price Index, year to year change, *Economic Report of the President*, 1981 (Bureau of Labor Statistics data).

with mandatory rate regulation have 3.7 percent lower costs per diem and 3.2 percent lower costs per admission. Further, this study found that even the mature rate programs (such as the New York program, established 1971, and the Rhode Island program, established 1975) did not exhibit cost-savings effects until 1976. The empirical studies questioning the effectiveness of regulation will be reviewed in Chapter 8.

The next section reviews the special properties in the hospital industry that insulate it from the normal checks of price-competition, the rationale for competition among hospitals for prestige and prestigious doctors, and how this desire for prestige leads the most inflationary and overequipped hospitals to flourish when unchecked by regulation or market competition.

Quality Disclosure: Consumers' Need to Know

Most economists argue that strengthening consumer participation in consumption decisions provides our only chance for efficient cost containment. The typical market-oriented approach, exemplified by Feldstein (1971) and his proposal to increase coinsurance rates, is that if consumers pay more they will consume less and costs will be contained. Another strategy would be to provide consumers with more quality of care information and close the resulting under-utilized facilities. The economist's rationale for providing consumers with more information regarding quality is that they might vote with their feet to avoid bad departments with high case-mix adjusted mortality rates. Given that the nation has an estimated 100,000 to 130,000 unnecessary acute care hospital beds (Institute of Medicine, 1976; Ensminger, 1976), it seems logical to support a program that closes the low-quality beds. Hospitals are not all bad or all good, but the services with very low quality ratings should be closed if any beds in an area are to be closed. The FTC has initiated a number of legal suits against the hospital industry because of presumably collusive arrangements to repress information about price and quality. Feldstein (1979) has suggested that limiting the rise in costs to 9.7 percent per year would result in a forced reduction in the quality of hospital services. However, this viewpoint has little or no empirical support. The nation's best hospitals, like Massachusetts General Hospital and Johns Hopkins Hospital, have costs rising at less than 8 percent per year. In short, a tight ship is usually a quality ship.

Quality disclosure is frightening to many people. For example, many physicians in southern Maryland did not like the recent public disclosure that 300 more Baltimore residents would have survived 1978 if they had been treated at Johns Hopkins instead of at the University of Maryland Teaching Hospital. However, the public has the right to clear and coherent information about service quality. Some progressive physicians have endorsed the concept of more detailed professional directories. However, most physicians appear to abhor commercial advertising and quality disclosure. The current editor of the *New England Journal of Medicine* has come out in favor of widespread dissemination of detailed information concerning only the availability of physicians and health services (Relman, 1978). More recently, the disclosure of open heart mortality rates at George Washington Hospital by the local Health Systems Agency caused many confirmed surgical candidates to cancel their appointments in December of 1979.

Blue Cross subscriber disclosure programs of quality measurement results might be the important first step in providing department-specific area-wide consumer information. More than 75 percent of all hospital bills are handled by Blue Cross for government and subscribers, and Blue Cross has three years of experience with Professional Standard Review Organizations (PSRO) concerning quality-reimbursement data linkages. Statistical profiles of provider quality would seem a superior alternative to ex-post assessments of consumer satisfaction. For example, an unwitting malpractice victim might be "satisfied" while being ignorant of the fact that the condition had an iatrogenic cause.

One potential danger of public disclosure of quality of care information is that it might adversely affect some 400 teaching hospitals. Medical students and residents operate under the educational philosophy of "see one, do one," increasing the chance of complications and iatrogenic death due to inexperience. Public outcry, if some teaching hospitals had very bad quality ratings,* might push American medical education back into the Anglo-Scandinavian mode. Western European medical students must follow their teachers through six to eight years of internship before treating patients.

---

* All outcome measures of quality of care must be standardized in such a fashion as to not penalize the hospital that treats the more difficult cases. The Stanford Center for Health Care Research has made significant methodological progress in adjusting such measures for the severity and complexity of the patient case-mix (Scott *et al.*, 1976; Flood and Scott, 1978; Schoonhoven *et al.*, 1980; and Scott *et al.*, 1980).

Alternatives to complete public disclosure of quality information include either only releasing the information for the worst 20 percent of hospitals, or encouraging better quality care by reimbursing hospitals at a higher level if mortality rates are low and the percentage of removed undiseased tissue is low.

The present payment system encourages unnecessary surgery by paying for all surgery, whether the pathologist finds that the removed tissue was diseased or healthy. The reimbursement incentives could stimulate better quality lower cost care if they continued to pay for every biopsy, but refused to reimburse the hospital or surgeon for care demonstrated to be unnecessary in an independent post-operative tissue committee assessment. The tissue assessment would have to be double-blind in order to protect society from potential conflict of interest problems. The PSRO tissue committee could be responsible for identifying the sampling frame. Hospital lobbyists have increasingly pressured reimbursement agents to justify their operations in terms of cost containment and quality benefits relative to paperwork costs. The construction of a rational sampling frame that maximizes information gain is a powerful tool in containing regulatory costs.

Health System Agencies (HSAs) could play a part in the consumer disclosure process if they survive the critical 1982 Congressional vote concerning future funding. Consumer disclosure activities might be expected to produce greater behavioral change in the more competitive urban markets. In smaller regions, with lower doctor to population ratio, the differential ability of clinicians is more likely to be known by the population. The present probability of hearing word-of-mouth evaluation of your doctor's past performance is lower in urban environments; consumer behavior might be more likely to respond to new information. To make the argument clear, let us postulate two consumers, each having 100 friends, in two different cities. One consumer lives in a small city of 10,000 with 10 doctors and (assuming independent probabilities) ten percent of his friends (or 10 friends) could provide information concerning a given doctor. The other consumer lives in a city with 1 million citizens and 3,000 doctors, and few, if any, friends who would be in a position to evaluate any given doctor. This hypothetical example is oversimplified, but the important point to consider is that the consumer information search costs are likely to be substantially higher in urban environments. The less-informed urban residents are more likely to be responsive to HSA-PSRO information disclosure than the rural resident who is more likely to have a significant sample of opinion, from trusted friends. Within any given area, the better-informed classes of citizens (those more likely to have doctors and other professionals as friends) would likely be more responsive to consumer disclosure PSRO materials than the less-informed subsets of the population; that is, better-informed individuals would have more opportunities to discuss it in informal social settings.

The issue of increasing or decreasing the scope of CON activities or other HSA implementation and planning activities must be kept distinct from the issue of consumer disclosure. The administrative issue of agency responsibility for coordinating disclosure activities, HSAs and/or PSROs or some third party, is a political decision that can be handled separately. The tougher issue of whether HSAs have produced a negative or positive net impact on the hospital cost containment effort is addressed in Chapter 8. One potential benefit of comprehensive consumer disclosure of provider cost information is that consumers might shop for the best buy, all factors considered. If we allow the physicians to disclose only basic charge information, like the cost per initial office visit, the information might be misleading. For example, the physicians with the cost-effective clinical decision-making mindset mentioned in Chapter 4 are more likely to provide services at lower total costs (including drugs, tests, hospital care).* Consumer disclosure in the public interest should involve publication of the net total cost of treatment, adjusted for case-mix, to identify the providers with the most efficient modes of treatment.

The physician community may attempt to counter any potential reduction in income that might result from consumer disclosure activities. For example, one possible supply-side response to not paying for unnecessary surgery would be that surgeons would require patients to pay the fee that insurance would not cover. However, if too many patients had to pay a fee for an unnecessary and unproductive service, they would spread skepticism about that surgeon's competence. The demand for the surgeon's service should be somewhat dependent on posterior estimates of diagnostic and therapeutic accuracy. Low quality surgeons might stop doing surgery, and the average level of surgical quality would be improved. It seems beneficial from a cost and quality perspective to

---

* The fees of such cost-effective clinical decision-makers might sometimes be higher than average, to compensate the individuals for their time, but total costs should be lower.

pay the surgeon much like we pay professional basketball players, on the basis of baskets made, rather than shots taken. This gives the professional more incentive to take careful aim before throwing, rather than shooting too frequently. The surgeon would have more financial incentive to obtain a better pre-operative assessment of his/her patient's condition rather than operate or hospitalize at will.

Entering an Era of Total Revenue Control

The capital cap and revenue cap approaches to total revenue control are anathema to most hospital administrators. They may be too busy trying to meet their institutions' financial requirements to dwell on social issues like unnecessary surgery, excessive numbers of beds, or unnecessary equipment. There are two possible scenarios for the implementation of total revenue controls. The administrators fear a "run the inefficient into bankruptcy" scenario. However, the planners support an alternative scenario: "Force the hospitals to contain costs." In the eyes of the medical community, both scenarios appear intended to bludgeon hospitals into submission under the heavy hand of federal bureaucrats.

Under the bankruptcy scenario, administrators fear that revenue controls will lead to submarginal cash flows, underutilization, poor employee morale, and lack of capital for equipment and plant maintenance. If hospital capital is eroded and management is not allowed to accumulate reserves for capital replacement, as is the case under the New York formula approach to total revenue control, debt financing will become increasingly important and default due to overextension of debt will become more prevalent. Sixteen percent of New York hospitals have gone bankrupt between 1975 and 1979. In 1979, 79 percent of New York State's voluntary hospitals had net operating losses totaling $181 million (Hospital Association of New York State, 1981). This operating margin is calculated by subtracting total costs from total revenues exclusive of non-operating revenues (for example, income on endowments, contributions, bequests). A second basis for measuring the financial health of these hospitals is bottom-line losses or profits, including non-operating revenues. Including non-operating revenue in the calculation either increases the operating profit or decreases the size of the operating loss. In 1979 some 129 voluntary New York hospitals (58.6 percent) experienced bottom-line operating losses totaling $130 million. One third of these voluntary hospitals reported bottom-line losses each year from 1975 to 1979. In fiscal year 1982, the 220 voluntary and 25 public hospitals in New York State are projected to have a net operating loss of $300 million and a net bottom-line loss of $225 million. If we restrict the projections to voluntary hospitals, they are expected to have a net operating loss of $220 million and a net bottom-line loss of $147 million in 1982. These estimates would be approximately 75 percent higher if the Reagan Administration's $1 billion limitation (5 percent annual increase cap) on the federal contribution to state Medicaid is implemented for fiscal 1982.

The problem with the "weakest up against the wall" bankruptcy approach to solving the cost containment problem is that it exacerbates the maldistribution and capital replacement problems. Civil rights groups fear that hospital closings will affect mainly municipal facilities and will be in the ghetto neighborhoods, where the need for care is the greatest. Forcing the highly leveraged, older, basic service hospital out of business would result in a maldistribution of services and an increased average cost per hospital episode if patients migrate to high-priced medical centers. As hospitals are forced to empty endowment and depreciation funds in order to meet the payroll, eventually all capital equipment will deteriorate to the point where rebuilding and replacement are more expensive than the customary process of gradual replacement (refer to Chapters 9 and 10). By running hospital reserves into the ground, forced deficits create much larger capital updating and replacement expenditures in the future for the 80–90 percent of hospitals that do not go bankrupt.

Under the second scenario, planners postulate that hospitals will be forced to contain costs, rather than run large deficits, as their revenues are brought under external control. By underfunding hospital departments, planners hope to force hospitals into slight deficit positions. The rationale is that short-run deficits may provide the necessary incentives to contain costs and tighten up operations. Many analysts realize that the pressure caused by a deficit crisis creates a heightened atmosphere of discord within the hospital, particularly between department managers and medical staff. Obviously, department managers and hospital administrators have more influence on the physician group in an atmosphere of tight money. Planners hope that in a state of crisis, managers will monitor the ratio of fat to lean, receive fewer demands for capital expense projects from physicians, and trim the fat from their budgets.

Both scenarios suggest that hospitals should be forced to run deficits. Under scenario one, hospitals are expected to run large deficits until the right number of hospital wings have gone bankrupt. Under scenario two, stimulating small deficits is considered a necessary evil to contain costs by containing physician demands for equipment and new programs. Most economists would not find this a persuasive argument for further regulation in industry. However, in the arena of hospital economics, market failure and lack of price competition is the rule rather than the exception. Competition exists in the hospital industry, but not between hospitals trying to attract sick people. Instead the competition is for the best doctors, with the newest expensive equipment acting as the lure. Consequently, hospital competition breeds higher expense. The "best" hospital becomes the one that caters to doctors by providing expensive machines. Fuchs (1974), Carlson (1975), and others have questioned the ability of an increasingly technological style of medicine to improve the health status of Americans. Physicians and administrators will no longer always be successful in parrying assaults from consumer interests and government. The days of easy money and soft management are over.

Potential Approaches to Rate Regulation

The 1970s trend away from cost-plus reimbursement to total revenue control and cost reimbursement has caused some hospital administrators to cannibalize their long-term reserves. While reimbursement is undoubtedly deficient in some hospitals within tough rate-setting states like New York, it is a highly difficult question as to whether hospitals can continue in their position as a growth industry. The future fiscal environment will provide administrators with incentives for a reduction in the number of beds, supplies, and services. Any future cost containment bill could be improved if it embodied more of the Maryland budget review approach to regulation, rather than the New York state formula approach to regulation. It was hard to support the Carter Administration contention that New York State should provide a model for the nation in the area of hospital cost containment. New York State hospital cost increases are the lowest in the nation. One could argue that the impressive low inflationary rates in New York are less a product of effective regulation, and more a result of a deteriorating state economy and state treasury that could support only a 4.07 percent increase in voluntary hospital employee wages in 1977, compared to a national increase of 7.4 percent.

New York and Maryland rank first and second in the nation for containing hospital costs since 1975. The Maryland regulatory approach monitors only marginal year-to-year changes in costs, limiting annual increases in expense per admission to 8.68 percent. Very few Maryland hospitals complain about the regulations and only 4 percent run deficits. Contrast the harmony of Maryland to New York State, where the New York increases in expenses have been 1 percentage point lower, but a majority of the hospitals operated in the red during 1977, 1978, and 1979. The more aggressive New York style of regulation monitors both marginal (year-to-year) and baseline inefficiencies in costs. The Carter Administration proposal did borrow one aspect of the Maryland approach to cost control, in that it monitored only marginal changes, in the hope that baseline inefficiencies are inconsequential relative to the total cost escalation problem.

Both the Carter and Kennedy cost containment proposals accepted a basic equity principle from the Maryland system, that all payer categories (Blue Cross, commercial insurance, self-pay, Medicare, Medicaid) should be regulated equally. The unregulated charge paying patients, self-paying or commercially insured, were previously forced to pay higher rates to finance deficits created by regulated cost paying reimbursement shortfalls. Cost-only payers reimburse at below true cost or in a "cost-minus" fashion because the cost formulas in all states, except Washington, do not recognize the need to finance working capital (Dowling, 1977). Maryland is currently the only state where all patients, both cost payers and charge payers, pay for hospital services on the same basis, regulated by a single state commission.

Regulation has often been criticized by economists for buffering producers from consumer demand for a "better" product, that is, one of lower price or higher quality. However, disclosure of mortality and PSRO quality of care statistics and/or linking reimbursement to quality measures would provide consumers with the means to shop for a better product. The better quality hospital department would experience an increase in demand, and could lower charges because they could spread fixed costs across a larger patient census. In addition to an anticipated improvement in the average quality of hospital care, the public can expect their disposable incomes to rise following enactment of a federal cost containment bill. The estimated total five-year savings was $31.7 billion for the Carter bill (H. R. 2626) and $26 billion for the Kennedy bill (S. 570).

Hospital industry spokesmen argue that hospital revenue control legislation is shortsighted. The resulting deficits produce a reduction in capital reserves that will cost society much more to replenish in the future, as failure to invest in the present will mean capital underdevelopment in the long run. Planners argue that between 100,000 and 130,000 beds at some 1,000 hospitals should be underdeveloped and eventually closed. The American medical establishment faces agonizing choices about closing hospitals and dismissing nurses and other employees. These twin problems of capital underdevelopment and excess bed supply should be addressed in the federal cost containment legislation in the 1980s. The basic ethical question one faces is whether the nation should have 50,000 planners trying to close beds, or 230 million consumers armed with quality of care information deciding which beds are unnecessary. How effectively planners operate at closing beds and containing additional plant asset acquisitions is the subject considered in Chapter 8. The quasi-market mechanism of quality disclosure to consumers offers the advantage of protecting 80–90 percent of the hospitals from capital underdevelopment, whereas the planned economy solution might leave a majority of hospitals with severe deficits and diminished ability to provide annual wage increases.

New Professionals: Physician Extenders

Recently new professionals have emerged to provide more medical care in a fashion that is more conducive to serving consumer needs than traditional solo physician practice. Since 1971, federal support of physician extender (PE) training programs has been the primary federal response to the perceived shortage and maldistribution of providers of primary care. The term physician extender includes both nurse practitioners (NPs) and physician assistants (PAs) with formal training that has equipped them for functions beyond the scope of the traditional nurse. The rapid growth in PE training programs in the 1970s was a byproduct of the unmet consumer demand for primary care and the perceived neglect of the human side of medicine. PEs frequently take the family approach to health education and contact the spouse or relative of the patient in an attempt to improve patient compliance with treatment and to convince the individual that a healthier life style is attainable. With the growth in concern for the caring function, prevention, health promotion, and care of the chronically ill has come a five-fold increase in the supply of PEs since 1970. In the current era of governmental retrenchment, concern over the nation's $240 billion 1981 medical bill should not a priori lead to a freeze at the current annual level of the number of PEs trained. Physician fears of competition will not change the fact that patients increasingly demand nonphysician personnel to act as counselor, educator, and ombudsman.

The promise of PEs is best described in terms of improved access to care, improved practice productivity, health education counseling, comprehensive planning in patient care management, and lower unit costs. PEs are meeting a previously unmet need in two basic senses: They are more likely than physicians to reside in medically underserved areas and they specialize in often neglected areas of medical practice. Physician resistance to employing more PEs has called into question the service delivery rationale for federal funding of training programs. The intent of the following sections is to suggest that PEs can increasingly become a medically and economically popular solution to the problem of providing health care in underserved rural and inner city areas.

For nearly two decades the terms "doctor shortage" and "primary care shortage" have been bandied about. The "crisis" was defined in the 1970s as one of both geographic and specialty maldistribution. One of the most vexing questions asked by labor economists is whether, and to what extent, PEs act to improve productivity and decrease average costs by performing delegable tasks (Zeckhauser and Eliastam, 1974), or whether they free physician time to perform less necessary and more costly complex tertiary medical care. In the parlance of economics, to what extent do PEs act as substitutes and/or complements for physician time? Another, less tangible, unanswered question is to what extent have PE training programs had a positive spin-off effect on physician education, that is, making physicians more aware of primary care and the need for the caring function and preventive counseling. Any benefit-cost framework for assessing the projected expansion in the supply of PEs should not underestimate the tangible benefits to society of health promotion, self-care, and prevention activities.

Current Levels of Manpower Supply and Training Support

In January 1980 there were an estimated 11,000 physician assistants, including 1,000 certified PAs who did not graduate from a formal training program. The class of 1980 will add an additional 1,600 PAs to the existing supply. An estimated 70–80 percent of certified PAs are presumed active. Most PA programs are university-based and require two years' training. Between 1972–1980 approximately 7,200 PA students received $66 million in direct and indirect federal support (Eastaugh, 1981). However, the level of federal support per annum has been frozen at approximately $8.5 million for the past four years.

Certificate and master's NP training programs vary in emphasis over a range of disciplines: family medicine, pediatrics, maternity care, midwifery, and psychiatric care. In January 1981 there were an estimated 18,000 NPs that had graduated from formal training programs. An estimated 85–90 percent are presumed to be active.* The American College of Nurse-Midwives estimates that 2,000 of the NPs are actively engaged in midwifery. Between 1972–1981, approximately 12,000 NP students and about half of the NP programs received $88 million from the Nurse Training Acts of 1971 and 1975. The level of federal support from the 1975 Nurse Training Act has been frozen at $13 million for the past four years. Only $1.1 million per annum has been awarded in direct traineeship support. Since 1978, the traineeships were awarded to individuals who were willing to perform postgraduate service in areas designated as underserved by DHEW.

One seldom mentioned benefit resulting from the emergence of PE training programs was the public questioning of the resistance of organized medicine to task delegation. Since 1847 the American Medical Association has committed itself to the trade union objective of promulgating restrictions upon nurses or would-be doctors (Kessel, 1958). According to the report of the Macy Commission (1976), the continued success of PEs will not only have a positive impact on the quality of health care, but will also encourage the development of other nonphysician competitors to physician sub-

---

* Data provided by the Bureau of Health Manpower, Division of Nursing, Public Health Service, DHEW.

specialist and solo practitioners. If consumers prefer high accessibility to care and cost containment, then training PEs seems a better bargain than training physicians at five times the cost.

Physicians Supply and Reimbursement Issues

An Institute of Medicine (1978) study questioned the need to train additional PEs if the anticipated supply of physicians in 1990 is at least adequate and if the projected specialization trend is a return to family practice and primary care. While recognizing the need for a comprehensive strategy that coordinates the supply and distribution of PEs and physicians, it seems a shortsighted policy to presume that physicians in oversupplied areas will suddenly decide to serve the poor and less profitable locations. If the Congress suddenly resolved to reimburse physicians on the basis of negotiated charges rather than on the basis of prevailing charges, then the financial disincentives to work in a region of low physician density (charity fee) would be diminished. A mass exodus of physicians from the suburbs under this new reimbursement climate would seem highly unlikely. Despite the fact that personal life style preferences dominate the physician's location decision, it seems poor public policy to pay more in areas where doctors are needed less and to pay less in areas where they are needed most. The Institute of Medicine study also fails to recognize that PE manpower policy should be made independently of physician manpower policy to the extent that PEs deliver a service that is different in scope and nature.

Current Medicare part B legislation provides coverage for the services of a PE only when those services are delegated by and performed under the direct supervision of a physician. Medicaid regulations typically permit reimbursement for PE services that are performed under "general" physician supervision. Some states are more liberal on this point, for example, the South Dakota legislature required health insurers to cover all PE services starting in 1980. Since 1976 the state of Nevada has directly reimbursed PAs at 100 percent of physician rates and NPs at 55 percent of physician rates. To liberalize the reimbursement climate among insurance payers in areas of physician shortage, the Congress passed the 1977 Rural Health Clinic Services Act (P.L. 95-210) which provided Medicare and Medicaid reimbursement in certified clinics for PE services rendered without direct physician supervision. However, because the DHEW has certified fewer than 400 clinics, the reimbursement climate for PEs has not significantly changed in three years.

Although one-fifth of PEs are employed in HMOs and clinics, the great majority of PEs are employed by physicians in private practice. A number of outside surveys have suggested that physicians' reluctance to hire PEs might be accounted for by conflicting perceptions about the PE role (Prescott and Driscoll, 1979). Five rationales have been suggested to explain why physicians may hire PEs. First, they may wish to improve the quality of care by creating a less crowded and more comprehensive schedule. Second, they may want to increase the quantity (minutes) of care delivered per visit. Third, they may indulge in the purely economic desire to expand practice profits. Fourth, physicians may desire more leisure time and a shorter work week. Last, employment of a PE may result in lower malpractice premiums in the long run, if improved patient rapport diminishes the incidence of nuisance suits.

Productivity and Cost Considerations

Many previous comparative cost studies have tried to portray PEs either as a financial windfall or as a liability. Some of the earliest pro-PE studies came from HMOs in which nonphysician personnel provided care in a majority of the visits. Other studies were flawed because they loaded a large amount of overhead unnecessarily onto PE practices only (Nelson *et al.*, 1975). The recent Systems Science (1978) study avoided such methodological pitfalls. The productivity component of their analysis focused on an economic efficiency measure, the number of ambulatory visits per $1,000 of cost. When the study considered group practices it found no differential in economic efficiency between PE and non-PE comparison practices; both kinds of group practice produced 66 visits per $1,000 of cost. However, the Systems Science study found that solo physician practices produced 81 visits per $1,000 of reimbursable cost (cost to society) when a PE was part of the team, compared to 57 visits per $1,000 of cost in solo physician practices without a PE. Three other major conclusions of the study were that (1) the average charge per visit was lower in PE practices, (2) physician job satisfaction increased in PE practices as the perceived workload decreased, and (3) process measures of quality of care were better on average in the PE practices.

The demand for PEs is a function of the consumer demand for

medical services, physician supply, physician reimbursement policy, PE reimbursement policy, and the willingness of physicians to hire PEs. For example, legal constraints, such as requirements for direct supervision of PEs by physicians, are cited by physicians as a rationale for not employing PEs. Another rationale for not employing PEs is the American physician's distaste for staff management. In estimating that physicians could profitably employ one to five PEs, Reinhardt (1972) suggests that physicians react with rather high psychic costs to employing a larger staff, that is, they hate to manage people. It is difficult to generalize these study results over time, but if we update the figures to 1980 dollars, Reinhardt estimates the marginal disutility of each additional PE employed to be between $200 and $260 per week. If the economic conditions of the 1980s erode a physician's ability to maintain a high living standard, the medical community may increasingly discount the marginal disutility of employing additional extenders and hire more PEs. However, the anticipated productivity gains may be overstated. For example, a recent study by Hershey and Kropp (1979) suggests that the productivity gain from employing a PA may be as small as 20 percent and the increase in net income may be negligible. However, the authors optimization-simulation model does not consider the possibility that shifts in the patient mix following addition of a PA might cause the measured productivity improvement to be understated.

Manpower Projections and the Appropriate Federal Role

The manpower projections in Table 5.2 are simple linear projections extrapolated from the points in time, 1973 and 1979. The projections are consistent with a study by Wallen (1980) suggesting that 8,000 more PEs or 4,000–5,000 physicians would be necessary to bring DHHS medically underserved areas up to the minimum supply ratios. It is overly simplistic to suggest, however, that the problem of a shortage of primary care is solved if the 1973–1979 growth rate in PEs is matched in the 1979–1985 period. Manpower projections and demand analysis cannot be done in a vacuum, independently of concerns for retention and employment rates, licensure, and alternative future methods of reimbursement. If the public continues to ask for deregulation and cost containment, these 1985 projections might easily be underestimates. Moreover, these projections will be

Table 5.2 **Population Distribution and Supply Ratios per Population of Phys-
cians, Physician Assistants, and Nurse Practitioners by Community
Size, Projected for 1985**

Community Size	Physicians per 10,000	PAs per 10,000	NPs per 10,000	Percent of U.S. Population
Under 10,000	10	.77	.54	18
10,000–49,999	22	.82	.54	16
50,000 plus	26	.42	1.14	66
National Average	22	.56	.90	
Projected Total Supply in 1985	525,000	13,250	21,250	

SOURCE: Eastaugh (1981) and Perry (1976).

underestimates if the recent restrictive legislation against foreign
medical graduates, representing at present one fifth of the physician
labor force, forces the physician supply to contract. In addition, if
specialists are increasingly successful in attracting PEs away from
the underserved areas and into institutional or private specialty
group practice, the total demand for PEs could be severely underestimated. PEs might learn from their physician colleagues that
higher incomes can be earned serving the overserved rather than
caring for the medically underserved.

The future policy direction of the federal government is beset by
uncertainties. Continued federal support of PE programs will be
necessary if the supply is to keep pace with the demand. Congress
appears more sympathetic to providing support for PEs than for
medical students, simply because the PEs are subject to a much
lower level of remuneration following graduation.

The federal government might better serve the public interest by
concentrating a higher proportion of PE funds into traineeships with
a service obligation. As an added inducement to increase retention
of PEs after completion of the service pay-back requirement, DHHS
might subsidize the malpractice premiums and office equipment
costs of individuals remaining in medically underserved regions.
The DHHS could further target direct grants and contracts to programs that offer curricula that track students into primary care.
Finally, the federal government should have an increased concern
for research in the area of primary care manpower. For example, we
need to ascertain the volume or critical mass of population necessary
to allow an independent PE practice to attain financial self-
sufficiency after three to five years of growth in an isolated rural area
(Moscovice and Rosenblatt, 1979). Specifically, PAs have a proven

ability to decrease per-visit costs by up to 20 percent in large urban practices (Greenfield *et al.*, 1978), but the introduction of PAs into smaller practices has not led to an equal reduction in unit cost or increase in patient volume (Frame *et al.*, 1978).

Another potential area for further research is the difference in productivity between PAs and NPs. A recent study of 455 matched paired comparison practices suggested that PAs are 6–36 percent more productive than NPs depending on practice arrangement (Medenhall *et al.*, 1980). The NPs in this study were employed in larger practices, practices with an average of 9.5 physicians compared to 4.7 in the average PA practice situation. However, the cause of the productivity differential was not explained by practice size.

The wisdom of increasing support for PE programs depends on judgments about future reimbursement incentives, PE responsiveness to required service location, PE retention in underserved areas following completion of the service requirement, and assumptions about competition in health care markets. In the short run if PEs merely add to the aggregate level of demand, they will, acting as an add-on, produce a net inflationary impact on medical costs. As a hypothetical example, expert opinion may differ as to whether $100 million of PE services yield merely $50 million in patient benefits (benefit to cost ratio equals 50/100) or $80 million in patient benefits plus a $40 million reduction in physician service [benefit to cost ratio equals $(80/(100 - 40) = 1.33)$].

Conclusion

The period 1965–1980 has provided a renaissance of interest in nonphysicians as providers of primary care. Although there are many reasons for the emergence of PEs as a profession, a dominant one is the concern for efficiency. Why must a $40 per hour physician spend 30 minutes with the anxious patient, when a $10 per hour PE can do an equally good or even better job in one hour at half the cost? Rather than spend a few rushed minutes with the physician, that patient can spend more time with a PE who can take the time to emphasize the caring function, yielding greater patient self-respect and improved rates of compliance.

Increased funding for PE traineeships and program development could be a powerful lever for influencing the geographic and specialty distribution of PEs through admissions policies and curricula. The worst possible scenario would be for the federal government to withdraw all support, thus eliminating all negative incentives for PEs to settle in attractive suburban specialists' offices. If the federal government expects PEs to act as a pool of gap-filling manpower in medically underserved areas, then DHHS must maintain the positive incentives for PEs to locate where physicians infrequently tread.

The other small scale reform strategy we reviewed in this chapter involved the dissemination of more information to the consumer concerning various medical providers. In 1981 the Public Citizen Health Research Group issued a policy statement calling on the federal government to assist Medicare beneficiaries in avoiding high-priced physicians. Consumerism should extend beyond simple price disclosure activities to include expanded information on quality and availability of care. The libertarian-conservatives in the Reagan Administration should be supportive of any efforts designed to promote informational equality between providers and patients. Improved informational equality is a necessary condition for stimulating competitive markets. However, the traditional-conservatives in organized medicine may resist any efforts to supply patients with more information concerning cost, quality, and access.

References

ARROW, K. (1972). "Problems of Resource Allocation in United States Medical Care," in R. Kunz and H. Fehr (eds.), *The Challenge of Life: Biomedical Progress and Human Values*. Basil, Switzerland: Roche.

BILES, B., SCHRAMM, C., and ATKINSON, G. (1980). "Hospital Cost Inflation Under State Rate-Setting Programs," *New England Journal of Medicine* 303:12 (September 18), 664–667.

CARLSON, R. (1975). *The End of Medicine*. New York: Wiley.

COELEN, C., and SULLIVAN, D. (1981). "Analysis of the Effects of Prospective Reimbursement Programs on Hospital Expenditures," *Health Care Financing Review* 2:3 (Winter), 1–40.

DOWLING, W. L. (1977). "Washington State," in *Prospective Rate Setting*, Chapter 3. Germantown, Md.: Aspen Systems.

EASTAUGH, S. (1981). "Physician Extenders: Potential for Improved Productivity," *Hospital Progress* 62:2 (February), 32–45.

ENSMINGER, B. (1976). "The $8 Billion Hospital Bed Overrun," Public Citizen's Health Research Group Report.

FELDSTEIN, M. (1971). "A New Approach to National Health Insurance," *The Public Interest* 46 (Spring), 93–105.

FELDSTEIN, M. (1979). Testimony before the Senate Health Subcommittee (March 15).

FLOOD, A., and SCOTT, W. (1978). "Professional Power and Professional Effectiveness: The Power of the Surgical Staff and the Quality of Surgical Care in Hospitals," *Journal of Health and Social Behavior* 19:3 (September), 240–254.

FRAME, P. S., WETTERAV, N. W., and PAREY, B. (1978). "A Model for the Use of Physician Assistants in Primary Care," *Journal of Family Practice* 7:12 (December), 1195–1204.

FUCHS, V. R. (1974). *Who Shall Live?* New York: Basic Books.

GREENFIELD, S., KAMAROFF, A., PASS, T., ANDERSON, H., and NESSIM, S. (1978). "Efficiency and the Cost of Primary Care by Nurses and Physician Assistants," *New England Journal of Medicine* 288:6 (February 9), 305–309.

HERSHEY, J. C., and KROPP, D. H. (1979). "A Re-appraisal of the Productivity Potential and Economic Benefits of Physician's Assistants," *Medical Care* 17:6 (June), 592–606.

Hospital Association of New York State (1981). *Ninth Annual Fiscal Pressures Survey, 1979* (March). HANYS, Albany, New York.

Institute of Medicine (1976). *Controlling the Supply of Hospital Beds*, National Academy of Sciences Report (October).

Institute of Medicine (1978). *A Manpower Policy for Primary Health Care*. Washington, D.C.: National Academy of Sciences.

KESSEL, R. A. (1978). "Price Discrimination in Medicine," *Journal of Law and Economics* 1:1 (October), 20–53.

Josiah Macy Foundation (1976). *Physicians for the Future: Report of the Macy Commission*, p. 27. New York.

MENDENHALL, R. C., REPICKY, P. A., and NEVILLE, R. E. (1980). "Assessing the Utilization and Productivity of Nurse Practitioners and Physician's Assistants: Methodology and Findings on Productivity," *Medical Care* 18:6 (June), 609–623.

MOSCOVICE, I., and ROSENBLATT, R. (1979). "The Viability of Mid-Level Practitioners in Isolated Rural Communities," *American Journal of Public Health* 69:5 (May), 503–505.

NELSON, E. C., JACOBS, A. R., CORDNER, B. A., and JOHNSON, K. G. (1975). "Financial Impact of Physician Assistants on Medical Practice," *New England Journal of Medicine* 293:11 (September 11), 527–530.

PERRY, H. B. (1976). "Physician Assistants: An Empirical Analysis," unpublished doctoral dissertation, Johns Hopkins University, Department of Social Relations.

PRESCOTT, P. A., and DRISCOLL, L. (1979). "Nurse Practitioner Effectiveness," *Evaluation and the Health Professions* 2:4 (December), 387–418.

President's Commission for the Study of Ethical Problems in Medicine, Morris B. Abram, Chairman (1981). *First Report: Ethical Problems in Medicine and Biomedical and Behavioral Research* (Summer). Washington, D.C.: U.S. Government Printing Office.

RECORD, J., BLOMQUIST, R., BERGER, B., and O'BANNON, J. (1977). "Quality of PA Performance at a HMO," in A. Bliss and E. Cohen (eds.), *The New Health Professionals*, Chapter 12. Germantown, MD.: Aspen Systems.

REINHARDT, U. (1975). *Physician Productivity and the Demand for Health Manpower*. Cambridge, Mass.: Ballinger.

REINHARDT, U. (1972). "A Production Function for Physician Service," *Review of Economics and Statistics* 54:1 (February), 55–66.

RELMAN, A. (1978). "Professional Directories—But Not Commercial Advertising—As a Public Service," *New England Journal of Medicine* 299:9 (August 31), 476–478.

SALKEVER, D. S. (1978). "Will Regulation Control Health Care Costs?" *Bulletin of the New York Academy of Medicine* 54:1 (January), 73–83.

SCHOONHOVEN, C., SCOTT, W., FLOOD, B., and FORREST, W. (1980). "Measuring the Complexity and Uncertainty of Surgery and Postsurgical Care," *Medical Care* 18:9 (September), 893–915.

SCOTT, W., FORREST, W., and BROWN, B. (1976). "Hospital Structure and Post-operative Mortality and Morbidity," in S. Shovrell and M. Brown (eds.), *Organizational Research in Hospitals*. Chicago: Inquiry Book, Blue Cross Association, 72–89.

Systems Sciences, Inc. (1978). *Survey and Evaluation of the Physician Extender Reimbursement Experiment*, Contract No. 55A-600-76-0167, Social Security Administration, Washington, D.C.

United States Congress (1978). House Commerce Oversight and Investigations Subcommittee Final Report, "Unnecessary Surgical Procedures," Compendium of Hearings 1976–78.

WALLEN, J. (1980). "Considerations in the Use of Nonphysician Health Care Providers in Physician-Shortage Areas," unpublished report, Division of Intramural Research, National Center for Health Services Research, DHEW.

ZECKHAUSER, R., and ELIASTAM, M. (1974). "The Productivity of the Physician Assistant," *Journal of Human Resources* 9:1 (Winter), 95–116.

Chapter 6

COMPETITION HEALTH PLANS

> *We do see hospitals competing for doctors and for prestige. But because of the way that health insurance connects to health services, with few exceptions there is no true economic competition in health services. The competition that now exists is not of a kind that rewards economy in the use of resources. . . . Fair economic competition of alternative delivery systems would force the health services industry to be more responsive to the desires of consumers. In the long run the surviving plans would be the ones that offered a good value to their customers. . . . I do not recommend a return to a completely free market in health insurance. The desirable competition I am referring to would be focused on the quality, accessibility, and economy of care and not, for example, on the ability of insurers to select only healthy people to insure.*
>
> —ALAIN C. ENTHOVEN

> *The ultimate purpose of pro-competitive proposals is to motivate doctors, hospitals, and other providers to compete with each other to offer health care in less costly ways. There is merit in this theory.*
>
> —WALTER J. McNERNEY

Most countries view the United States health care system as being very market-oriented and competitive. Some of these nations look to the United States approach for alternatives to total government regulation. The preference in Canada and Western Europe is for some degree of private management of the national health service or national health insurance plan. In the United States, physicians and administrators who distrust regulatory approaches are advocating the injection of more competitive relationships between health care providers. However, not all physicians have a truly pro-competitive bias.

The public policy question is not simply one of whether to allow competition or regulation, but rather, what is the proper balance of regulation and competition and how much price and non-price competition should be encouraged. As we have observed in Chapter 1, the strongest argument for regulatory limits on competition, significant economies of scale leading to excessive monopoly power, does not exist in the medical sector. We shall review in Chapter 8 the rationale and benefit-cost of a number of regulatory activities. The major question for consideration in this chapter is to what degree should we promote competition in the market for health services.

The basic rationale behind the competitive model is to keep the insurance companies, and hopefully providers, under constant pressure to find the means to provide care at lower costs. Third-party payers and HMOs will on occasion make management mistakes, create long patient queues or unacceptable patient care conditions, but the strength of competitive markets is that the good-quality lower-cost operators will grow. Advocates of competition recognize consumer ignorance, insured consumers' indifference to costs, and strong physician influence on demands as three strong arguments for regulatory activity. Granted that government has a role in providing information and preventing fraud, many analysts are increasingly advancing the concept of consumer choice health plans as a competitive alternative to more regulation (Enthoven, 1980).

Advocates of competition have attempted to convince physicians that competition health plans are the only defense against expanding federal regulations instituted in the name of cost containment. This is a rather negative promotional approach for the competitive ideal. Before we review some proposals for injecting competition into the health arena, let us review other markets that have faced the dilemma of choosing between further regulation or deregulation.

Oftentimes an industry will reject competition in favor of a planned solution. In the mid-1970s the airline industry had a problem of excess capacity, much like the current state of affairs in the hospital industry. The planners' solution, to fight the problem by reducing the number of flights, was a failure. In 1977 Civil Aeronautics Board Chairman Alfred Kahn suggested a radical old idea: competition. The approach that finally cured the excess-capacity problem was to deregulate and let price competition fill up empty planes. The analogy between the airline and hospital industry breaks down for one very important reason: There is more of a social cost involved in filling hospitals with unnecessary patients than filling planes with discount-paying vacationers. However, before forsaking the analogy one should point out that both sectors benefit from a degree of regulatory licensure. Society has made a decision to set a minimum standard that all airlines and hospitals must meet in order to minimize the intangible collective regret that we might feel if "something goes wrong." The deregulatory advocates have not convinced society that the public role in operating each industry should simply be dissemination of information on risks and costs, and let the buyer beware.

Consumer Choice

Wide variation in consumer tastes is one major argument for advancing competition health plans; that is, if planners knew what individuals wanted we could mandate the result and be done with it. Many ideas have been suggested to increase consumer choice and competition in the medical care sector. All of these pro-competition ideas are designed to affect consumer decisions at either the point of consumption or the point of enrollment. Feldstein's (1971) Major Risk Insurance, requiring consumers to pay 100 percent of their medical bills annually until total bills exceed 10 percent of family income, is designed to make the public, and consequently the providers, more interested in cost containment. Such risk co-payments at the point of consumption would increase the provider incentive to experiment and implement new management techniques. Physicians might change the style of medical practice by selecting more cost-effective options, such as generic drugs or outpatient surgery. Because providers have a long-term interest in maintaining their reputations, one would not expect any significant or dangerous reduction in the quality of care while pursuing short-term cost-minimization goals.

Not all pro-competition health plans assume that individuals should purchase their medical care from a single organization such as an HMO. Newhouse and Taylor (1970) have proposed a Variable Cost Insurance plan whereby the consumers select the expense level (high, medium, or low cost) for hospitals they will utilize in the coming year. Premiums increase in proportion to the expense level of the eligible hospitals (low-expense hospitals have low-cost premiums, high-expense hospitals have high-cost premiums). The consumer can decide to purchase an average-cost hospital insurance option, and then pay cash to have heart surgery at a very expensive hospital. The providers might begin to get the message, through revealed consumer preference, that medical consumers would prefer to purchase the moderately priced American car to the expensive Mercedes. Basic service hospitals would flourish and tertiary care medical centers might have to streamline their product line. Currently there is little restraint on the consumption of health services if the premium cost is linked only to the aggregate costs of the insured group rather than to the more controllable elements in the given individual's consumption preferences.

To defer the financial hardship of high co-payments, the insurer or physician might offer the patient extended terms for payment. Consequently, the patient would remain concerned with cost, but would not be so financially pressured as to be unable to budget for necessary medical care. The insurer might only lend money to cover the co-insurance if a second opinion confirmed the necessity of the care. The patient would find the out-of-pocket costs more bearable if paid on an *ex post* rather than *ex ante* basis. It is highly unlikely that Congress would increase consumer co-insurance rates to the 33–50 percent level as advocated by Feldstein. Yet the real need persists to increase cost sensitivity among consumers and providers in order to protect the public from unbearable insurance-driven inflation, while protecting the individual from catastrophic out-of-pocket costs.

Most of this chapter will emphasize promoting competition, on the basis of price and benefits, at the point of enrollment in a health plan. In this context, the Reagan Administration can be expected to stimulate a lively policy debate concerning the promotion of HMOs as a method of injecting more price competition into health services delivery. Consumers have become increasingly insensitive to the price of medical services as insurance coverage has become more comprehensive and cost-sharing requirements have declined (Table 6.1). In addition, consumers have become less sensitive to insurance premium costs because employer benefits are excluded from the individual's taxable income. Under the current tax system the incentives favor purchasing excess health insurance (Feldstein and Friedman, 1977). For example, currently the employer can pur-

Table 6.1   Consumer Co-payment Rates for Hospital Care or Physician Professional Service, Selected Years 1964–1980

	Effective Co-payment Rate (Out-of-Pocket) *Payments as a Fraction of Total Cost* *(percent)*	
Year	*Hospital Care*	*Physician Services*
1964	27.7	63.4
1966	23.1	59.8
1968	15.5	46.1
1970	16.6	44.2
1972	13.5	41.7
1974	11.8	37.6
1976	11.1	34.9
1978	14.2	34.1
1980 (est.)	14.0	33.8

SOURCE: Health Care Financing Administration data, DHHS.

chase for the employee $1,400 of health insurance as a tax-free fringe benefit. If the employee were in the 33 percent tax bracket and had to purchase $1,400 worth of insurance annually, he would have to earn an additional $2,090 of before-tax annual income (ignoring the $150 of insurance cost that would be tax deductible). The employer could alternatively utilize that $2,090 to purchase $1,700 of insurance and increase the employee's annual wages by $300 (minus the added tax for social security and unemployment insurance). The employer would be $100 better off (before corporate taxes), and the employee would have $300 of excess insurance and $170 additional after-tax disposable income. This is a hypothetical example of a range of employer choices. The employee is better off if the insurance is bought with before-tax dollars. In summary, tax policy distorts consumption decisions and encourages the purchase of excess health insurance.

Barriers to Competition

There are a number of barriers to competition in the health field. While there is sufficient time to shop for maternity care, there is seldom enough time to shop in most hospital "purchase" situations. Conventional analysis says there is seldom a real "purchase" choice to be made, since the consumer, acting with minimal knowledge of medicine, goes to the doctor and says "save me." One might counter-argue that an economist who purchases a jacuzzi has less knowledge of the equipment than the typical high school graduate has concerning medicine. Yet the economist, with the aid of *Consumer Reports*, can make the best purchase decision for his needs. The ignorance problem does not preclude competitive markets in the case of high technology consumer goods. However this problem is compounded in the medical sector when "rival" providers and hospitals act in a collusive fashion, for example, they restrict advertising or quality disclosure activities.

In Chapters 5 and 6 we have already listed a number of examples of market failure in the health industry. We should add to the list the question of potential natural monopoly situations in the case of the most inflationary of all health providers, the hospitals. In contrast to the steel or airline industry, the competitive nature of hospital service markets has been called into doubt. Not only is the price elasticity of demand for hospital services very low (Phelps, 1975), but many hospitals have a natural lock on the market because of the high fixed costs to enter the market and compete. The "blue-sky" estimates of the percentage of hospitals residing in a natural monopoly situation vary from 30 to 60 percent. One should refer to the American Hospital Association Annual Survey to get an idea of the scope of the problem. Of the 3,100 distinct counties and regions in the country, 18 percent have no hospitals and 48 percent have only one hospital. However, these hospitals are small and low cost, representing no more than 10–25 percent of the beds and 7–14 percent of total hospital expenditures.

New Health Maintenance Organizations are seldom found in a natural monopoly situation. To ensure some degree of competition, Enthoven (1980) suggests that no HMO be allowed to enlist more than half the physicians in a community. The one exception to this guideline would be the rural community which, in order to attract a critical mass of patients and physicians, must either remain atomistic and uncoordinated or organize into a one-HMO town where the one HMO is the dominant provider. Antitrust regulations might be employed to ensure that the one HMO or the one hospital in an area does not exert excessive monopoly power on the public. One could imagine the various parties involved in litigation—the public versus the hospital, the public versus the HMO, the HMO versus the hospital, and the hospital versus the HMO.

Many analysts fear that the "cream skimming" alluded to by Enthoven in the introductory quotation would be encouraged by promoting competition among health plans. Academic theorists have not solved the problem of how to police the health plans to ensure that they are not skimming off the healthy low-risk enrollees. Another problem is that the more healthy individuals might themselves be encouraged to select an insurance option with higher co-payments and consequently lower premiums. Some would argue that the poor might be most likely to select these high cost-sharing insurance plans, risking "gambler's ruin," and then expect society to bail them out of bankruptcy. This raises an equity issue, because the poor would face greater financial barriers to needed care if they select the lower coverage insurance plans. The poor may be more susceptible to misleading advertising from competing health plans. Needless to say, no system of competition health plans would be completely self-regulating, but government regulation would be substantially curtailed.

The competitive model runs the risk of increasing the incidence of cream-skimming the easy (healthy) section of the population, but carries the benefit of minimizing the incentive to overutilize. However it seems reasonable to suggest that it might be more costly to police unnecessary care than to monitor potential bias in membership. Some of these issues will be discussed in Chapter 12.

HMOs have also been accused of cream-skimming activities. There is some evidence that HMOs selectively market their plan to the healthiest people. An HMO can cream skim by selectively marketing its plan to the suburban elderly and by avoiding the elderly from poor neighborhoods. A 1980 report from the Health Care Financing Administration to the Senate Finance Committee concerning 12,000 elderly members of the Puget Sound HMO reported that elderly new-enrollees to the plan are much healthier than the non-HMO elderly of Seattle. This study had an adverse effect on the national drive by HMOs to improve Medicare reimbursement policy. The HMOs would prefer a risk contract that reimbursed 95 percent of what would be expended by the average patient in the fee-for-service system,* rather than the present system of retrospective cost reimbursement. However, the aforementioned report from the Group Health Cooperative of Puget Sound raises concern

---

* In 1972 this idea was advanced in a proposal by President Nixon to reimburse HMOs at a rate equal to 95 percent of annual per capita Medicare costs for non-HMO beneficiaries. In 1979 Medicare actuaries estimated that the extra cost of the basis of reimbursement would be an additional 7 percent drain on the Hospital Insurance Trust Fund or $1.6 billion in fiscal 1980.

as to whether an HMO could unfairly reap a profit by selecting "healthy" elderly individuals who always utilize a significantly smaller fraction of health services than the "average" elderly person. Cost reimbursement has inhibited HMO growth, but risk contract reimbursement, even without the means of easily monitoring new enrollee health status, would benefit cream-skimming behavior. Some analysts could argue that the administrative costs for assessing health status and determining whether cream skimming behavior exists exceed the potential benefits of changing the basis of reimbursement.

HMO Growth

President Nixon's vision of 40 million American HMO enrollees by 1980 has not been realized. The nation has approximately 236 HMOs and 9.5 million enrollees in the most recent DHHS National HMO Census (Table 6.2). More than half of the HMO enrollees are in the state of California. One of the most frequently cited benefits of HMO market penetration (in areas where the HMO has achieved a greater than 10 percent share of the total market) is the positive impact that these organizations can have on containing hospital costs. For example, Goldberg and Greenberg (1979) report that Blue Cross responded to HMO competitive pressure by establishing their

Table 6.2 **National HMO Census Data from the Office of Health Maintenance Organizations—Public Health Service**

Year	Prepaid Health Plans (PHP)	Enrollment (in millions)	Percentage of U.S. Population Enrolled
1970	39	5.0	2.4
1975[1]	166	5.8	2.7
1976	169	6.2	2.9
1977	183	6.9	3.2
1978	208	7.8	3.6
1979	224	8.8	4.0
1980	236[2]	9.5	4.3
Projected 1983	327	12.4	5.5
Projected 1988	442	19.1	8.1

SOURCES: DHEW (1979), DHHS (1980).

[1] The HMO Act, P.L. 93-222, was passed in 1973.
[2] Of the 94 percent responding, 64 percent are group-staff model HMOs with the physicians acting as contracted employees. The remaining 36 percent are Individual Practice Associations (IPAs) with the physicians operating out of their own offices to serve HMO enrollees and non-member patients.

Table 6.3 Growth in HMO Members, Change in HMO and Non-HMO Monthly Premium Rates, Detroit, 1979–1980

	1979	1980
Enrollment in the Health Alliance Plan (HAP) HMO by Big-Three Auto Workers in Detroit[1]		
• Number of Families	10,638	12,973
• Number of Plan Members	34,881	38,831
Monthly Premium Rates for Chrysler Employees		
• HAP	$148.17	$160.24
• Blue Cross–Blue Shield	201.84	171.32
Monthly Premium Rates for General Motors Employees		
• HAP	$149.91	$162.99
• Blue Cross–Blue Shield	169.38	175.46
Monthly Premium Rates for Ford Employees		
• HAP	$142.52	$154.03
• Blue Cross–Blue Shield	150.26	152.60

[1] Hourly workers for all three companies only have the dual choice of HAP or Blue Cross–Blue Shield. Salaried workers at Chrysler and General Motors have a choice of three HMOs (HAP, Independence Health Plan, Group Health Plan) or Blue Cross–Blue Shield. At Ford, the salaried workers have the dual choice of HAP or Blue Cross–Blue Shield.

own HMOs and altering traditional reimbursement procedures in northern California and Hawaii. McClure (1978) reports that Blue Cross and other insurance plans constrain hospital rate increases to make their premiums competitive relative to HMOs in California, Hawaii, Minneapolis, and the District of Columbia. The benefits of increased competition between closed-panel HMOs and traditional Blue Cross plans include: lower insurance premiums due to price competition between insurance organizations, improved benefit packages, and the stimulation of innovative delivery ideas that save money (for example, preadmission testing and ambulatory surgery centers).

No one is sure how high the HMO market penetration rate has to be to lower Blue Cross/Blue Shield premiums in the region for all employees. However, even in markets where the HMO market share is below the 10 percent level, Blue Cross has lowered premiums for individual companies as a competitive response. These actions are consistent with findings by McGuire (1981) in Connecticut, where each $1 per month drop in Blue Cross premiums decreased the expected employee probability of joining the HMO by 3 percent. The data in Table 6.3 demonstrate the degree to which the non-HMO insurance plan opted to lower its company-specific premium rates in response to an aggressive marketing campaign by an HMO and the injection of two new HMO options into the market. Another interesting aspect of this example is that the employee has a choice of plans, but the burden of his or her choice rests on the employer who must pay 100 percent of the premium. The Enthoven health plan would offer a tax credit of $110 per month, and make the consumer price-conscious for every dollar in excess of $110, causing individuals to bear the costs of their decisions.

Havighurst and Hackbarth (1979) have argued that when individuals select the lower cost insurance plan, they should be given the savings tax free. By eliminating the practice of requiring the employer to pay the entire premium, society can end the forced subsidy of traditional solo practice fee-for-service medicine at the expense of the more efficient modes of practice. The Federal Employees Health Benefits Program is the oldest prototype of a consumer choice health plan with a fixed dollar contribution on behalf of the employer. This program was originally promoted in 1959 by public officials in the name of fair market competition, and has served both the taxpayer and federal employees well.

Competition Health Plan Proposals

The most comprehensive and well-documented strategy for implementing competition health plan is the one advanced by Enthoven. Enthoven's health plan offers some rather progressive features relative to other "competition" health bills. Current poor and elderly government insurance recipients would receive direct subsidies in the form of vouchers to purchase insurance. It is a moot point among economists whether these individuals should simply be given cash rather than vouchers. It is more of a relevant moot point among politicians as to whether consumers should be allowed to make a "profit" if their voucher amount exceeds the insurance premium. The non-poor employee would be provided with a limited tax credit with which to shop for the best available insurance option. The tax credit would equal 60 percent of the average per capita cost for covered services. Consequently, the individual might be faced with the decision of paying an additional 16 percent of the per capita regional average to join an HMO or an additional 40 percent to join the Blue Cross/Blue Shield option.

Enthoven (1980) attempts to address the cream-skimming issue by saying that the government will monitor a fair form of competition where competing health plans cite premiums by demographic category. Each health plan would practice community rating, that is, charging the same premium to all persons in the same demographic risk group enrolled for the same benefits. One way we could justify the subsidization implicit in community-rated insurance is that everyone eventually becomes sick, so that the healthy low-risk individuals who currently subsidize high-risk patients will one day also receive a subsidy from the healthy low-risk working population.*

None of the theoretical competition plans developed by academicians have been introduced as a legislative bill before Congress. Of the three competition plans in Congress, the most publicized bill in 1980 was Senator Durenberger's (R.–Minn.) Health Incentives Reform Act (S. 1968). The bill avoids the issue of directly mandating or promoting HMOs, but most faithfully incorporates the ideas of Enthoven and McClure—to give the employee financial incentive to shop for insurance. The hope is that health insurers would compete on the basis of price, quality, and scope of benefits to attract consumers. Employers would be required to contribute equally to each insurance plan. If the individual selected a low option plan with a premium below the employer contribution level, the employee would receive the differential as a rebate. The bill offers a "carrot" to business in the form of making business expense income tax deductions conditional on the two aforementioned requirements of the bill, but mandates linking the tax breaks to a requirement that firms with more than 100 workers must offer three or more insurance options to their employees. The Durenberger bill could receive some support from the administration, given that the present secretary of DHHS, former Senator Richard Schweiker, was also the author of a competition health plan bill in the 96th Congress (S. 1590).

---

* This same argument cannot be advanced against the Newhouse and Taylor (1970) proposal for linking consumer preferences for expensive hospitals to their premium rates. For example, if the author refuses to be cared for by any facility less expensive than the Mayo Clinic and New York Hospital, he should have to pay for the cost of this decision. One could not argue against making him pay top dollar premium rates with the suggestion that we all end up in the most expensive facilities eventually.

The Durenberger and Schweiker* competition health proposals were designed to transform the Enthoven (1980) suggestions for changes in the tax code into a format that may be more palatable to the Congress. Since all such proposals provide some net increase in the tax laws, it is hard to imagine that such measures will be passed in the near future. The tax code is seldom changed because too many groups benefit from current deductions and exclusions. Collectively Americans will reduce their tax burden by $3.6–$3.9 billion in 1982 through deductions from personal income of insurance premium costs plus out-of-pocket health expenditures exceeding 3 percent of net income. In 1982 business will save between $12–$13 billion by deducting from income the expenditures they make to employee health benefit plans. A few business groups have decided to take a long-range view and support the competition health plan concept. The rhetoric of injecting competition into the unmanageable health care system is conceptually tidy for some groups, but how long will it take the uncertain savings in future fringe benefit cost to justify making the move to competition health plans? There are other major obstacles to building a coalition for competition health plans. Labor groups will resist any attempt to equalize and/or reduce employer contributions to health benefit options. In the collective bargaining process unions traditionally negotiate health benefits per employee, not health dollars provided per employee. Two other groups that may openly oppose competition reforms are the Council of Teaching Hospitals, and the nation's 125 medical schools (survey in Chapter 11), as teaching hospitals can ill afford to provide services for health plans at competitive rates. The health plans that ally with nonteaching hospitals would grow, and the plans that ally with teaching hospitals for any routine admission would price themselves out of the market. These obstacles are not totally insurmountable, but adoption of the competition idea will be a slow evolutionary process.

We have already made a national commitment to the HMO concept, which underlies all competition health reform proposals. The federal government has promoted HMOs since 1973 by requiring "dual choice" under section 1310 of the HMO Act (P.L. 93-222) and that employers offer at least one HMO if it is federally qualified and has requested to be included in the employee benefits program. In

---

* In 1981 Senate Labor and Human Resources Committee Chairman Orrin Hatch (R–Utah) reintroduced the Schweiker proposal (S. 1590). The new bill (S. 139) requires insurance plans to include catastrophic benefits for medical expenses in excess of 20 percent of annual family income.

addition to having federally assured marketing access, HMOs are eligible to receive grants, loans, loan guarantees, and technical assistance. A developing HMO can receive a maximum $75,000 feasibility grant, a $200,000 planning grant, and a lifetime maximum $2 million development grant. Loans and loan guarantees are available to cover initial operating deficits up to a maximum of $4.5 million. Loans are also available for the modernization, construction, or purchase of ambulatory facilities (not to exceed $2.5 million per facility acquired or renovated). In the next section we shall review the growth pattern of HMOs.

The History and Performance of HMOs

HMOs experienced very slow growth in the three years following enactment of the HMO bill (P.L. 93-222) in 1973. Subsequent amendments in 1976 and 1978 stripped away a number of progressive but costly elements of the original HMO Act. The required benefit package was reduced in scope and the plans were allowed to charge indigent groups above-average rates. The number of federally qualified HMOs has increased to 115. In the four years since 1976 the total number of HMOs grew by 39 percent and the enrollment expanded by 54 percent (Table 6.2). In the period 1974–1980 the federal government invested $111 million in grants for HMO development and $193 million in loans.

As with all business ventures, there have been some failures in the HMO field. Only eight of the 123 federally stimulated HMOs have gone bankrupt as of October 1980. This 6.5 percent failure rate is substantially lower than the failure rate among the 1300 commercial insurance companies. All eight failures in the HMO field carried insolvency insurance to allow the orderly dissolution of the plan members into alternative insurance plans. This failure rate might be reduced in the future as more health administration programs offer specialized courses in HMO management. Recently, poorly managed HMOs have been swallowed up by large, well-established HMOs. For example, in September 1980 the Georgetown Community Health Plan became the Kaiser-Georgetown HMO (55,000 enrollees).

There are many types of HMOs. Group and staff model HMOs are frequently not differentiated. Staff model HMOs hire physicians as salaried employees. In the case of a group model HMO, a physician group contracts with the HMO management and insurance entity to provide patient care. The physician group is a partnership, association, corporation, or other group composed of licensed health professionals. As outlined in the Federal Register (1978), the members of such a group "as their principal, professional activity (over 50 percent individually) engage in the coordinated practice of their profession and as a group responsibility have substantial responsibility (over 35 percent in the aggregate of their professional activity) for the delivery of health services to members of an HMO." Typically, the physician group shares in the risk for cost overruns if actual utilization exceeds enrollee revenues. A third type of Health Maintenance Organization eligible for federal support is the so-called Independent Practice Association (IPA). The term "independent practice association" refers to the physician component of this third type of HMO. The IPA is a separate legal entity from the HMO that contracts with individual professionals, who practice out of a traditional setting. The differentiating factor between the physician group in a group model HMO and the IPA in an IPA-model HMO is the "principal professional activity requirement" described above. If a medical group of an HMO cannot meet the principal, professional activity requirement, the HMO will be an IPA-model HMO as opposed to a group model HMO. HMOs are prepaid health insurance plans where the organization and participating physicians accept contractual responsibilities for the delivery of a stated benefit package of covered health services available to the enrollees. Group and staff model HMO physicians are organized on a closed-panel (restrictive) basis and paid on a salaried or capitation basis, whereas IPA physicians are open-panel and reimbursed fee-for-service.

Perrott (1971), Gaus *et al.* (1976), and others (Luft, 1979) have reported that group and staff model HMOs achieve their 10–30 percent "savings" through lower hospital utilization rates than the fee-for-service sector (solo, group, or IPA). The incentives to contain services and aggressively review utilization habits are not as strong in an IPA as compared to a group or staff model HMO. In the case of the IPA, the physicians bear none of the risk if the plan goes bankrupt from in-patient service costs exceeding enrollment premium revenues.

Some of the more recent unpublished cost studies (DHHS, 1980) confirm the aforementioned economies of closed-panel HMOs and the relative improvement that some IPAs have made in closing the differential between IPA and HMO (group or staff) premium rates.

The size of the cost-savings differential between the group, staff HMO, or IPA plan and traditional insurance (Blue Cross/Blue Shield) depends on the area of the country, demographic characteristics of the population, and the maturity and size of the HMO operation. IPAs still produce less significant cost savings than group or staff model HMOs. Comparable paired comparisons of IPAs and group or staff model HMOs with 20,000 enrollees reveal that IPAs save (relative to Blue Cross/Blue Shield) 15–20 percent less than group or staff HMOs (DHEW, 1979). As the organization increases in size, group and staff model HMOs are increasingly less costly per capita than IPAs. At 50,000 enrollees, IPAs save 40 percent less than group or staff model HMOs of the same size. Not surprisingly, the federal government emphasizes the development of nonprofit group or staff model HMOs rather than IPAs. Another rationale cited by the federal government for promoting HMO models other than IPAs in target communities in the 1980s involves the competitive response from traditional providers to new entrants in the market. When group or staff model HMOs enter the market, fee-for-service physicians often respond by establishing IPAs; there is a multiplier effect rippling through the marketplace causing two or more individuals to sign up for some form of IPA for every one closed-panel HMO enrollee. However, the direction of the multiplier effect is not symmetrical. IPAs do not stimulate group practice HMO development, although HMOs certainly stimulate IPAs.

Controlling Hospital Utilization

In the instances where IPAs have instituted strong utilization review programs and restructured the reimbursement incentives to place the physicians at risk if the plan overutilizes services, the premium costs and hospital admission rates have been comparable to closed-panel HMOs (Moore, 1979; Egdahl et al., 1977). The two principal positive attributes of IPAs are that they avoid the large start-up costs of group or staff model HMOs and offer a mode of reimbursement, per unit-of-service, that is more attractive to private practitioners. Physicians prefer IPAs because they offer the benefits of utilization controls without the discomfort of closed panels and the economies of scale of a large group without foregoing the convenience of private offices. Physicians do not like being placed under a financial risk. However, the IPAs that survive and grow reimburse physicians at only 70 or 80 percent of customary fees during the fiscal year as a hedge against potential operating deficits. If the control of utilization was stringent enough to allow a year-end budgetary surplus, then a fraction of the 30–20 percent discount fees is returned to the physicians. However, seldom is an IPA profitable enough to allow the physicians to receive their full customary fees.

Why do physicians join IPAs? Most of the 100 existing IPAs were started by the local medical society in response to declining patient volumes induced by the introduction of successful HMOs in the area. Some of the larger corporations have provided seed money for IPA development programs, typically with the conditions that the clinicians are paid on a capitation rather than fee-for-service basis. Most physicians are unwilling to abandon fee-for-service free enterprise unless the activities of a competing HMO make the IPA an attractive option.

There is conflicting evidence as to whether consumer access to a physician is better or worse in prepaid group or staff model HMOs versus fee-for-service IPAs. Held and Reinhardt (1980) report that prepaid groups have a statistically insignificant 5 percent longer average queueing time to an appointment than fee-for-service group practices. In contrast, Luft (1979) reports that prepaid groups have 10–20 percent shorter queue duration, as measured by average wait to appointment, than fee-for-service groups.

Problems with the actual, as differentiated from perceived, quality of patient care cannot be considered a barrier to HMO development. A recent study by Cunningham and Williamson (1980), reviewing quality of care, reported that group or staff model HMOs and a few IPAs provided superior care to that in fee-for-service settings in 53 of 80 instances. None of the studies reviewed in the literature, 1958–1980, reported HMO care to be inferior to fee-for-service care overall. These findings suggest that HMOs are providing good quality care in order to avoid losing enrollees to the competition (other HMOs, IPAs, and fee-for-service solo practitioners).

It is not clear that cost reimbursement of Medicare patients has inhibited HMO growth to the degree that some HMO managers have claimed. A federally designated HMO receives incentive payments equal to one-half of one percent for each percentage point below the adjusted average per capita cost. The comparison between HMOs and non-HMOs is made with appropriate actuarial adjustments for differences in race, age, sex, and chronic medical impairments. Consequently, a typical HMO operating at 76 percent of adjusted per capita costs would receive an incentive payment of 12 percent of the per capita amount. The typical HMO in our hypothetical example would receive an incentive payment under current reimbursement conditions equal to 16 percent (88 divided by 76) above its own actual costs. Needless to say, this 16 percent "profit"—revenues in excess of costs—is better than the net profit margin of the 1200 commercial insurance companies and 80 Blue Cross plans. HMOs have a number of disincentives concerning enrollment of the poor. Poor people require more health services, exhibit high rates of turnover in eligibility for Medicaid, and a consequent high risk of retrospective denial of reimbursement.

Business Involvement in HMOs

It is important to remember that while HMOs may represent a minor share of the market, they can represent a major share of the employees in a single corporation. For example, in the five-year period 1976–1980 the HMO enrollment at General Mills increased from 40 to 72 percent. A majority of the employees cited economy and dependability of care as the most attractive aspects of HMOs. Other consumer advantages include continuity of care (one medical record follows the individual through the system), total absence of claims forms and other paper work, and the comprehensive nature of the HMO benefit package (for example, a family need not budget for mundane or recurring ambulatory visits).

Big business is beginning to invest in the HMOs. The John Deere Company of Moline, Illinois, invested $600,000 in fiscal 1979–1980 for development of a group HMO and IPA. The subsequent 50 percent reduction in the rate at which employee health benefits had been inflating more than covered the cost of the initial investment during calendar year 1980.

The Safeco Corporation, through its United Health Care subsidiary, has been successful at attracting underworked practitioners into a unique capitated IPA arrangement. Some 600 primary care practitioners in Washington state and California have agreed to participate in a plan that places the physician at risk. Each physician serves as the sole manager of all medical services for the enrollee and family. The practitioner receives a fixed annual capitation payment based on the demographic characteristic of the enrollees, with higher payments allotted for blacks, women, and the elderly. From that fund the physician must pay for all normal medical costs, including hospitalization, prescriptions, and surgeon's fees. At the end of the enrollment period, after earning a capitated salary, the physician-gatekeeper splits any residual profit 50/50 with the United Health Care Corporation. This unique IPA arrangement offers some elements of the British experience (with the physician acting as a gatekeeper to the hospital system, and the physician playing the role of a mini-HMO in providing for all ambulatory care needs). However, the parallel with Britain is less than perfect; the Safeco doctors are allowed to treat the patients in the hospital rather than leave them totally in the hands of the hospital's specialists, as in Britain. Second, British physicians do not have to pay for, or control, the institutional care of the patients on their practice lists.

The recent major jumps in insurance premiums have persuaded a number of corporations to co-sponsor new HMOs. One of the most highly publicized examples was the R. J. Reynolds HMO investment in Winston-Salem in 1976. More recently, Burlington Industries invested in an HMO in Greensboro, North Carolina. In some cases IPA development is supported as a joint venture by business and insurance companies. The Mead Corporation managed to enlist 46 percent of their employees in one Dayton IPA during 1980. One commercial insurance company, INA, has recently sponsored two new IPAs in Milwaukee, Wisconsin, and Gary, Indiana. Kaiser has also entered into a joint venture in Dallas developing a large HMO with the aid of Prudential Insurance. Prudential has also contributed $22 million in development money for the creation of five additional HMOs in Austin, Atlanta, Houston, Oklahoma City, and Nashville. However, there are risks associated with business alignment with any type of HMO, especially federally nonqualified HMOs. For example, Hewlett-Packard in Palo Alto had aligned with three nonqualified HMOs that went bankrupt in the late 1970s. Nationally, twenty nonqualified HMOs have gone bankrupt since 1974, as opposed to the failure of eight federally qualified HMOs between 1975 and 1980.

Large employers are more capable of absorbing the search costs associated with shopping for the insurance option that offers the best long-term value. Institutions provide information to large employers that is not typically allowed in advertising campaigns. The less-informed consumers or consumer groups could benefit by observing the negotiations and behavior of the informed large employers and unions. Private individuals lack the resources and time required for an adequate search of the options. Not all individuals will agree with any group consensus concerning medical care, because it is in many ways an "experience good," that is, a good that must be experienced in order to value its intangible and tangible attributes.

Advertising and Demand Creation

Most medical providers have been slow to realize that marketing principles can be successfully applied to service industries like health care. The most frequently misunderstood concept concerning the marketing process is that consumers are so ignorant and gullible in the health care business that they can be duped into asking for services that they do not in fact need. No study has demonstrated that advertising merely stimulates medically unnecessary utilization. Some surveys have indicated that the public is currently oversold on the benefits of medical technology. The Chicago Mount Sinai Medical Center market survey report, published in the Chicago edition of *Time* (January 1977), suggests that area residents are well informed about health and hygiene matters, but feel that modern medicine has the miracle techniques and spare parts to fix them no matter how they live their lives. Future research should consider the question of whether the excessive faith the public has in technology makes them susceptible to misleading advertising campaigns or whether public faith is on the wane. Malpractice stories in the media might be eroding the public faith in medical technology.

One should not suggest that advertising will induce consumers to suddenly shop for health plans and providers as methodically as they shop for automobiles. It is clear that many individuals will opt for the protection and security of the status quo, and not shop among competition health plans. Most consumers will not immediately abandon their current providers, even after being convinced that a new health delivery option will save the family a few dollars per week. However, over time if the family has a "bad" experience with their doctor or hospital, they will be more likely to upgrade the importance of cost considerations in their future annual enrollment decisions and move to the plan that provides the best buy with all factors considered. Enthoven (1980) was the first to admit that competition health plans are a 20-year cost control strategy that will slowly affect consumer behavior. Advertising is simply one method of providing consumers with the facts concerning lower cost health plans or better providers.

In principle, to inform the public is the essence of advertising.

Expanded services or new inclusive pricing packages should be promoted in a well-managed institution. The perceived style of advertising is important in the health arena. Noncompetitive "natural" advertising, sometimes labeled "social marketing," is generally more acceptable to health providers than competitive advertising ("buy our product"). Hospitals should go beyond the product orientation of selling in-patient or hospital-based services, and realize that their one chance for expansion may reside in taking a broader market orientation. The hospital could then better serve the latent demands of the community with independent ambulatory surgicenters, home health care services, and health education and promotion. HMOs have taken a broad market orientation, but have suffered by allowing providers' values to dominate the advertising function. In Chapter 7 we shall review the topic of marketing applications in health care.

Health Care Alliance (HCA) Concept

Ellwood and McClure (1979) have suggested an alternative to the traditional group, staff, or IPA model HMO mode of practice. Insurance companies or employers could enlist efficient providers to join their Health Care Alliance (HCA) plan. In contrast to the HMO concept of a single organization insuring and providing care, the HCA would offer a clear separation between insurer and provider. The HCA, like the IPA, would not place the physicians at financial risk if the plan were to fail. This newly labeled concept of competition among HMOs–HCAs offers obvious advantages to consumers and insurance companies. The consumers are now presented with a larger choice of insurance options for selecting the "best buy" each year. The insurers can deal only with the providers willing to practice cost-effective medicine, rather than simply pay the bills of any and all providers. Perhaps with time the medical care business will become so competitive that providers will have an incentive to bind together in HCAs, but currently the power of insurers to create HCAs or the incentive for physicians and hospitals to join HCAs seems weak.

Under a capitated IPA, the physicians are placed at financial risk for the total cost of their enrollees' care. Consequently, the incentive to more efficiently review utilization patterns is substantially higher in a capitated IPA than the traditional IPA. In those areas of California, Minnesota, and Washington state where capitated IPAs have started, the physicians' fear of losing current patients to IPAs is always cited as a critical factor in plan development.

IPAs would become more competitive relative to group or staff model HMOs if they would implement stringent utilization review controls or move to a capitated method of physician reimbursement. In Chapter 12 we shall review utilization controls. One very recent successful example of an IPA implementing tough controls involved the Physicians Health Plan of Minnesota (DHHS, 1980). This IPA realized in 1976–1977 that their survival depended on initiating a utilization control effort. Fewer than a dozen IPA physicians dropped out of the plan when the mandatory controls were installed. In the first year of controls, hospital days per 1,000 IPA enrollees declined 16 percent. In the second year of controls (1979), hospital days per enrollee declined an additional 9 percent, to the level of the average HMO in the Midwest. Sixty percent of the decline in hospital utilization was attributable to a decline in lengths of stay and 40 percent was attributable to a decline in hospital admission rates. According to the authors (DHHS, 1980), most IPA physicians applauded utilization review efforts and some expressed satisfaction over the voluntary retirement of the doctors who were most prone to overutilize resources. One might speculate that the IPA doctors in other areas of the country, where there is little fear of competition, would have been less supportive of utilization controls. However, in the Minneapolis–St. Paul area, the physician could either join a group practice or face the prospect of losing more patients to the eight HMOs in the area.

If the third-party insurance agency wishes to minimize costs, and preserve a level of quality that ensures repeat business, they will need to make critical decisions concerning the selection of providers with whom to ally. In this context, the evidence on the long-term viability of IPAs is not clear. We have already cited one example of an IPA success story when physicians cooperated in aggressive utilization review programs—for example, monitoring both the length of stay and admission-decision appropriateness of hospital episodes. More recently, Sorensen *et al.* (1980) have reported on the failure of an IPA to survive for longer than three years in the Rochester area. The failed IPA suffered from an incentive structure that weakens all such physician foundations: the IPA avoided placing its physicians at financial risk. Further research is needed to discover the most effective strategies for promoting IPAs and alternative delivery systems.

Generalizability of the Success Stories

HMO growth areas (Table 6.4) are typically socially progressive, youthful, overdoctored areas, with few unions, a growing economy, and highly fragmented local medical societies with many disparate factions. For example, in the Minneapolis–St. Paul area, which has 23 percent more physicians per capita than the national average, there are eight competing HMOs, including two IPAs, two staff model HMOs, two group practice HMOs, one hospital-based HMO, and one network-primary-care based HMO. Minneapolis–St. Paul was a receptive climate for HMOs. The Group Health prepaid group practice had increased in enrollment consistently since 1957. Some would argue that the growth and competition between HMOs caused the creation of disparate physician factions, and others would argue on behalf of the other causal direction. Certain demographic groups are more predisposed to join HMOs. The failure of regression models (reported in unpublished consulting reports) to explain the cross-sectional variation in HMO market penetration rates is disappointing. These results argue for suggesting that the self-serving attempts of HMO advocates to generalize on the basis of a few successful anecdotes in selected areas may be misleading. One can say that the proportion of Minneapolis–St. Paul's two million citizens enrolled in HMOs has

Table 6.4 HMO Market Penetration Rates in Potential High Growth Target Markets for the 1980s

Projected Growth Areas	*Percent of Population in HMOs, Projected 1983*
Denver–Boulder, Colorado	9.2
New York, New York	8.4
Miami, Florida	7.7
Cleveland, Ohio	6.5
Anaheim, California	6.3
Albuquerque, New Mexico	6.0
Washington, D.C.	5.5
Milwaukee, Wisconsin	4.3
Ventura, California	3.8
Houston, Texas	3.3
St. Louis, Missouri	3.2
Baltimore, Maryland	2.6
Boston, Massachusetts	2.6

SOURCE: DHEW (1979).

grown from 2 to 20 percent between 1970 and 1980. It is unclear whether the marketing success of HMOs in a few areas can be duplicated nationwide in the 1980s. One might speculate that physicians, if they face a doctor oversupply in the 1980s, will increasingly express interest in joining fledgling HMOs and HCAs. If physicians become increasingly underworked, they may be more willing to take risks and engage in competitive behavior.

Two final caveats must be made concerning the competition advocates' assumptions that insurers will compete and that the number of regulations will decline. McNerney (1980) suggests that insurers almost never compete by negotiating with doctors and hospitals to contain costs. Instead, insurers are in the habit of diverting competition before it reaches the provider by competing on other grounds: packaging special benefits, risk selection, and experience rating. It will be hard for the government or the HMO and insurance industries to establish enough detailed rules to restrain these practices. It would be ironic if competition reformers created a climate in which enrollment scandals forced a net increase in regulatory involvement, because government had to monitor 2,000 HMOs and health insurers. The irony is found in the observation that many people become competition enthusiasts in reaction to excessive government regulation, for example, the publication of 12,000 pages of Medicare reimbursement rules since 1967.

Conclusions

None of the competition health plans promise substantial immediate relief from the medical cost inflation problem. However, with medical costs inflating at approximately the same rate as the Consumer Price Index, advocates of competition argue that society should not rush to a judgment on behalf of a more traditional regulatory approach. Many analysts see better potential long-run effectiveness in pro-competition incentive schemes than in quick-fix, short-term regulatory intervention. Many liberals still argue that long-term regulation in the form of global (health sector) regional budgets is the better alternative (Fein, 1980).

Less spectacular strategies, such as the dissemination of information to consumers suggested in Chapter 6, stand some chance of being encouraged by Congress in the name of competition. It is doubtful that Congress would be willing to remove the current tax incentives regarding promotion of health insurance, and redirect the incentives to promote group, staff, or IPA model HMOs and HCAs. The insurance industry that currently represents some 200 million Americans would lobby against any such tinkering with the tax incentives. The mood of the country seems to be drifting in the direction of small-scope strategies, such as increasing consumer cost-sharing provisions in insurance contracts.

Hopefully this chapter has shed some light on the incremental proposals to restructure the health services industry into a system of competitive markets. One of the reasons why "competition" rhetoric is currently popular is because the idea connotes so many different things to different people. However, if competition begins to make things rough for some providers, or if it fails to contain costs, a large fraction of the pro-competition camp will become embittered. The competition mind set has one political advantage: If you go bankrupt you cannot blame it on external regulations. Bankrupt service institutions in a competitive environment have only two scapegoats: poor management or poor provision of service.

References

CUNNINGHAM, F., and WILLIAMSON, J. (1980). "How Does the Quality of Health Care in HMOs Compare to Other Settings?" *Group Health Journal* 1:1 (Winter), 2–23.

Department of Health, Education and Welfare (1978). *Federal Register* 43:176 (September 11), Part II, Public Health Service, Health Maintenance Organizations, Proposed Requirements, p. 40378.

Department of Health, Education and Welfare (1979). *National HMO Development Strategy Through 1988*, PHS 79-50111. Washington, D.C.: U.S. Government Printing Office.

Department of Health and Human Services (1980). "The Physicians Health Plan of Minnesota: A Case Study of Utilization Controls in an IPA," PHS 80-50128. Washington, D.C.: U.S. Government Printing Office.

EGDAHL, R., TAFT, C., FRIEDLAND, J., and LIND, K. (1979). "The Potential of Organization of Fee-for-Service Physicians for Achieving Significant Decreases in Hospitalization," *Annals of Surgery* 186:9 (September), 288–396.

ELLWOOD, P., and McCLURE, W. (1979). "Health Care Alliances," InterStudy Memorandum. Excelsior, Minnesota: InterStudy.

ENTHOVEN, A. C. (1980). *Health Plan.* Reading, Mass.: Addison-Wesley.

FEIN, R. (1980). "Social and Economic Attitudes Shaping American Health Policy," *Milbank Memorial Fund Quarterly* 58:3 (Summer), 349–385.

FELDSTEIN, M. (1971). "A New Approach To National Health Insurance," *The Public Interest* 23:1 (Spring), 93–105.

FELDSTEIN, M., and FRIEDMAN, B. (1977). "Tax Subsidies, The Rational Demand for Insurance and the Health Care Crisis," *Journal of Public Economics* 7:2 (April), 155–178.

GAUS, C., COOPER, B., and HIRSHMAN, C. (1976). "Contrast in HMO and Fee-for-Service Performance," *Social Security Bulletin* 39:5 (May), 3–14.

GOLDSMITH, J. C. (1980). "The Health Care Market: Can Hospitals Survive?" *Harvard Business Review* 8:5 (September-October), 100–112.

GOLDBERG, L., and GREENBERG, W. (1979). "The Competitive Response of Blue Cross and Blue Shield to the HMOs in Northern California and Hawaii," *Medical Care* 17:10 (October), 1019–1028.

HAVIGHURST, C., and HACKBARTH, J. (1979). "Private Cost Containment," *New England Journal of Medicine* 300:23 (June 7), 1298–1305.

HELD, P., and REINHARDT, U. (1980). "Prepaid Medical Practice: A Summary of Recent Findings From a Survey of Group Practices in the United States," *Group Practice Journal* 1:2 (Summer), 4–15.

LUFT, H. S. (1979). *Health Maintenance Organizations: Dimensions of Permanence.* New York: Wiley.

MARSHALL, A. (1922). *Principles of Economics.* London: Macmillan.

McCLURE, W. (1978). "On Broadening the Definition of and Removing Regulatory Barriers to a Competitive Health Care System," *Journal of Health Politics, Policy and Law* 3:3 (July), 303–327.

McGUIRE, T. (1981). "Price and Membership in a Prepaid Group Medical Practice," *Medical Care* 19:2 (February), 172–183.

McNERNEY, W. J. (1980). "Control of Health Care Costs in the 1980's," *New England Journal of Medicine* 303:19 (November 6), 1088–1095.

MOORE, S. (1979). "Cost Containment Through Risk-Sharing by Primary-Care Physicians," *New England Journal of Medicine* 300:24 (June 14), 1359–1362.

NEWHOUSE, J., and TAYLOR, V. (1970). "The Subsidy Problem in Hospital Insurance," *Journal of Business* 43:10 (October), 452–456.

NIXON, R. (1971). "President's Message on Health and Hospitalization," *Congressional Record*, 92nd Congress, First Session, 117, Part 3: 3015–3021. Washington, D.C.: U.S. Government Printing Office.

PERROTT, G. (1971). "The Federal Employees Health Benefits Program: Enrollment and Utilization of Health Service 1968–69," DHEW Report. Washington, D.C.: U.S. Government Printing Office.

PHELPS, C. (1975). "The Effects of Insurance on Demand for Medical Care," in R. Anderson (ed.), *Equity in Health Services: Empirical Analysis in Social Policy.* Cambridge, Mass.: Ballinger.

ROVETI, G., HORN, S., and KREITZER, S. (1980). "ASSCORE: A Multi-attribute Clinical Index of Illness Severity," *Quality Review Bulletin* 6:7 (July), 25–31.

SORENSEN, A., SAWARD, E., and WERSINGER, R. (1980). "The Demise of an IPA: A Case Study of Health Watch," *Inquiry* 17:3 (Fall), 244–253.

STIGLER, G. (1961). "The Economics of Information." *Journal of Political Economy* 69:3, 213–225.

Chapter 7

HEALTH MARKETING

The interest that policy makers and administrators in the health care field are currently showing in marketing stems in part from their sympathy with its basic principle: the identification and satisfaction of consumer needs. Marketing activity should not be regarded as an expensive, speculative drain on the resources, but rather as a planning process that can guide the allocation of these resources toward a more effective result. At the same time, marketing practitioners must clearly understand the value system of the health care professionals with whom they are collaborating; the existence of different criteria for the measurement of success; and the unique problems of consumer behavior.

—JOHN A. QUELCH

Marketing is not selling, rather marketing is improving consumer satisfaction. The AMA, American Marketing Association, recognizes this fact and has given its highest award to two studies that have resulted in socially desirable declines in sales of a very precious commodity: energy resources.

—PHILIP D. COOPER

Pressure on health service providers to control costs and close facilities has stimulated interest in health marketing activities. Marketing consultants take the public stance that their activity can help the firm provide better service and be more responsive to consumer's demands. Marketing is defined operationally as the set of activities designed to satisfy consumer needs and wants, including delivery, advertising, selling, and pricing. In the past, providers seldom considered measuring and satisfying consumer preferences. During the mid-1970s consumer groups in a few states initiated programs for bland informational advertising in "Medical Yellow Pages," giving schedules, fees, and location. In the late 1970s a few large urban hospitals, facing increased competition from suburban hospitals, bad debts, and the added responsibility of having their emergency rooms serve as the sole source of primary care for the poor, initiated competitive advertising schemes. The approach was usually linked to quality: "Buy our product (for example, open-heart surgery) or our service (for example, maternity and pediatrics) and you'll have a better chance of survival, thanks to our experienced staff and teaching hospital physicians." In one case, the publication of differential survival rate statistics at two institutions caused the closing of the higher mortality suburban service and slight expansion of the previously underutilized urban hospital's service, much to the delight of the medical school officials who needed additional patients for the education of their students and residents.

Marketing activities will become increasingly popular in the 1980s, especially if the medical economy grows more competitive. Many hospital administrators have adopted a plodder strategy to pursue "quiet" competition, for example, to accept slight changes in customer mix as a fait accompli that should not result in open predatory reaction among hospitals, because no single competitor is strong enough to disturb the silence. Proprietary hospitals were the first to question the wisdom of a plodder strategy.

Proprietary corporate hospital chains have been the biggest promoters of competitive advertising. The chains typically target their marketing to self-pay patients or employers and argue that their competitive advantage lies in the provision of lower cost care. Proprietary hospitals argue that they provide a wide range of services at lower cost and equal quality, due primarily to better management (such as group purchasing and product specialization).

Many health professionals balk at the term *marketing* because it runs counter to their feelings that health care is "special"—not to be treated like a marketable commodity or service. The non-profit hospital industry has been criticized by Carlson (1975) and by other advocates of holistic medicine for having a static, limited-scope, product orientation that does not provide the consumer with the necessary information concerning the product (health services). The proprietary hospitals, one tenth of the total hospital market (beds), are exempt from this criticism in that their marketing efforts provide the consumer with this information through effective advertising, publicity, and promotion (elements of the marketing communications mix).

Conflicts between Marketing and the Non-Profit Ethos

Many non-profit managers have the misconception that marketing is simply selling a fixed given product. Selling is only one aspect of the marketing process. Marketing is a process of assessing consumer wants by changing the product and/or the distribution channels. Marketing is not always a process designed to increase demand.

Marketing involves managing demand and improving consumer satisfaction. For example, a public utility may decide to decrease (demarket) demand for their product in the name of energy conservation. In the case of health care, a given institution or Health Systems Agency may wish to demarket nursing home care while promoting home care, or demarket in-patient surgical or psychiatric care in order to promote the substitute product—ambulatory care. The largest potential benefit from health marketing may reside with a local health planning council developing a regionalized integrated health marketing plan. Marketing activities performed on a macro scale by a regional planning council will be less costly and more efficacious than those performed by individual institutions. If many institutions bind together as a cooperative group, duplication of marketing research efforts is avoided. To achieve the best allocation of resources, the group can divide the service area among themselves and develop a vertically integrated sharing agreement where each institution provides the service at which they are the most proficient.

One could postulate that the invisible hand and competitive pressures might induce a given firm (for example, a nursing home) to demarket their product to some extent and to promote substitute products (home health care). However, due to institutional inertia, the invisible hand often turns out to be all thumbs; nursing homes might prefer to maintain the status quo rather than to face charges of predatory marketing behavior that pulls demand away from their neighbors.

Marketing activities that are designed to communicate with and motivate the public to consume health care services have some unique problems in health services delivery. First, the consumption of health services is frequently remembered in negative terms; pain is often a deterrent to seeking medical care. Second, even if the physicians make the major consumption decisions, health managers should increasingly treat patients as customers and potential sources of return business or word-of-mouth advertising. If the emphasis of the marketing program is to redirect the locus of care to less costly sites and to improve patient education and compliance, society benefits. A regional marketing effort by the local Health Systems Agency need not negatively affect the cash-flow position of the individual hospital if the decline in in-patient volume is more than compensated for by an increase in out-patient volume. The rise in out-patient volume directly results from the activities of the out-patient department, hospital-based clinics, and the emergency room. The progressive hospital can also manage three types of captive, corporately independent distribution channels: freestanding outpatient clinics, freestanding emergency rooms, and the leased adjacent physicians' office building.

Hospital marketing is not simply the maximization of hospital admission rates or patient census. Marketing tailored to this industry, often called "social marketing," implies a service orientation (better health), not a product orientation (more patient bed days). The smart administrator need not decrease firm size or net revenues by diversification away from in-patient care to other services. The three major rationales for diversification are (1) to acquire profit making services (such as laboratory, radiology, alcohol rehabilitation care, and inhalation therapy); (2) to increase production volume, and consequently decrease unit costs, by contracting with other firms to supply services (such as laboratory, laundry, and food services); and (3) to develop a feeder system into the hospital. Although ambulatory care clinics are loss leaders, most institutions operate clinics as a feeder system into the hospital. Further, the product portfolio of the hospital can be diversified to include health promotion and health education activities designed to improve patient compliance. The problem of patient compliance and health education is a major growth area in our health care system. Problems with patient compliance to medical regimen was a contributing factor to 21 percent of the hospitalizations in one recent study (Mason *et al.*, 1980).

If enough health providers pursue marketing techniques, the health services industry might be capable of recapturing some semblance of self-regulation. The hospital that ignores marketing considerations will be relegated to a "plodder" or negative growth existence. Those hospitals most frequently employing marketing techniques, proprietary hospitals, have almost doubled their market share of hospital beds over the past five years, while the rest of the industry talks of retrenchment. Most of the hospitals currently employing marketing concepts are investor-owned or contract-managed hospitals. Such facilities tend to offer a broader range of services and offer lower cost per patient stay (Biggs *et al.*, 1980). One unquestioned benefit of health marketing activities is the resulting increased sensitivity to consumer needs for amenities, information, and emotional support. Some fear that marketing health care as a commodity will ultimately demean it. In transplanting marketing techniques from the business sector, one must be careful to avoid hucksterism while pursuing competitive consumerism.

There are a number of reasons why marketing activities aimed at potential health care consumers are necessary. First, people concerned with day-to-day living often underestimate the value of early diagnosis and preventive medicine, and have to be reminded of the potential benefits of screening activities (Lezer, 1977). Second, the daily news accounts of malpractice suits and second opinion surgery studies have shaken the public faith in the medical establishment. While some skepticism is in order, unbridled skepticism can keep some people away from the health care system for too long a period. Some of the health care providers can regain public trust through customer preference analysis and integrated market planning. For example, Humana Corporation performed a market survey of patient preferences and concluded that: (1) people want to see a triage nurse or physician within minutes of their arrival at the emergency room and (2) people resent being hassled for financial and insurance coverage information upon arrival. Consequently, the 90 Humana hospitals guarantee that a triage nurse will see the patient within 60 seconds after arrival at the emergency room and that the financial information will be collected in due time (10, 20, or 60 minutes later).

Non-profit institutions might borrow their marketing principles from the three basic points in the "Penney Idea," adopted by J. C. Penney in 1913. The three points are listed below:

1. To serve the public, as nearly as we can, to its complete satisfaction.
2. To expect for the service we render a fair remuneration and not all the profit the traffic will bear.
3. To do all in our power to pack the customer's dollar full of value, quality, and satisfaction.

Most health managers are surprised to learn that a proprietary concern has adopted and implemented such humanistic principles. The spirit of these principles is consistent with traditional ideals of non-profit institutions. The non-profit manager needs to achieve a sufficient rate of return to cover total financial requirements while not appearing to reap a profit. Achievement of the precarious balance between too much profit and not enough profit to refinance the future capital needs of a non-profit institution is the subject of Chapter 9. The J. C. Penney Company will go so far as to fire a store manager for earning too great a profit. Excess profits are considered unfair to consumers, whose trust—and repeat business—Penney seeks to establish and maintain.

Market Analysis

Marketing is a multi-stage process with many potential audiences. A hospital's marketing audience might include patients as consumers, physicians as direct customers of the institution, and physicians as middlemen. The first step in any marketing program is the assessment of market structure. One needs to assess the distinctive role the facility plays in meeting consumer demand in various market segments (market positioning). The existing and potential catchment area and service mix should be identified. The attractiveness and specificity of the service or product line must also be defined (market definition). The analyst should also partition the market into fairly homogenous segments, any one of which can be expanded as a primary target market with a marketing strategy tailored to the situation. This concept of market segmentation may imply multiple marketing efforts or marketing to only one segment area.

The second step in the typical marketing effort involves an analysis of consumer tastes and attributes. The provider of service should assess the intensity of demand for various products, perceptions of specific services and the entire facility, and the causal link between consumer behavior and image. Consumer satisfaction and multi-attribute consumer preferences should be determined through conjoint measurement techniques. The next three steps in building a marketing approach involve assessment of the product line, presentation of differential advantages relative to the competition, and development of the initial marketing program design (integrated market plan).

The seven stages in evaluation and periodic re-examination to be considered by the management before making decisions about promotion, pricing, product, and place (location) are listed below.

1. Market Catchment Area Definition. What demographic and geographic areas are served or could be served.
2. Physician Customer Preference Analysis. What physicians require and desire for a health care facility.
3. Patient Customer Preference Analysis. What potential patients seek in a health facility.
4. Product Definition Objectives. Assessment of the present and future product line of the health facility.
5. Differential Advantages Marketing. Definition of what services and reputation are marketable to advance facility prestige in the eyes of customers (doctors and potential patients), including providing different messages to different customers or regulatory agencies to best project the facility image.
6. Integrated Market Planning. Coordination of actions resulting from assessment in Steps 1–5. For example, we might conclude that integration between uncoordinated hospital departments is necessary to achieve a reliable and more efficient organization. The forthcoming management ideas are often quite simple, for example, placing nuclear medicine next to the x-ray department so that patient transporters in each department can assist the other during peak demand periods. Efficient transportation and scheduling can significantly contain costs and increase consumer perception of the quality of the institution.
7. Market Activity Evaluation. Assessment of the costs and benefits of marketing activities and making timely corrective action. Management and trustees must ultimately decide whether the long-run intangible benefits and discounted cash flows justify reorganizing priorities. If the hospital can profit from increased head-to-head competition, they might develop a more homogeneous product line relative to the competition. It is not always worthwhile to chase or confront the competition in a reactive fashion. The institution might better profit from a pro-active solution, such as the development of a more heterogeneous product line.

The first stage, market catchment area definition, is a familiar process for most health care facilities. Hospitals have been performing this element of the marketing process under the title of needs assessment for over twenty years. However, certain elements of the marketing function, such as informing the public of the availability of new services and departments, is a task that most administrators fail to perform effectively.

In performing a physician customer market survey (Stage 2), the hospital must make basic decisions as to which preferences they should weight highest. If the objective function of the hospital is to maximize the patient census, then they should give highest priority to the preferences of physicians who admit the largest number of patients—general surgeons and family practitioners. If the objective function is to operate the hospital as a feeder system for the hospital-based specialists, then general surgeons who require less assistance from these specialists would have a lower priority relative to internists and other specialists.

Historically, market research of consumer preferences (Stage 3) has been done by the health planners. While the old style health planners of the 1950s and 1960s did not use marketing jargon, their mission was to assess consumer needs, promulgate new product lines, and open new service points. Planners utilized the jargon of needs assessment and increased accessibility, but the approach was vintage health marketing. Consumers value access, but they also value amenities such as well-decorated rooms, better food, and friendly personnel. Ease of exit can also help provide the patient with an overall positive impression of the institution. A courtesy discharge policy that avoids stops at the accounts receivable department on the final day of hospitalization is one potential approach.

Although price elasticity of demand for hospital care is low, price decisions are still important to some consumers. Consumers might be attracted by a more liberal credit policy, health education programs, or single-priced "packages" for underinsured services (for example, maternity care). One major threat to the success of hospitalization package pricing is the possibility of excessive variation in resource costs across patients. For example, the facility could unwittingly attract a biased sample of admissions that represent the more complex and costly cases because they perceive the price as a bargain.

Some analysts tailor the marketing approach to the physician as the ultimate client, while others emphasize studying the preferences of consumers. A dual approach of studying both groups is probably warranted. The Humana Corporation applied a two-pronged approach in Louisville, Kentucky. Initially they performed a market survey of consumer preferences by telephone and interview. After discovering that over one-third of the families did not have a physician, they published an ad in the paper stating: "If you need help finding a doctor fill out this coupon." The consumers' referral coupons were provided only to the doctors affiliated with Humana. As a result of the coupon referral program the patient census increased almost 10 percent. In the second prong of their market survey they assessed physician preferences by asking existing Humana affiliated physicians and potential new physicians how Humana may satisfy the physicians' needs.

A facility should look at the product-market competencies of neighboring facilities in the process of assessing internal product definition objectives (Stage 4). Some product lines may need to be expanded, contracted, or phased out of existence. The decisions are seldom simple, for example, the maternity or emergency room services are seldom cost-beneficial unless one includes off-setting revenue from estimated return business and ancillary services. If diversification of the product line seems in order, the decision should be made in consultation with the four internal publics (trustees, physicians, volunteers, employees) and the numerous external publics (bankers, unaffiliated physicians, philanthropists, suppliers, consumers, regulators, competitors). New product lines for consideration might include, depending on the service area demographics: rheumatology, multiphasic annual physicals, alcoholism treatment, prenatal clinics, nuclear medicine, nephrology, and mental health services.

Targeting more resources to certain segments of the market where you have a differential advantage (Stage 5) and contracting resources from other segments can reap a larger market share for facilities that previously provided a whole range of services. In the recent era of more stringent forms of reimbursement, to ignore market segmentation increases the risk of falling behind in the purchase of state-of-the-art equipment. In other words, the rate regulators may allow a facility the slack to purchase expensive updated replacement equipment in three to five departments, but not in all areas. More aggressive rate regulation programs provide incentives for increased specialization in the hospital industry.

The amalgamation of the information acquired in Steps 1–5 must be synthesized in the development of the Integrated Market Plan (Step 6). To be effective the market plan must consider the needs of the surrounding community, patients, physicians, employees, insurers, donors, planners, and other regulators. Ultimately the plan should lead to a better distribution of services and intermediate products (such as pre-operative tests) through distribution channels and access points across the catchment region. Both the customer of the intermediate products (the physician) and the customer of the final product (the patient) should benefit. The opportunity cost of both the physician's time and the patient's time should be taken into account when determining access point locations. Physician productivity can be improved by providing convenient office space, thus minimizing wasted travel time. Consumer time can be saved by performing more ambulatory surgery and pre-admission workups. Decisions will have to be made in some areas because both target groups of customers cannot be satisfied simultaneously. For example, it is impossible to design a clinic scheduling system that minimizes waiting time for both physicians and patients.

Integrated market planning, with its emphasis on exchange relationships, implies eliciting the preferences of the facility staff, in addition to the preferences of physicians (Stage 2). Marketing surveys of staff can educate the administration and physicians as to the wants and desires of other staff members. In this era of a rising sense of professionalism among nonphysician staff, the administrators should be increasingly sensitized to staff members' needs to be recognized and rewarded for their contribution to the institution. A number of hospitals in Maryland and Florida have offered employees bonus pay for productivity improvement and cost containment ideas. Ideas include closing certain departments, sharing services with a competitor or local school, and expanding services and selling them to other providers (clinics, hospitals, nursing homes).

Marketing Applications

One of the major reasons why proprietary hospital groups can produce basic medical and surgical services at 5–10 percent less costs (Biggs *et al.*, 1980), even after allowing for a profit margin, is because the administrators are believers in market segmentation. Contrary to the view of non-profit administrators who offer specialization in any area, the proprietary hospitals believe in specialization in some subset of the universe of medical services. Marketing segmentation involves identifying those services and consumers most likely to demand care from your institution. Detractors of the market segmentation approach claim that such cream-skimming is unethical and places the burden on non-profit hospitals to do the unprofitable services such as maternity care and open-heart surgery. However, what is unprofitable under bad administration can be made very profitable under good management if a market segmentation approach is taken. Humana converted one hospital in Tampa into an Obstetrics and Gynecology Hospital, upgraded the price and quality of the service, and found that, as their market survey had predicted, women would flock to this specialized center as the "only good place in town." The non-profit hospital administrators claimed that maternity care could never be arranged in a profitable fashion, but this Tampa hospital is the most profitable facility of the 90 Humana hospitals. It should also be pointed out that as low occupancy rate competitors closed their maternity services, the quality of care—as measured by perinatal and other mortality statistics—increased in the region: Underutilization breeds lower quality due to out-of-practice effects among staff.

The relevant consumer preferences may not be limited to the opinions of the average consumer in the region. When selling a service, selling effort should be directed at the individual(s) in a position to control the purchase decision. As we learned in Chapters 1 and 2, the amount of insurance coverage is a major factor in determining the demand for health services. Employers like to provide visible fringe benefits such as group health insurance. Union leaders might be the dominant voice in selecting which benefits are preferred. Undoubtedly the union members do not have homogeneous preferences, but the relevant preferences to poll if one is concerned with maximizing union market share are those of the senior union decision makers. The leadership is generally older than the average union member and more interested in purchasing excessive amounts of insurance, relative to the taste of the average worker. Because they comprise the high-risk, high-utilization group, it is in the interest of the older leadership to select the most comprehensive benefit package. Implicit in this line of reasoning is the assumption that majority rule does not prevail, and the elite in the union are likely to pressure the employer for a more comprehensive benefit package than the average worker would select. The union leadership knows that if they had to purchase the more comprehensive benefits on an experience-rated or individual basis, the older workers would have to pay higher premiums.

For the hospital initiating a program, one natural place to begin a marketing research effort is in the patient representative department. The institution will benefit more from a survey of the needs and values of its consumers than listening to planners or consultants speculate on what they think market preferences should be.

HMOs that have taken heed and listened to potential new enrollee preferences have grown substantially. Historically, innovation in the area of health marketing for HMOs has been retarded for fear of retaliation by organized medicine. For example, in the mid-1970s the HMOs in Boston and New York would promote only the physician perception of what consumers value: good, comprehensive care. Beginning in 1979, these same HMOs ran ads mentioning the major advantage of their product from a consumer viewpoint: cost savings, reduced out-of-pocket premiums, and less paperwork than fee-for-service billings procedures. The advertising had a positive effect on consumer response; that is, the HMO had an increased enrollment.

For customer preference surveys to be usable to management, some aggregation of individual responses has to be made. The customers can be algorithmically clustered according to similarity in benefits preferred. Alternatively, they can be *a priori* clustered according to observable demographic or utilization characteristics, for example, urban-rural or high-user versus low-user, or physician-referral versus self-referred.

Physician preferences also need to be aggregated into clusters. Physicians could be partitioned into four basic groups: clinicians who are hospital based, clinicians who frequently utilize their privileges at hospital X, clinicians who seldom utilize their privileges at X hospital, and area physicians who have never sought treatment privileges at hospital X. The hospital can organize a marketing program after identification of the sources of physician dissatisfaction. Some physician complaints may not be easily resolved: unacceptable nursing care, demands for additional equipment, or unpredictable availability of same-day surgery. Frequently the hospital attracts new physicians with a capital project: satellite clinics, inclusion of a family practice department, providing part-time office space, and ambulatory surgicenters. The marketing ideas need not involve capital acquisitions; marketing the hospital with coupons in the newspapers for families can act as a practice-building source for the physicians.

HMO administrators seldom have problems in dealing with physician preferences. Fortunately, the number of physicians interested in salaried employment has not limited HMO growth, even in areas with a shortage of doctors. For example, the HMO serving the R. J. Reynolds Plant in Winston-Salem, North Carolina, had no problem attracting clinicians to serve the initial 11,000 enrollees in 1980. HMOs have a number of attributes that are increasingly valued by younger physicians: regular hours, scheduled vacations, and no responsibility for malpractice premiums or office management.

One of the positive benefits of a physician preference analysis is that marketing techniques can be utilized to cut costs by suggesting ways of smoothing irregular demands functions, such as scheduling less elective surgery during peak periods. An automated operating room block booking schedule system assigns weekly periods of time for each physician with privileges in the hospital. Physicians who perform more surgery or have higher seniority receive better time slots. The elective cases are scheduled in their surgeon's time slot prior to entering the hospital. The advance bookings, sometimes weeks in advance, allow for a smoothing of the operating staff workload and increased patient flexibility in scheduling their domestic life. Most hospitals utilize block booking in combination with two or more rotating operating rooms.

In a service industry, such as health care, consumption and production typically occur in the same location. Consequently vertical pricing decisions within distribution channels are seldom relevant except in the case of Independent Practice Associations or other contract service situations. Horizontal pricing decisions are made at the retail level by commercial insurance plans or Blue Cross plans paying negotiated charges. Governmental payers and half of the Blue Cross plans simply pay cost or the health industry equivalent of wholesale prices.

Physicians as Customers and Middlemen

The hospital can meet the needs of its office-based physician-customers in a number of ways. The oldest physician marketing technique is to provide low-rent office space next to or within the hospital grounds. A more recent technique is to set up a loan fund from philanthropic funds to attract physicians. The monies from the loan fund are "loaned" to fill the gap between the actual annual income of the physician and the individual's targeted yearly income. In highly competitive areas, hospitals make no attempt to collect the loan. A more traditional technique is to grant low interest start-up loans to new physicians. Another time-honored technique for increasing physician referrals is to set up satellite clinics in the surrounding areas to act as a feeder system to the hospital. Research funds and gifts of office equipment are two more ways to attract physicians, and consequently more patients. A few Southern hospitals have gone so far as to offer new homes at deferred low-interest mortgage rates. Young physicians are the best targets for loans or equipment gifts, because they work the longest hours and can provide a steady, high flow of patients to the hospital over the coming years. These "perks" or inducements for physicians are seldom formalized in a written agreement, since such behavior would be considered unethical and sometimes illegal in most states. This situation leaves physicians in the enviable position of being able to request new equipment and take advantage of underutilized facilities, while retaining the flexibility to break the unwritten agreement with the hospital if they get a better deal elsewhere. With the increasing cost of new equipment and medical education, physicians can be expected to make decisions among competing offers on a financial basis. Most physicians cannot be expected to stay with a poorly equipped and poorly staffed neighborhood clinic for altrustic reasons, and some of those that do stay end up doubting the marginal value of their services.

Clinics should be considered in market terms as middlemen or facilitating intermediaries. Satellite clinics seldom have a written agreement with the individual hospital that financed much of their development. However, in providing money and management expertise, the hospital would be foolhardy not to demand a return on its investment. Typically the clinic is managed by an individual who represents the hospital by informing physicians whenever the occupancy level is low and by providing information regarding which type of beds are most underutilized. In some cases the clinics are not placed where the patient need is higher, such as a poorly insured neighborhood of the working poor (too wealthy to qualify for Medicaid and too poor to afford commercial insurance). Instead, the clinics are placed where the population has the best insurance coverage for hospital reimbursement, or in a location near a competitor's clinic to prevent potential hospitalization cases from straying to another facility. There is legitimate skepticism in the nonprofit sector as to whether location decisions should be made in a fashion that dumps unprofitable poorly insured patients on the facilities with an open door policy.

The most frequently mentioned "carrot" for pleasing hospital-based physicians is the purchase of new medical equipment.* Hospital-based specialists are in many ways a franchised monopolist. Increasingly, state rate-setting authorities are establishing their authority to regulate hospital-based physician fees. The original court cases were waged by the Maryland Health Services Cost Review Commission. Publications of the lucrative annual incomes of hospital-based specialists relative to office-based clinicians have increased public interest in containing the fees of radiologists, anesthesiologists, and pathologists.

Marketing experts unfamiliar with health care require some orientation about the peculiarities of physician reimbursement. There are six basic methods by which hospital-based specialists are reimbursed for professional services: fee-for-service billings to the patient, fee-for-service compensation from the hospital, salary from the hospital, salary negotiated with the department chief or specialty group practice unit, a fixed percentage of net department revenues, or a fixed percentage of gross department billings. These six methods of reimbursement often exist in hybrid form; salary plus percentage provides the comfort of a minimum guarantee for the clinician. There are differences in the popularity of these methods of reimbursement. Pathologists prefer straight salary or fee-for-service billings done by the hospital. Radiologists are increasingly entering into leasing arrangements with the hospital whereby they compensate the hospital radiology department for the rental of staff and equipment, and all billings are generated from the specialty group. Historically, radiologists preferred a fixed percentage of billings or revenues, but over the last five years fee-for-service reimbursement has become more popular. Cardiologists are more likely to be reimbursed on a percentage of gross billings basis, after deductions for bad debts, discounts, and charity.

Hospital-based specialists are interested in maintaining distribution channels that ensure "interesting" product assortment, efficiency (whenever possible), and progressiveness (including the ability to foster technological change). Elimination of a service or department should be analyzed in light of risks and benefits,

---

* An equally important carrot in the case of proprietary hospitals is that hospital privileges do not carry the usual obligations of rotation responsibility such as covering the emergency room and clinics once a week. Proprietary hospitals tend to avoid such unprofitable services, and consequently have no need to thrust such social obligations on their physicians.

response from the competition, and alienation of internal hospital-based vested interests. The hospital-based physicians frequently lobby for revitalization rather than elimination.

Marketing decisions, or their analog in the Health Systems Agencies, demand-sensitive planning, do not occur in a political vacuum. For example, in 1972 the trustees of the one general hospital in Tompkins County (New York) had to make a decision as to location of the new (replacement) facility. They could place the new facility next door to the existing hospital and meet the preferences of the local medical society for a location near their existing office buildings. Alternatively, they could meet the preferences of the public and bring the hospital back into the city. Building the hospital in the city would increase the project cost by 4 percent but decrease the average consumer travel time by 80 percent. The decision was made in favor of the physicians' preference.

Statistical Techniques

The majority of quantitative studies in the hospital setting have focused on non-consumer issues such as materials management. Statistical techniques might increasingly be directed at causal modeling of consumer behavior. For example, how long is a consumer willing to wait at a clinic without seeing a contact person of any sort before deciding not to return or to repeat elective service? Path analysis is one technique that might be applied to such consumer behavior problems. The technique of path analysis allows the analyst to decompose the correlation between any two relevant factors into a sum of compound and simple paths (Wright, 1960). The decomposition of the correlation has three basic components: direct effects, indirect effects, and spurious effects from compound paths that are not interpretable but are mathematically part of the decomposition. For example, the finding that more liberal maternity benefit packages attracts more enrollees to an HMO (Hudes *et al.*, 1980) may or may not be a spurious relationship. However, if one had built a path model, the efficacy of liberalizing maternity benefits might be found to be spurious if the correlation between benefits and number of enrollees vanished when the effects of income and other socioeconomic variables were controlled.

Customers' preferences and objectives are multifaceted, and consequently require very sophisticated methods of analysis. Custom-

ers providing preference judgments about a set of hypothetical questions may produce errors in the responses provided. In considering
the percentage of error variance in the criterion variable, one would
expect an inverse relationship between errors and individual involvement in the process of providing preference judgments. One
would expect lower degrees of error if the choice is among alternatives of substantial importance to the individual, for example, among
potential customers for open-heart surgery or among radiologists
concerning preferences toward purchasing CAT scanners. High
rates of error probably result from situations where the decisions
have minimal impact, such as patients' decisions concerning vaccinations or pediatricians' preferences concerning whether the hospital
should have a CAT scanner.

No single technique is appropriate for all marketing problems.
One technique, conjoint measurement, is probably the most underutilized and promising technique in the health services marketing
arena. Conjoint analysis is a major technique used to assess what
combination of service or product attributes the users, consumers,
or providers most prefer. It summarizes the preference ranking information as an index that is easily understood by non-quantitative
decision makers. Wind and Spritz (1976) were the first to utilize
conjoint measurement techniques in a health service market to
analyze the effect of a number of independent variables on a single
(response) dependent variable: "consumers' hospital selection decision." The authors cite the previous work of Green and Rao (1971)
concerning conjoint techniques for quantifying judgmental data. In a
conjoint measurement study, the respondent (hypothetical consumer) is presented with a set of multi-attribute alternatives and is
asked to rank or rate combinations of attributes on the basis of some
desired dependent variable (intention to buy, preference to utilize).
Contrary to traditional attitude measurement approaches in psy-
chology, the respondent is asked to provide an overall evaluation of a
product basket or combination of various attributes, rather than
simply providing only the relative rating on each individual attribute. The resulting internal trade-offs that each respondent makes
among the various attributes can be decomposed into internal,
scale-derived, utility judgments of given attributes and recon-
structed to impute the consumer's predicted preference for new
combinations of attributes.

Of the few applications of conjoint measurement techniques in
the health sector (Green and Srinivasin, 1978), all have presented

rather naive interpretations. For example, most hospital administrators would be amused at the assumption of Wind and Spritz that the consumer has a large role in the hospital selection decision for cases of single elective surgery or serious surgery. The vast majority of patients select physicians, not hospitals. The individual's physician makes the decision to do the operation, or refers the patient to a surgeon, who in turn makes the hospital choice decision. The surgeon or physician has a limited pool of hospitals at which he has privileges to treat patients. Despite the fact that Wind and Spritz misconstrued the typical aspects of the purchasing dynamics in hospital markets, their data provides insight into what consumers value. The consumer's three most important factors in evaluating a hospital were, in order of importance: proximity to home, prestige of the physician(s), and physical appearance of the hospital. It may be surprising to some that the least important factor was whether the hospital was a teaching hospital or had some affiliation with a major university. This corroborates the anecdotal testimony of many multi-hospital system managers, that consumers place a slightly positive miniscule value on whether or not a hospital is a teaching facility.

Conjoint analysis has more recently been applied to an HMO marketing problem in a large Northeastern metropolitan area (Acito and Jain, 1980). HMO attributes were described to prospective enrollees along parameters of convenience, scope of benefits covered, cost, method of selecting a physician, and type of facility. These two techniques, conjoint analysis and path analysis, hold promise in application to health markets.

The health care industry could benefit from the techniques and imagination of marketing specialists. If hospitals go beyond a single product orientation to think in terms of a service orientation, they may discover new markets in the areas of health promotion or home health outreach care. After selection of the product mix is completed, advertising is the next step. The advertising component of marketing does not have a good record among professionals. One unpublished study by Frazier of dental advertisements concludes that 43 percent of the information presented was "inaccurate, misleading, or fallacious" (Robertson and Wortzel, 1978). Advertising has a bad reputation in fields on the periphery of the health care system, such as the pharmaceutical industry and its drug firm representatives. For many health professionals, advertising is the surreptitious influencing of the potential consumer into using more medical services than necessary. However, in the case of one Las Vegas hospital that went to the extreme of offering a chance to win a free cruise for patients scheduling weekend surgery, the major effect was to smooth the demand evenly across the week rather than induce unnecessary surgery.

The Role of Advertising

The Federation of American Hospitals in a 1977 policy statement identified five rationales for advertising: public education about health care, information on service availability, accounting to the community, seeking support, and employee recruitment. The industry also lists guidelines for acceptable advertising content: truth and accuracy, "fairness" in avoiding any quality comparisons with the competition, and avoiding "claims of prominence." The hospital industry is going to be rather slow in recognizing the need for differential advantages marketing. In the minds of the authors of the advertising code, the public has no right to know if a competitor has less modern facilities, a less well-trained staff, or inferior quality of care. This anti-consumerist philosophy will erode in the future as bans on professional advertising are overturned in the courts. Havighurst (1980) has reviewed a number of recent court decisions where prohibitions on advertising have been overturned by the courts. Hospitals should still seek the permission of physicians to use their names in advertising. A hospital may benefit from promoting the fact that they have a highly regarded individual specialist, but such advertising might prove too embarrassing for some physicians.

Physician attitudes toward advertising are in a period of transition. The 1980 American Medical Association Code of Ethics, revised for the first time since 1957, contained language designed to promote competition and limited advertising. The Federal Trade Commission had been pushing a number of suits against the AMA on behalf of chiropractors and advertising, and against the old code that "physicians should never solicit." The new code also recognizes the role of government as a prudent buyer of physician services. As we argued in Chapter 5, the government is interested in stimulating advertising and information sharing because these activities should lead to cost containment.

Advertising and public relations activities were pioneered by the four large investor-owned hospital companies. Advertising has helped recruit physicians and acquire lower cost capital financing. The average age of the affiliated physicians, and public relations image of the hospital, are two parameters that bankers consider in assessing the riskiness of a capital project. Aggressive marketing programs are a major reason for the five-year (1975–1980) doubling (from 446 to 900) in the number of hospitals managed or owned by proprietary hospital systems. The following four companies have revenues in excess of $1 billion: Humana, Hospital Corporation of America,* National Medical Enterprises, and American Medical International. Humana and American Medicorp (acquired by Humana in 1977) were innovators in the field of health marketing. The focus of their marketing effort was an aggressive pursuit of satisfying the wants and needs of the physician community. As has been mentioned a number of times in this text, physician preferences are usually emphasized in marketing because the majority of patients go to the hospital of the physician's choice. Hospitals can still compete for the self-referral patient who comes without a physician, but the expected probability of a bad debt is higher (as is the chance that you can charge the patient on the more profitable basis of charges, rather than merely costs).

Summary

Advocates of marketing and injecting competition into the health delivery system argue that smoothly working market forces will better reflect the preferences of consumers than planning and regulation. Skeptics argue that constructing cost consciousness and price competition among providers requires unbearably high copayment rates (33–50 percent), with little guarantee that the consumer and his preferences will dominate. These opponents of deregulation argue that the competitive dream of setting up the "consumer as king" in the marketplace is a false expectation in health care markets because of the informational imbalance: You need to visit a physician to know if you need to see a physician. Health policy makers and management may be surprised to learn that customers

---

* In 1981, following the acquisition of the INA health subsidiary (Hospital Affiliates International), the Hospital Corporation of America (HCA) became the largest of the "big four." HCA currently owns 28,000 hospital beds in 175 hospitals. HCA also provides contract management services at 159 hospitals, 107 of which they both lease and manage.

do not place health services high on their priority list or that patient values diverge sharply from physician values. For example, one of the reasons why elective surgical queues are months long in England is that consumers are called up frequently to come in for surgery on the weekend, and the customer responds: "My weekend is more important," or "I'll only have it done on workdays, or not at all, so put me back on the revolving queue." In other words, even in cases when the service has no dollar cost, free care for simple surgery seldom is valued as equivalent to that 48 hours of free time. Increasing consumer power to tell providers their values and preferences will be one very important byproduct of health marketing activities.

In Chapter 5 we argued that advertising information concerning quality and access (hours and types of service) could play a significant role in aiding the consumer's choice process. In addition, other marketing activities can promote diversification, better product development, and increased market penetration. Most of this chapter has emphasized these micro-marketing techniques for individual institutions. It could be argued that the greater social good might be achieved by macro-marketing activities at a higher level of aggregation. The social marketing activities of 200 Health Systems Agencies or a few hundred large regional consumer organizations might provide the most important prerequisite to competition: the better-informed consumer.

Organized medicine has consistently criticized marketing and advertising activities as being just another additional cost to be paid by the public. Such an attitude ignores the fact that the net effect of such promotional activities in other sectors of the economy has been to decrease consumer prices. It is difficult to find examples of health markets that have allowed any form of advertising. Traditionally, professional groups have required that members refrain from advertising to consumers on the price or scope of available services. Medical providers often have a simplistic distaste of advertising and consumer information dissemination because they assume that such activities increase rather than decrease prices. Stigler (1961) was the first to point out that this viewpoint is fallacious. More recently, in a health services context, Feldman and Begun (1980) report that after correcting for service quality differentials and optometric case-mix, the regions that have not imposed a ban on optometric and optician price advertising have prices that are 11 percent lower for optometric examinations. The authors also conclude that advertising has decreased the variance in prices for vision examinations. In the case of non-emergency medical services that offer sufficient time for consumer search, advertising may reduce the mean and variance in out-of-pocket prices.

Provider arguments against giving the consumer more information because it would cost too much are also highly questionable. The recent report of Martin *et al.* (1980) concerning the Massachusetts Medicaid Second Opinion Consultation Program for elective surgery revealed the significant downward effect that additional information can have on surgical demand. Only 72 percent of the referred patients had the originally proposed surgery and 22 percent had no surgery. The likelihood of the consumer having surgery was related to the financially unbiased opinion of the external consultant: Only 30 percent of the patients whose need for surgery was not confirmed by the second opinion had the operation or any form of related surgery. The benefit-cost ratio of the consultation program for Massachusetts Medicaid was 4:1, and surprisingly the greatest decline in surgical rates occurred in the inner city areas of Boston that also had the lowest surgical rates prior to the program. The poor are as capable as the middle class in processing information and avoiding unnecessary care.

With the current push for at least a 10 percent reduction in the number of hospital beds, hospital competition appears to be emerging, especially in the 12 largest urban areas, which comprise 17 percent of the U.S. population and have a mean of 81 hospitals per city. For the unprepared hospital administrators, competition and fiscal stringency are frightening developments. However, what hospital management abhors as fiscal stringency and cost containment is what American business has labeled "normal competitive market conditions," that is, "if you don't cut costs, don't expect to survive." Survival also requires strategic planning and anticipation of future market conditions. For example, if promotion of HMOs in a region decreases the demand for hospital beds, an individual hospital should consider negotiating a monopsony arrangement with an HMO.

Health marketing is a new field. Ignoring health marketing is an increasingly hazardous style of management that frequently leads to retrenchment of services or fiscal insolvency. However, refinements will be required to sell the industry on marketing techniques. As increasing numbers of health services administration students are being introduced to marketing, these activities will increase and the public and the managers will be better able to assess needs and improve efficiency. As with any management science technique, poorly applied marketing can be a disaster for the institution. The reasons why health marketing is underdeveloped range from a lack of adequately trained manpower to the hesitancy of trustees to support marketing efforts due to pejorative "business world" connotations. The health institutions that grow in the 1980s will be forward-looking and market-wise; these institutions will not be simply reacting to the immediate demands of regulators and local physicians. A good marketing program can increase consumer satisfaction, improve efficiency, and deliver better quality health services.

References

ACITO, F., and JAIN, A. (1980). "Evaluation of Conjoint Analysis Results: A Comparison of Methods (HMO Example)," *Journal of Marketing Research* 17:1 (February), 106–112.

BIGGS, E. L., KRALEWSKI, J. E., and BROWN, G. D. (1980). "A Comparison of Contract-Managed and Traditionally Managed Nonprofit Hospitals," *Medical Care* 18:6 (June) 585–596.

CARLSON, R. J. (1975). *The End of Medicine.* New York: Wiley.

CLARKE, R. N. (1978). "Marketing Health Care: Problems in Implementation," *Health Care Management Review* 3:1 (Winter), 21–77.

COOPER, P. D. (ed.) (1978). *Health Care Marketing.* Germantown, Md.: Aspen Systems.

EGDAHL, R., and WALSH, D. (1978). "Health Care Advertising and Marketing: The Lady or the Tiger?" in *Health Services and Health Hazards: The Employees Need to Know,* Chapter 2. New York: Springer-Verlag.

ELLWOOD, P., and ELLWEIN, L. (1981). "Physician Glut Will Force Hospitals to Look Outward," *Hospitals* 55:3 (January 16), 81–85.

ENTHOVEN, A. (1980). *Health Plan.* Reading, Mass.: Addison-Wesley.

EVANS, R. (1977). "Add Soft Data to Product Elimination Decisions," *Industrial Marketing Management* 6:2 (April), 91–94.

FELDMAN, R., and BEGUN, J. (1980). "Does Advertising of Prices Reduce the Mean and Variance of Prices?" *Economic Inquiry* 18:3 (July), 484–492.

GREEN, P. E., and RAO, V. R. (1971). "Conjoint Measurement for Quantifying Judgment Data," *Journal of Marketing Research* 8:3 (July), 355–363.

GREEN, P. E., and SRINIVASIN, V. (1978). "Conjoint Analysis in Consumer Research: Issues and Outlook," *Journal of Consumer Research* 5:9 (September), 103–123.

HAVIGHURST, C. C. (1980). "Antitrust Enforcement in the Medical Services Industry: What Does It All Mean?" *Milbank Memorial Fund Quarterly* 58:1 (Winter), 89–124.

HELD, P. J., and REINHARDT, V. (1980). "Prepaid Medical Practice: A Summary of Findings from a Recent Survey," *Group Health Journal* 1:2 (Summer), 4–15.

HUDES, J., YOUNG, C., SOHRAB, L., and TRINH, C. (1980): "Are HMO Enrollers Being Attracted by a Liberal Maternity Benefit?" *Medical Care* 18:6 (June), 635–648.

KOTLER, P. (1979). "Strategies for Introducing Marketing into Nonprofit Organizations." *Journal of Marketing* 43:1 (January), 37–44.

LAUBACH, P. B., RAND, R. L., and LAUBACH, P. A. (1979). "Marketing Management for Health Care Executives," monograph. Chicago: American College of Hospital Administrators.

LEZER, L. (1977). *Community Medicine.* New York: Vantage.

MACSTRAVIC, R. E. (1980). *Marketing by Objectives for the Hospitals.* Germantown, Md: Aspen Systems.

MARTIN, S., SCHWARTZ, M and COOPER, D. (1980). "The Effect of a Mandatory Second Opinion Program on Medicaid Surgery Rates," *Grants and Contracts Reports.* Washington, D.C.: DHHS, Health Care Financing Administration.

MASON W. B., BEDWELL, C. L., ZWAAG, R. V., and RUNYAN, J. W. (1980). "Why People Are Hospitalized," *Medical Care* 18:2 (February), 147–163.

MISENETH, P. (1978). "Marketing Ambulatory Care," *Hospital Progress* 59:3 (March), 58–61.

NESLIN, S. (1978). "Linking Product Features to Perceptions: Applications and Evaluation of Graded Paired Comparisons," *Proceeding of the American Marketing Association.* Chicago, Ill.: August Educators Conference.

QUELCH, J. A. (1980). "Marketing and Preventive Health Care," *Milbank Memorial Fund Quarterly* 58:2 (Spring), 310–347.

ROBERTSON, T. S., and WORTZEL, L. H. (1978). "Consumer Behavior and Health Care Change: The Role of Mass Media," Volume 5 in C. H. Lovelock and C. B. Weinberg (eds.), *Readings in Public and Nonprofit Marketing.* New York: Scientific Press, 206–220.

ROTHSCHILD, M. L. (1979). "Marketing Communications in Nonbusiness Situations, or Why It's So Hard to Sell," *Journal of Marketing* 43:2 (Spring), 11–20.

SEAVER, D. (1977). "Hospital Reverses Role, Reaches Out to Cultivate and Capture Markets," *Hospitals* 51:11 (June 1), 59–62.

SIMON, J. K. (1978). "Marketing the Community Hospital: A Tool for the Beleaguered Administrator," *Health Care Management Review* 3:2 (Spring), 11–23.

STIGLER, G. (1961). "The Economics of Information," *Journal of Political Economy* 69:3, 213–225.

SWAN, J., and COOMBS, L. J. (1976). "Product Performance and Consumer Satisfaction: A New Concept," *Journal of Marketing* 40:2 (Spring), 25–35.

URBAN, G. and HAUSER, J. (1980). *Design and Marketing of New Products.* Englewood Cliffs, N.J.: Prentice-Hall.

VENKATESAN, M., and KEOWN, C. (1979). "Awareness of Attitude of Employers and Marketing of HMOs," *1979 Educators' Conference Proceedings.* Chicago: American Marketing Association.

WILSON, A., and WEST, C. (1980). "The Marketing of Unmentionables," *Harvard Business Review* 59:1 (January-February), 91–102.

WIND, Y., and SPITZ, L. K. (1976). "Analytical Approach to Marketing Decisions in Health Care Organizations," *Operations Research* 24:5 (September-October), 973–990.

WRIGHT, S. (1960). "Path Coefficients and Path Regressions: Alternative or Complementary Concepts?" *Biometrics* 16:5 (June), 189–202.

ZUCKERMAN, A. (1977). "Patient Origin Study Profiles Service Area, Evolving Patterns," *Hospitals* 51:14 (July 16), 83–86.

Chapter 8

HEALTH REGULATION TO CONSTRAIN CAPITAL EXPANSION

> *We have no system for closing out excess capital. We don't let hospitals fail, which keeps the pathology in the system, and that drives the costs up.*
>
> —ELI GINZBERG

> *Regulation inevitably operates at the periphery of the decision-making process.*
>
> —ALFRED E. KAHN

The excessive growth in hospital expenditures has increased the burden of health care costs on employees, employers, and both federal and state governments. Since 1970, three administrations have sought to impose mandatory cost controls on hospitals while simultaneously trying to deregulate the general economy. The presence of market failures in the health economy is the most common justification given by economists for placing controls on physicians and hospitals. The most frequently cited example of market failure is the way consumers become myopic about price-consumption decisions in this highly insured sector of the economy. The physician is in the unique position of affecting both supply and demand. Acting as an input broker for his patient, he demands service from the hospital; at the same time he is the supplier of personal service to the patient. Most consumers have little interest in cost, since the insurance carrier pays the bill. The success of price controls in curtailing costs and prices from August 1971 to April 1974 was the major

179

reason why the Republican administration was slow to remove the controls from the health sector after concluding that they were unsuccessful in the other sectors of the economy (Congressional Budget Office, 1979).

The two basic modes of health regulations surveyed in this chapter are planning and rate regulation. Before we review the efficiency and effectiveness of existing cost control regulations, some economic theories for analyzing regulation in other sectors of the economy will be introduced. The chapter ends with an econometric model for assessing the impact of two planning programs, Certificate-of-Need (CON) and Federal-State review Section 1122 of the Social Security Act (SS1122) signed under P.L. 93-641, on hospital costs in the period 1974–1978.

The Federal Rationale

From the federal perspective in the United States, the increasing subsidization of medical care compels accountability to justify the medical sector's stewardship of increasing amounts of public money. The nominal dollars increase from 1977 to 1978 in Medicare and Medicaid reimbursements ($5.7 billion) was greater than the entire HEW budget for all other health activities ($5.5 billion). To government officials, cost containment means spending less tax money for Medicare and Medicaid, irrespective of whether the cost escalation is increasingly shifted to private insurance companies, state and local governments, and ultimately the consumers.

The real growth in resources devoted to the health sector is most significant in the hospital industry, where percentage of GNP devoted to hospitals has grown from 1.0 percent to 3.8 percent since 1950. The explosion in real resources devoted to Medicaid hospital patients, combined with the popular demand for shrinking government, has placed an added burden on state governments to lobby for shifting the tax burden of the poor man's medical care onto the federal government by passing national health insurance (NHI). In response to such pressure, the White House and many leaders in Congress have supported the concept of national health insurance, with the caveat that mandatory price and/or revenue controls of hospitals are the necessary precursor to NHI. Whether one supported the Carter bill to contain hospital revenue increases per annum to 9.7 percent, or the Kennedy proposal for a 10.9 percent cap, both approaches implicitly assumed that economies would be obtained through fiscal starvation (that is, administrators would not run deficits for long periods), thereby forcing economic discipline upon a highly undisciplined market that exploits the current anarchy of multiple payers.

With cost containment as the number one health policy issue in the 1980s, it is obvious that there will be some changes in the scope and form that medical regulation takes over the coming years. The medical establishment is increasingly being forced to cooperate with the National Center for Health Care Technology, and eleven other medical technology assessment advisory councils in the executive branch, in studying the cost and efficiency of new or unproven tests and therapies. Recent documentation of inefficient utilization of diagnostic tests seems to harbinger increased federal regulation of medical practice (Kassirer and Pauker, 1978). This signals a more aggressive government intervention into areas previously left to professional self-discipline. Although the Professional Standards Review Organization (PSRO) program clearly places responsibility for the evaluation of clinical decision making in the hands of the doctors, in accordance with the principle of peer review, there is a likelihood that government will take more responsibility.

The scope of regulation in the health field is broad and complex. This section focuses on the types of controls favored in the Carter Administration's hospital cost containment proposal, which employed neomarket principles to control costs by containing revenues. This orientation, derived from economic theory and techniques, is perceived by many to be at odds with the type of consensus planning favored by political scientists. Consensus planning in health care was begun in this country in 1966 with the passage of the Comprehensive Health Planning (CHP) Act, and strengthened in 1974 by passage of the National Health Planning and Development Act that created 203 regional Health Systems Agencies (HSAs). The Carter Administration's assumption that revenue starvation would curtail hospital cost inflation and force management to get tough with doctors was not supported by the behavioral response of hospitals to price controls (1971–1974). The physician community is in a stronger position as captain of the ship than the typical hospital administrator. Fiscal starvation through revenue controls to date has only produced an explosion in deficit spending and debt financing. For example, the percentage of new capital dollars financed through debt instruments has grown from 25 percent in 1965 to 75 percent in 1978 (see Chapter 11). Hospital management has avoided conflict with the physician community by increasingly borrowing money from the private sector. Hospital administrators thus face the risk of default if debt service payments are eliminated as an allowable expense in regulatory rate formulas, but avoid the risk of being "sacked" as a result of physician dissatisfaction. We begin with a survey of two economic arguments concerning the efficacy of regulation and conclude with an econometric study of the impact of two hospital capital containment strategies.

The Theory of Rational Expectations

The theory of rational expectations has been widely heralded in the popular press as one of the most exciting advances in economic theory. However, older economists have always considered anticipatory behavior and announcement effects as being key hypotheses within the classical theory of the firm. Social scientists will find this "new" theory of the firm entitled "rational expectations" to be similar to a more familiar concept of the self-fulfilling prophecy. Simply stated, the theory of rational expectations postulates that people and institutions will take action based on how they expect outsiders, including government, to behave. In the process of attempting to predict or foresee the timing and details of new regulations, hospital administrators, commensurate with the theory, are believed to behave with anticipatory actions. There is concern within the Congress that the sharp double-digit annual increases in hospital expenses might represent an attempt by the industry to build up its revenue bases in anticipation of a stringent national control program that monitors only those marginal percentage changes in revenues after the base year.

Critics of hospital controls argue that a nationwide cap on revenues will unduly benefit hospitals that were provoked to add new fixed-cost items in order to inflate cost profiles before regulations take hold (Eastaugh, 1979). However, in support of revenue control efforts, Bauer (1977), in reviewing the experience of the twenty-seven states with some form of rate setting or monitoring program for hospitals, has forewarned federal policy makers about the cost of delays in the implementation of a nationwide cap. Moreover, administrators who rush into new purchases of hospital equipment are eschewed as "irrational" by regulators, but if their behavior stems from anticipatory actions designed to increase the reimbursement base, such behavior may be considered a rational measure of self-protection. The smart administrator learns to anticipate future edicts from the rule makers, and merely devises a new set of games for co-optation of future rules. For example, Hellinger (1977) suggested that hospital administrators invested in a large amount of new capital the year before enactment of state Certificate-of-Need legislation that would regulate purchases above $100,000. Another rational game to engage in is to raise per diem hospital room rates excessively prior to federal price controls and the enactment of local price controls. However, some administrators, feeling that per diem prices are an overly publicized number, opt to double the laboratory and x-ray prices in order to keep per diem increases under 10 percent per annum. Another strategy for administrators in the nine states where in-patient prices are highly controlled is to increase out-patient charges at rates that are far in excess of the national average, in order to compensate for any shortfall in in-patient revenues.

Hospital administrators are not the only health professionals to engage in anticipatory defensive behavior. Many physicians raised their prices excessively in 1971 to anticipate a federal price control program designed to cap increases at below 3–3.5 percent per annum. Physicians and administrators behave idiosyncratically in the eyes of the regulators, when in fact their behavior should be viewed as rational because it is governed by a best estimate of how the government and the insurance industry intend to change the reimbursement rules. The nationwide trend in the early 1970s from cost-plus to simple cost reimbursement rendered it difficult for any hospital to survive intact if it did not play games. The lag and indecision in achieving a concerted public policy over how to contain health spending contribute to misunderstanding of the cost crisis and increased distrust of government in a time of weakening confidence in social institutions in general. It is surprising that the regulators complain of anticipatory co-optive behavior. After all, the value system of the regulatory strategist exhorts hospital administrators to behave more like businessmen, which is what in fact they are doing.

Capture of the Regulators by the Regulated

The capture theory of regulatory behavior is the most prevalent regulatory model among American economic theorists. According to the capture notion, the regulated group gradually comes to dominate the decisions of the regulators until the watch dog agency is converted to an ally, or even subsidiary, of the private sector group. Truman was one of the first to point out that capture is a natural process in the life of any federal agency (1951). Truman argued that the regulated have more cohesion than the bureaucrats, that they keep closest track of the agency, that they are sure to reveal any malfeasance by the agency at the annual budget hearings, and consequently little will be done by the agency beyond what is desired by the regulated group.

Bernstein (1955) carried the Truman argument further and suggested that all agencies pass through a lifecycle from early zeal to a period of debility and decline in which the regulators become the captive of the regulated. Capture is not necessarily bad if efficient decision making requires cooperation between industry and government. Effective cooperation must be a two-way street, rather than a one-way dominance of the industry by regulators. Social reformers who often get carried away by the one-way street view of regulation should pause to reconsider the value of regulators as adversaries (Battistella and Eastaugh, 1980). The social and economic cost of an antagonistic relationship between regulators and the industry may be much higher than society is willing to bear. If you destroy the motive of the regulated to cooperate, what is the result? More regulation and lower productivity?

Three new variants of the capture theory have appeared recently in the literature. One moderate variant of the capture concept advanced by Peltzman (1976) postulates "bureaucratic survival through politics" in observing that agencies respond primarily to the politicians in control of their budget. Maintaining the proper balance in the relationship is not always easy. There is a danger that the regulated can become the determining voice at the budgetary hearing, especially in the current era of anti-regulatory spirit. In this regard, Cohen (1975) has suggested a second variant to the capture theory. He postulates that after initial popular support for regulation has waned, the regulated become the only substantive and ongoing interest group concerned with the agency. Thus, over time, some degree of capture is inevitable if the industry exercises its monopoly power. A third theory of regulatory behavior as advanced by Hilton (1972) is "minimal squawk," or, in other words, the "squeaky wheel gets the grease." The key idea is that the regulator acts to minimize complaints. Bureaucrats are viewed as rational economic individuals operating in a complex political environment and attempting to minimize the sum total of government-consumer-industry dissatisfaction with regulatory policies. According to this view, the regulatory agencies and staff that experience the longest tenure pursue the most purely reactive policy possible. Agencies that follow the path of least resistance are destined to become less combative, and avoid the ire of politicians on whom their survival depends.

Evidence as to whether the capture theory holds for regulation in the health field is mixed. Evaluation of programs that attempt to limit capital growth are criticized for two reasons. First, the regulators are often thought to be under the thumb of the hospital industry. Second, the Salkever and Bice (1976) study found no regulatory effect on total investment dollars, as dollars not used on new beds were shifted to the purchase of new equipment. This discouraging evaluation of regulatory effectiveness has provided impetus for price-revenue caps and other neomarket controls. Biles *et al.* provides some evidence that rate regulation has been more effective than health planning. The states with mandatory hospital rate regulation had a rate of inflation that was 4.6 percent lower per diem and per admission in 1977 when compared to the states without mandatory rate regulation. We have already surveyed some of the positive aspects of state rate setting programs in Chapters 1 and 5. However, one must balance the short-term direct cost savings against the cost of regulation, increased debt financing, cannibalization of endowment, and the intangible cost of reduced employee morale. For example, state government will be ill-served if tough health regulation bankrupts hospitals heavily in debt to the state treasury. One example of the harm done by regulation is New York, the state with the most effective (least inflationary) record of cost containment, where two thirds of the 220 voluntary hospitals ran deficits totaling nearly $470 million between 1977 and 1979. Few regulators have considered studying the costs associated with forced postponement of maintenance and capital investment during a period of fiscal starvation. The neglect of equipment and facility maintenance will probably require larger future expenditures of resources simply to revitalize the surviving hospitals.

Another contributing factor to the possible conservatism of regulatory agencies with experience and tenure is the fear of court reversals. Recently, the hospital industry has utilized their due process safeguards, along with the overcrowded court calendar situation, to engage in lengthy legal delaying tactics to wear the regulators down. The word is out in the hospital industry that it is better to get even than to get mad. For example, a hospital can tie up state revocation of its license for more than a decade in court (Kinzer, 1977). Rather than experience the high opportunity costs of lengthy legal proceedings, perpetually understaffed regulatory boards prefer to negotiate a quick settlement, almost always to the advantage of the hospital industry. In addition to the dollar costs of court appeals, regulators fear the loss of credibility and erosion of public trust resulting from court reversals. Thus the major effect of due process safeguards is to foster conservatism among the regulators. Ironically, the more technological and less consumer-responsive hospitals are better situated to withstand the legal costs and win the court battles with the regulators. The financially weak hospitals providing a disproportionately higher share of primary patient care in the region are the least likely court participants, and consequently hold less clout in the eyes of the regulatory forces.

Rationale for Evaluation of CON

Despite widespread support for CON program effectiveness among health care officials, the evidence has been highly anecdotal, theoretical—"CON reduces duplication so it must save millions"— and inevitably leads to the conclusion that CON saves money. A highly publicized example of the latter phenomenon was provided by the American Health Planning Association (AHPA) February 1979 report that CON activities saved $3.4 billion. The General Accounting Office (1980) was quick to point out that $1.2 billion of that total was attributed to one consultant's estimate of the capital expenditures avoided in the Los Angeles HSA region during the study period 1976–1978. It should be pointed out that during this period there was little CON program activity and no stable HSA active in the region.

The AHPA questionnaire contained biased statements asking for urgently needed cost savings estimates to help get a larger budget for HSAs from the Congress. The HSAs responded by including many questionable items as savings. The GAO report estimated that 45 to 65 percent of the $3.4 billion savings was not supportable. The four basic types of errors in the AHPA tabulation of "savings" identified by the GAO are

1. Projects initially disapproved, then later approved.
2. Projects built despite the disapproval.

3. Projects withdrawn because of an inability to acquire debt financing.
4. Multiple counting of projects disapproved each time they were disapproved.

As an example of the first and second type of errors, the GAO reports that of the 16,000 hospital beds saved (not built), more than half were actually built in the period 1976–1978. The AHPA report also includes 114,000 nursing home beds as saved by planning, when in fact 60 percent were built.*

Some planners are under the delusion that "analysis" consists of wild overestimates of what projects would have been undertaken in the absence of CON. Likewise, economists should not underestimate CON program benefits by acknowledging only the dollar-and-cents effect it has on total plant assets and beds. However, as a first approximation we shall consider whether this form of regulation has proven effective as a cost control device. This approach neglects the fact that CON programs have indirect benefits. For example, the high status teaching hospitals in Boston and New York may get 95 percent of what they requested in the CON application, but the CON agency slows the process for 18–24 months until the hospital agrees to a "low status" primary care satellite project for the poor. It would be difficult to assess in dollar terms the intangible benefit of doing "something extra for the poor" as a *quid pro quo* requirement for the hospital getting the CON approval. Richard Nathan at the Brookings Institution is one of the few economists to take a case-by-case approach to this type of question, in another context (community development block grants) (Nathan and Dommel, 1978). This approach deserves further research, and has been encouraged by Rashi Fein† and others (Institute of Medicine, 1980). The case study approach should examine small areas within HSAs across the nation to evaluate the degree to which hospitals collude or compete for regulatory favor in the CON process.

In the evaluation of capital expenditure controls, we first should set aside the presumption that planners are "special" and need to be evaluated only on the basis of activities, irrespective of outcomes. Bureaucrats have a tenacious notion that what counts is the act of

---

* The GAO report was not above reproach. The irrational stratified sampling design that was employed violated all established statistical principles.

† Rashi Fein suggested the Nathan case study approach to the author.

pushing paper or producing great plans, rather than providing re-sults. One must study the existence of any benefits (such as reduced assets or beds) across states with mature CON programs, new CON programs, new SS1122 programs, or no programs. A total of forty-three states had some degree of experience with regulatory attempts to constrain hospital capital expansion (CON and/or SS1122) prior to December 1978. The wave of enthusiasm for capital supply-side constraints has not been based on the available evidence. Salkever and Bice (1976) have reported on the 1968–1972 experience with CON programs, and concluded that the net effect of the program over the four-year period was to reduce the growth in beds by a meager 5–9 percent, while assets per bed increased by 15–20 per-cent. The authors were quick to point out that the study evaluated CON program effects at a very early stage of implementation: Only five states (New York, Maryland, Rhode Island, Connecticut, and California) had mature operating programs.

The national trend data on hospital assets in Table 8.1 (American Hospital Association, 1979) reflect changes in hospital accounting designed to provide a more complete accounting of asset values after 1969. Despite the lack of uniformity, two trends are discernible. First, the expansion of health insurance with the passage of Medicaid and Medicare allowed hospitals to continue expanding assets at the rate of 2–3 percent per year in real dollar terms. The tougher state and federal reimbursement policies and the growth of CON programs in the 1970s did not precipitate a decline in hospital assets. Further study of the cost containment impact of CON pro-grams is needed. If CON programs were effective, the states with long-standing active CON programs would have retarded asset ex-pansion in comparison to states without CON. The question posed is whether CON and Section 1122 programs constrained costs and achieved a more desirable allocation of hospital capital.

Historical Context

Planning has historically been regionalized in the United States. The Hill-Burton program (1948–1976) for hospital bed construction was implemented through forty-eight state hospital planning councils. The Regional Medical Programs (1966–1974), designed to diffuse new medical technological discoveries to the community physicians, were implemented by fifty-six Regional Advisory Groups. Concur-

Table 8.1 Plant Assets, Total Assets, Assets per Bed and the Five-year Percentage Increase, at Non-Federal Short-term General Hospitals, for Selected Years 1950–1979

Year	Hospitals	Plant Assets (in millions)	Total Assets (in millions)	Total Assets per Bed	5-Year Percentage Increase	
					Assets per Bed	APB in Real Dollars[1]
1950	5,031	$ 2,782	$ 4,349	$ 8,612	n.a.	n.a.
1955	5,237	5,188	6,985	12,298	42.8	28.4
1960	5,407	8,292	10,858	16,992	38.2	24.9
1965	5,736	12,316	16,364	22,084	30.0	22.0
1966	5,812	12,989	17,783	23,155	26.5	16.6
1970	5,859	18,132	26,674	30,766	39.3	13.2
1974	5,977	28,059	41,840	44,941	53.7	14.3
1975	5,979	31,655	47,256	49,901	62.2	17.0
1977	5,973	39,946	61,133	62,765	65.0	13.9
1978	5,935	42,141	68,248	70,004	74.2	18.7
1979	5,939[2]	45,937	76,151	77,076	71.5	16.5

SOURCE: *Hospital Statistics, 1978* (1979). The AHA stopped publishing data on assets in 1978. The 1978 and 1979 unpublished figures were provided by the AHA.

[1] Deflated by the Consumer Price Index, U.S. Department of Labor, Bureau of Labor Statistics.

[2] The AHA questionnaire was changed in 1978 and 1979. Consequently these figures are underestimates, since 1,150 hospitals chose not to report data concerning restricted funds.

rently, Comprehensive Health Planning (CHP) was attempted in the spirit of consensus planning through fifty state "a" agencies and 200 areawide CHP "b" agencies. Since passage of the 1974 National Health Planning and Resources Development Act (P.L. 93-641), the role of areawide planning fell to the 203 federally designated Health Systems Agencies (HSAs).

The HSAs are nonprofit corporations with boards comprised of representatives from the public, providers, third-party payers, and politicians. Marmor and Morone (1980) have recently questioned the assumption that HSAs, which are at least 51 percent consumers, can represent the wider public interest. There is little incentive for the local HSA to reduce health service production costs if the social costs are borne by that area alone; whereas the benefits are distributed nationwide and are not perceivable by the local citizens. Given the present mode of financing hospitals, local HSAs have many more disincentives to close facilities and increase unemployment if the benefits of these actions accrue largely to over 100 million Americans paying taxes and insurance premiums. In the language of economics, there is little incentive for HSAs to get tough if all the costs are internalized locally and most of the benefits are externalized nationwide.

The relationship between the HSAs and the fifty State Health Planning and Development Agencies (SHPDA) is analogous to the relationship between the CHP "b" and "a" agencies prior to 1974. The important differences in the current planning infrastructure is that P.L. 93-641 inserted two layers of new bureaucracy into the picture. The State Health Coordinating Council (SHCC) was inserted between the HSAs and the SHPDA to act as an advisory body to the SHPDA and the governor. The other layer of bureaucracy, inserted at the top of the bureaucracy, was the federal National Health Planning Council acting in an advisory capacity to the Secretary of the Department of Health and Human Services.

The 1979 three-year extension (P.L. 96-79) of the 1974 Health Planning and Resources Development Act has pushed health planning into a new phase. Planners have to face foreign new concepts such as "promoting competition" and "health marketing." Moreover, the HSAs are having trouble convincing Congress of their effectiveness. Most HSA board members are not vocal about the contradictory objectives contained in their lists of goals and objectives. For example, the process of plan writing and implementation creates new provider goals and consumer wants for a more inflationary style of medical care, yet all 198 fully designated HSAs in 1980 have cost containment as a major goal. In this regard, David Kinzer (1977), President of the Massachusetts Hospital Association, has cited the HSAs for spreading wants and adding to the hospital cost problem. A second paradox in the HSA mission is the goal of keeping new construction below a maximum level X without realization of the long-run inflationary possibilities implicit in that strategy: (1) freezing out new low-cost competitors such as HMOs and surgicenters and (2) allowing a nearly 95 percent rate of approval of expansion projects in existing facilities (Lewin, 1975). Concerning this second point, the Abt (1976) study corroborates Lewin's suggestion that local agencies have difficulty turning down high technology equipment requests from existing providers. One class of new entrants trying to break into the marketplace was exempted from the planning process by the 1979 Amendments (P.L. 96-79). Federally designated HMOs with more than 50,000 enrollees or new HMOs are now exempt from the Certificate-of-Need process. Small existing HMOs are still subject to the CON process, but at least one factor inhibiting new HMO development has been eliminated. Growth of existing small HMOs will still be inhibited to some degree by the planning process.

The major policy question in the late 1970s was not the overall effectiveness of CON or 1122 regulatory efforts. The big issue was whether such modes of providing regulatory teeth to the health planning movement were counter-productive in terms of restraining competition. CON regulation in particular was criticized for blocking entry of lower cost alternatives such as HMOs and ambulatory surgicenters (Havighurst, 1980). The anecdotal reporting of planners favoring the existing providers at the expense of new entrants is consistent with all variants of the capture hypothesis.

Defenders of capital expenditure controls would argue that the CON programs need more time, have only been half-heartedly supported, and are seriously understaffed. While the CHP boards and the early HSAs could argue that they were under-budgeted, the resource flow to HSAs more than doubled in the 1976–1978 period. Given that HSAs have attempted to meet an expanded list of functions during a recalcitrant anti-regulatory period between 1979 and 1981, it may be better to evaluate their performance between 1974 and 1978. Since planners and politicians have identified Certificate-of-Need (CON) activities as the most cost-beneficial element of HSA activities, it seems surprising that little quantitative evidence exists on the matter.

Impact of CON and Section 1122
Regulatory Controls

Tests of the investment impact of capital expenditure analysis (CON and SS1122) were derived from a cross-sectional multiple regression analysis. The data employed in the analysis pertained to fifty states. Three dependent variables were defined over the 1974–1978 period. The first dependent variable, plant assets,* was viewed as a total dollar value of investment. The second variable, beds, was considered a measure of the capacity of 5973 short-term general hospitals. The third variable, plant assets per bed, was viewed as an index of capital intensiveness or technological sophistication. The advantages of the four-year time period 1974–1978 were two-fold: (1) it included enough long-term exposure to CON and widespread exposure to SS1122 to retire the argument that "planners everywhere need more time to become effective" and (2) it excluded the confounding influence of the federal Economic Stabilization Program controls.

The regression approach taken was to estimate an investment function (K) for each of the three dependent variables as a function of six measures of the availability of funds (F), 14 measures of factors determining hospital demand (D), two regulatory factors (CON, $SS1122$), two structural factors ($MULTI$, AFF), and a cost-of-construction variable (CW) (Table 8.2). The equation estimated was of the general form:

$$K = \beta_0 + \beta_{1\text{-}6}F + \beta_{7\text{-}20}D + \beta_{21}CON + \beta_{22}SS1122 + \beta_{23}MULTI + \beta_{24}AFF + \beta_{25}CW + E.$$

The intercept term is β_0 and the error term is E.

Two specific forms of this equation were estimated: (1) linear percentage change and (2) linear logarithmic change. The major advantages of these two specifications were that they have been tried and tested in previous studies by Salkever and Bice (1976) and Muller *et al.* (1975), and they restrict the absolute impact on scale-free independent variables that are correlated with state size. Two of the scale-free variables that have not been previously analyzed are

---

* External accounting reports deduct depreciation to arrive at net plant assets. If there existed a centralized data source on annual depreciation charges, we could add depreciation back into net plant assets to get more accurate figures for capital investment trends.

SS1122 and *MULTI* (Table 8.2). The scale-free variable with the highest positive correlation with state size was per capita income. As the independent variables employed here were similar to those utilized in the two cited studies, they require little comment. The *SS1122* and *MULTI* variables were expected to have a negative impact on duplication of services and all three dependent variables. An attempt was made to improve the measurement precision of the two crucial regulatory independent variables *CON* and *SS1122*. For example, in the previously cited Salkever and Bice (1976) study, the crucial date of regulatory impact was the date of enactment of the legislation. However, a state like Kansas that passed a CON program in 1972 should not be counted as having CON in effect for year 1972 if the program was not made operational until 1974.

A telephone survey of the thirty-four states enacting a CON law prior to 1978 was attempted. The original intent of the telephone survey was to collect proxy measures for regulatory effort, for example, applications reviewed or full-time CON staff per hospital. The variability in program implementation was high and the inability of CON staff to provide data concerning their productivity was less than reassuring. We learned that some states with CON programs (Georgia is one) were designed to review only nursing homes and consequently could not be expected to have any impact on hospital investment. In the final analysis, the *CON* variable was taken as percentage of time the state actually had a CON program in operation during the 1974–1978 period (twenty-eight states). The telephone survey revealed that thirteen states started Section 1122 reviews prior to 1974, and seventeen states initiated Section 1122 review during the 1974–1978 period. The *SS1122* variable was taken as the percentage of time the state actually participated in 1122 review process during the 1974–1978 period (thirty states, fifteen of which did not have operating CON programs).

The regression results presented in Tables 8.3 and 8.4 are summarized below:

1. Capital expenditure regulation (CER) appeared ineffective in constraining plant assets, beds, and assets per bed. The CON program effect appears to significantly add to plant assets and assets per bed in two of the specifications. The sign of the *SS1122* coefficient was more uniformly negative, but still insignificant statistically. There is no evidence suggesting that CON or SS1122 activity is effective or efficient. On the other

Table 8.2 Variables Included in the Regression Analysis of the Impact of Planning Regulations on Hospital Investment

	Percentage Change Equations		Logarithmic Change Equations	
	Form of Variable	Name	Form of Variable	Name
Dependent Variables				
Change in Plant Assets, 1974–1978	a	D6PA	c	D6LPA
Change in Beds, 1974–1978	a	D6BD	c	D6LBD
Change in Plant Assets per Bed, 1974–1978	a	D6PAB	c	D6PAB
Availability of Funds Variables				
Ratio of Total Hill-Burton Allocations to 1974 Plant Assets				
1975–1978	b	R8HB	d	LR8HB
1971–1974	b	R1HB	d	LR1HB
1971–1978	b	RTHB	d	LRTHB
Ratio of Total Hospital Net Revenues to 1974 Plant Assets				
1974–1978	b	R6NR	d	LR6NR
1970–1974	b	R2NR	d	LR2NR
1970–1978	b	RTNR	d	LRTNR
Demand Variables				
Change in Population				
1974–1978	a	D6POP	c	D6LPOP
1970–1974	a	D2POP	c	D2LPOP
Change in Mean per Capita Income				
1974–1978	a	D6INC	c	D6LINC
1970–1974	a	D2INC	c	D2LINC
Occupancy Rate in 1974	b	OCC	d	LOCC
Change in Occupancy Rate, 1970–1974	a	D2OCC	c	D2LOCC
Change in Proportion of Population with Blue Cross or Medicare Hospital Coverage				
1974–1978	a	D6BCM	c	D6LBCM
1970–1974	a	D2BCM	c	D2LCBM
Change in Proportion of Population with Hospital Insurance				
1974–1978	a	D6PH	c	D6LPH
1970–1974	a	D2PH	c	D2LPH

Table 8.2 (continued)

	Percentage Change Equations		Logarithmic Change Equations	
	Form of Variable	Name	Form of Variable	Name
Change in Number of Physicians				
1974–1978	a	D6MD	c	D6LMD
1970–1974	a	D2MD	c	D2LMD
Change in Number of Specialists				
1974–1978	a	D6SP	c	D6LSP
1970–1974	a	D2SP	c	D2LSP
Other Independent Variables				
Percentage of the 1974–1978 Period with CON Program in Effect	b	CON	d	CON
Percentage of the 1974–1978 Period with Section 1122 Agreement in Effect	b	SS1122	d	SS1122
Percentage of Beds in a Multi-hospital System in 1977–1978	b	MULTI	d	MULTI
Annual Construction Wages in 1976 (in thousands of dollars)	b	CW	d	LCW
Residents and Interns per Hospital Bed, 1976	b	AFF	d	LAFF

a   Percentage of change
b   Level
c   Change in logarithms
d   Logarithm

hand, it is equally true that there is no indication that SS1122 regulation is inefficient.

2. Occupancy rate has a negative impact on total investment per bed, that is, the higher the occupancy, the smaller the investment per bed. This occupancy effect appears to be the result of significant increases in bed capacity combined with insignificant reductions in other types of investment in plant assets.

3. The supply of physicians per capita had a negative impact on all three measures of hospital investment. This agrees with the Salkever and Bice (1976) findings, and adds support for the theory advanced by Greer (1980) that specialists have more

Table 8.3 Regression Coefficients for Percentage Change, Hospital Investment Equations 1974–1978 (*t*-statistics in parentheses)

Equation No.	3.1	3.2[1]	3.3	3.4	3.5[1]	3.6	3.7	3.8[1]	3.9
Dep Var.	D6PA	D6PA	P6PA	D6BD	D6BD	D6BD	D6PAB	D6PAB	D6PAB
Constant	-0.071	0.237	-0.259	-0.267	0.104	-0.310	0.396	0.361	0.519
CON[2]	0.112 (0.84)	0.150[4] (1.49)	0.048 (0.45)	-0.006 (0.18)	0.019 (0.66)	-0.027 (0.91)	0.122[4] (1.31)	0.154[4] (1.62)	0.090 (0.89)
SS1122[2]	-0.018 (0.02)	-0.046 (0.39)	-0.085 (0.72)	0.011 (0.36)	-0.013 (0.43)	-0.009 (0.30)	-0.030 (0.24)	-0.039 (0.32)	-0.088 (0.86)
MULTI	-0.014 (0.28)			-0.010 (0.35)			-0.005 (0.09)		
D6POP	0.762 (0.95)	0.821 (0.79)	1.084 (1.00)	0.195 (0.53)	0.046 (0.09)	0.086 (0.39)	0.599 (0.71)	0.815 (0.68)	0.970 (0.82)
D2POP	0.847 (0.79)	0.216 (0.13)	1.292[4] (1.46)	0.552[4] (1.47)	0.626[5] (1.76)	0.145 (0.60)	0.316 (0.58)	-0.423 (0.39)	1.265[4] (1.31)
D6INC	-0.273 (0.64)	-0.428 (1.24)	-0.241 (0.61)	-0.018 (0.07)	-0.013 (0.09)	-0.016 (0.09)	-0.233 (0.96)	-0.470 (1.14)	-0.282 (0.86)
D2INC	-0.507 (1.08)	-0.258 (0.34)	-0.356 (0.94)	-0.154 (1.26)	-0.085 (0.43)	-0.004 (0.03)	-0.371 (0.57)	-0.223 (0.46)	-0.329 (0.74)
OCC[3]	-0.031 (0.41)		-0.008 (0.15)	0.017[4] (1.39)		0.047[5] (2.39)	-0.049 (0.61)		-0.063[4] (1.35)
D2OCC		-0.222 (1.17)			0.217 (0.74)			-0.436 (0.91)	
D6PH	0.320 (1.16)		0.478[5] (1.79)	-0.052 (0.36)		-0.040 (0.38)	0.415[4] (1.56)		0.466[5] (1.70)
D2PH	0.119 (0.45)		0.273 (0.88)	0.459 (0.50)		0.216 (1.11)	-0.348 (1.23)		0.094 (0.25)

Table 8.3 (continued)

Equation No.	3.1	3.2[1]	3.3	3.4	3.5[1]	3.6	3.7	3.8[1]	3.9
D6BCM		-0.735^4 (1.36)			-0.495^6 (2.81)			-0.159^5 (1.73)	
D2BCM		0.178^4 (1.40)			0.079^4 (1.66)			-0.090 (1.06)	
D6MD	-0.561 (0.38)			-0.227 (1.18)			-0.367 (0.26)		
D2MD	-1.378^5 (1.70)		-1.659^5 (1.81)	-0.363^4 (1.58)		-0.183 (1.02)	-0.881^5 (1.94)		-1.469^5 (2.02)
D6SP		-0.324 (0.75)			-0.385 (1.21)			0.117 (0.36)	
D2SP		0.524^4 (1.61)			0.275 (0.86)			0.247 (0.71)	
R8HB	-2.014^5 (2.37)			-3.017^6 (6.54)			0.890 (0.97)		
R1HB	4.874^5 (1.82)			4.162^6 (5.83)			0.689 (1.16)		
RTHB		1.217^5 (1.90)	3.632^6 (5.19)		-0.074 (0.57)	0.653^6 (2.88)		1.304^5 (1.76)	2.816^6 (3.32)
R6NR	0.157 (0.63)			0.064 (0.78)			0.103 (0.29)		
R2NR	-0.011 (0.03)		0.241 (0.57)	-0.034 (0.29)		0.041 (0.43)	0.014 (0.07)		0.180 (0.72)

Table 8.3 (continued)

Equation No.	3.1	3.2[1]	3.3	3.4	3.5[1]	3.6	3.7	3.8[1]	3.9
RTNR		0.199 (0.75)			0.058 (0.47)			0.136 (0.68)	
CW	0.009 (0.75)	0.014 (0.92)	0.022[4] (1.46)	−0.017[5] (1.94)	−0.019[5] (2.06)	−0.019[5] (2.17)	0.031 (1.10)	0.039 (1.26)	0.043[4] (1.31)
AFF		0.836[5] (1.69)			0.061 (0.53)			0.728[4] (1.45)	
R-Squared	0.464	0.451	0.487	0.642	0.719	0.748	0.423	0.406	0.450

[1] Nevada and Wyoming are excluded because of undefined values for independent variables.
[2] Coefficients shown are actual coefficients multiplied by 100.
[3] Coefficients shown are actual coefficients multiplied by 10.
[4] Significant at the 0.1 level (one-tailed test).
[5] Significant at the 0.05 level (one-tailed test).
[6] Significant at the 0.005 level (one-tailed test).

Table 8.4 Regression Coefficients for Logarithmic Change, Hospital Investment Equations 1974–1978 (*t*-statistics in parentheses)

Equation No.	4.1	4.2[1]	4.3	4.4	4.5[1]	4.6	4.7	4.8[1]	4.9
Dep Var.	D6LPA	D6LPA	D6LPA	D6LBD	D6LBD	D6LBD	D6LBD	D6LPAB	D6LPAB
Constant	−0.302	0.518	−0.490	−0.406	0.071	−0.561	0.575	0.597	0.723
CON[2]	0.054 (0.91)	0.071[5] (1.69)	0.025 (0.73)	−0.003 (0.16)	0.010 (0.52)	−0.013 (0.78)	0.046[4] (1.43)	0.062[4] (1.58)	0.035 (1.16)
SS1122[2]	−0.011 (0.09)	−0.024 (0.45)	−0.038 (0.81)	0.008 (0.24)	−0.005 (0.26)	−0.004 (0.20)	−0.016 (0.18)	−0.017 (0.21)	−0.036 (0.57)

Table 8.4 (continued)

Equation No.	4.1	4.2[1]	4.3	4.4	4.5[1]	4.6	4.7	4.8[1]	4.9
MULTI	−0.031 (0.45)			−0.020 (0.29)			−0.009 (0.15)		
D6LPOP	0.547 (0.48)	0.409 (0.38)	0.562 (0.72)	0.106 (0.78)	0.094 (0.30)	0.077 (0.65)	0.473 (0.59)	0.345 (0.29)	0.359 (0.40)
D2LPOP	0.620 (0.82)	0.082 (0.15)	1.284 (1.28)	0.535[4] (1.34)	0.758[4] (1.60)	0.196 (0.54)	0.084 (0.42)	−0.651 (0.87)	1.098 (1.23)
D6LINC	−0.255 (0.67)	−0.602[4] (1.45)	−0.267 (0.79)	−0.173[4] (1.40)	−0.104 (0.55)	0.012 (0.06)	0.091 (0.50)	−0.499[4] (1.33)	−0.256 (0.79)
D2LINC	−0.386 (0.89)	−0.079 (0.21)	−0.228 (0.80)	−0.163 (1.19)	−0.106 (0.61)	0.019 (0.05)	−0.227 (0.54)	0.024 (0.06)	−0.210 (0.63)
LOCC	−0.105 (0.47)		−0.054 (0.31)	0.085[5] (1.92)		0.060[5] (2.17)	−0.208 (0.85)		−0.074[4] (1.52)
D2LOCC		−0.152 (0.64)			−0.014 (0.10)			−0.139 (0.43)	
D6LPH	0.284[4] (1.37)		0.296[4] (1.53)	−0.051 (0.46)		0.008 (0.01)	0.277[4] (1.45)		0.296[4] (1.58)
D2LPH	0.107 (0.49)		0.315 (0.91)	0.482 (0.43)		0.197 (1.06)	−0.375[4] (1.32)		0.120 (0.43)
D6LBCM		−0.568 (1.27)			−0.385[6] (3.13)			−0.192[5] (1.85)	
D2LBCM		0.236[4] (1.50)			0.107[5] (1.84)			0.128[4] (1.45)	
D6LMD	−0.492[6] (0.36)			−0.231 (1.26)			−0.262 (0.57)		

Table 8.4 (continued)

Equation No.	4.1	4.2[1]	4.3	4.4	4.5[1]	4.6	4.7	4.8[1]	4.9
D2LMD	-0.898[4] (1.57)		-1.281[4] (1.65)	-0.329[4] (1.47)		0.195 (1.17)	-0.609[5] (1.76)		-1.487[5] (1.83)
D6LSP		-0.079 (0.37)			-0.148 (1.06)			0.068 (0.16)	
D2LSP		0.408[4] (1.59)			0.239 (0.68)			-0.176 (0.94)	
LR8HB	-0.475[5] (2.11)			-0.693[6] (4.97)			0.245[4] (1.42)		
LR1HB	0.516[4] (1.62)			0.445[5] (2.59)			0.087 (0.85)		
LRTHB		0.159[6] (2.94)	0.452[6] (4.76)		0.035 (0.69)	0.074[5] (2.60)		0.125[4] (1.67)	0.377[6] (2.94)
LR6NR[3]	0.153 (0.59)			0.090 (1.01)			0.062 (0.24)		
LR2NR[3]	-0.046 (0.10)			0.087 (0.42)			-0.135 (0.72)		
LRTNR[3]		0.127 (0.70)	0.157 (0.46)		0.031 (0.42)	0.093 (0.61)		0.096 (0.63)	
LCW	0.046 (0.92)	0.071 (1.03)	0.112[4] (1.57)	-0.067[5] (1.66)	-0.074[5] (1.89)	-0.076[5] (2.01)	0.115 (1.16)	0.148[4] (1.37)	0.210[4] (1.34)
AFF		0.614[5] (1.78)			0.106 (0.64)			0.513[4] (1.41)	
R-Squared	0.515	0.472	0.429	0.704	0.696	0.601	0.558	0.480	0.472

[1] Nevada and Wyoming excluded because of undefined values for independent variables.
[2] Coefficients shown are actual coefficients multiplied by 100.
[3] Coefficients shown are actual coefficients multiplied by 10.

[4] Significant at the 0.1 level (one-tailed test).
[5] Significant at the 0.05 level (one-tailed test).
[6] Significant at the 0.005 level (one-tailed test).

interest in hospital capital than the typical physician. If generalists appear to consider hospital investment as a substitute for professional service, specialists treat hospital capital as a complementary resource. The supply ratio of specialists has a significantly positive impact on plant assets in one equation and a uniform (but statistically insignificant) impact on assets per bed.

4. The coefficient to measure strength of affiliation and teaching activities (AFF) conforms to the expectation that teaching hospitals are more strongly concerned with assets per bed than number of beds. This is consistent with the previous work of the author (1980) and Salkever and Bice (1976).

5. The coefficient for percentage of beds in multi-hospital systems has the expected negative impact on beds, assets, and assets per bed. Unfortunately the coefficients are insignificant and disappointing. One would have hoped that multi-hospital systems would have stimulated enough sharing of services, and elimination of capital duplication, to significantly alter the hospital investment profile.

Returning to the question posed in the middle of the chapter, the results suggest that states with active CON programs have stimulated investment in sophisticated technology and modernization projects, without affecting the number of existing beds. The assessment of the SS1122 program is only a bit less pessimistic, in that the program has not had a significant effect on beds, assets, or assets per bed. Consequently, one can only conclude that these two regulatory efforts have been a failure in retarding hospital investment. The potential reasons why the Section 1122 program may have been less of a failure, in the sense that it stimulated no excess investment, are three-fold: (1) the uniform 1122 Social Security program was never successfully challenged in the courts, in contrast to a dozen CON programs that had sanctions invalidated in court, (2) Medicare auditors provided an established uniform national system of checkers to detect all facilities trying to avoid SS1122 review, and (3) SS1122 is as broad or broader in scope of expenditures reviewed than state CON programs. When the final revised SS1122 regulations are published for 1981, the overlapping inconsistencies between CON local activities and 1122 programs should be almost eliminated, thus reducing the costs involved in operating two duplicate review programs. However, the Congress and the public should question the value of operating any inflationary regulatory activity, much less one that operates with duplicate inefficiencies. Further study seems warranted concerning the efficacy and effectiveness of the other two functions of HSAs: health plan implementation and service appropriateness reviews.

Up to this point there has been minimal discussion of the adaptive responses that hospitals might pursue in highly regulated situations. Hospital administrators have three methods of co-opting the regulatory process. First, they can purchase equipment that is below the CON program review ceiling (section D, Figure 8.1), for example, depending on the state, these are items costing less than $100,000–$200,000. Second, if the administrators cannot spend money on new bed construction or modernization, they can bombard the CON agency with a number of capital equipment requests (Section F, Figure 8.1). Failing at either of these strategies, the administrator can hire an excessive number of LPNs or grant above-average wage increases (Section G, Figure 8.1). This third phenomenon is consistent with all non-profit models of hospital behavior and has been observed in a sample of 1228 hospitals, 1970–1975, by Sloan and Steinwald (1980). In summary, the compensatory response to regulation can occur on both the capital and wage side of the patient care production process. The regression results presented in this chapter only assessed the non-labor response and essentially support the earlier findings of Salkever and Bice (1976).

Regulation or Competition?

There is a lively debate beginning to develop concerning the question of whether competition will bring higher or lower capital costs in the hospital industry. Most analysts agree that the effect will be inflationary in the short run. If new competitors are to attract the speculative venture capital needed to enter the market, above-average rates of return will have to be forthcoming. Opponents of competition label such a conscious attempt to establish the opportunity for large profits as madness. How can one defend competition on equity grounds if the marketplace has always failed to provide sufficient resources in poor rural and inner city neighborhoods? Enthoven's (1980) response is that with a voucher system of universal insurance the poor will be placed on an "almost" equal footing with the affluent neighborhoods, and the market will respond by shifting resources to the underserved and smoothing out the maldistribution problem.

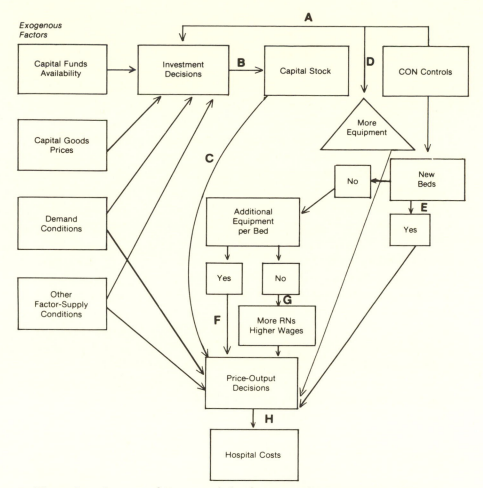

Figure 8.1 Conceptual Framework for the Hospital Investment Decision-Making Process.

Advocates of competition are less concerned with the liberal disdain for profits in a largely non-profit industry and counterargue that competitors will force inefficient providers to close up shop and sell their capital at low salvage prices, thus reducing the capital costs in the hospital industry. One might even go so far as to suggest a planned-competitive solution, whereby the new competitor would get an apportionment of capital at least equal to the new competitor's market share after five years of operation, and the HSA would reduce the capital apportioned to the existing non-profit providers. Society must face the two political questions as to how much short-term "excess" capital we will allow new competitors to purchase and how many inefficient providers we will allow to go bankrupt. The competitive solution may require "unacceptable" lead and lag times and hospital labor union unrest.

Most health policy makers doubt that the competitive market allocation of hospital capital is as effective as a fully planned allocation system based on the CON process. Unfortunately, regional planning in the United States has not achieved its goal. Planners have inadvertently kept many cost-containing competitors out of the market in the name of planning. Given the recent experience with CON, one still has reason to doubt the ability of planners to reduce costs while not adversely affecting the non-profit hospitals, and while not inhibiting surgicenters, HMOs, and new proprietary hospitals. There is a significant chance that Congress will abolish or limit HSAs in 1982. One potential argument for continuing a system of HSAs with reduced responsibilities, even if not cost-beneficial, is to assert that the start-up cost of reinventing planning boards after passage of national health insurance is too high. Planners are quick to argue that even if HSAs operate as an organizational "mess," with interrelationships among functions usually poorly defined and inadequately coordinated, they have identified some significant shortfalls or gaps in health resource supply.

Devotees of the health planning process would scoff at the notion that CON activities have been ineffective or cost-increasing. Planners have always argued that they are understaffed and constantly receive an expanded list of review responsibilities from the Congress every few years. However, the HSAs and CON agencies had significant staff budget expansions in the mid-1970s, and they cannot blame the budget cuts of 1980 for the failures of 1974–1978.

Caveats Concerning Other Regulatory Methods

One recent state hospital association report complained about the problem of excessive regulation in the health field. For example, the report cited the example of New York state hospitals' reporting to 164 different local, state, and federal bureaucracies. In view of the range and complexity of health regulations, one cannot hope to comprehend the totality of health regulation in any one chapter. Accordingly, the approach taken herein was to assess the impact of what planners cite as their most visible and cost-beneficial activity: capital expenditure controls. If a strong case cannot be made for

Certificate-of-Need (CON) and Section 1122 capital control regulatory programs, then perhaps the burden of proof concerning other regulatory endeavors must lie with the regulators. Recently, other regulatory instruments such as tax subsidies, training programs, and quality and utilization controls have been called into question. For example, the May 1980 Congressional Budget Office report on Professional Standard Review Organizations (PSROs) reports a savings of $40 for every $100 in PSRO program costs. State rate control programs have proved a modest success in six states (refer to Chapter 5), but in other states the program has been abolished (Colorado) or the hidden costs in cannibalization of assets have been enormous (New York).

References

Abt Associates, Inc. (1976). "Incentives and Decisions Underlying Hospitals' Adoption and Utilization of Major Capital Equipment," NTIS No. PB-251-631. Washington, D.C.: DHEW, Health Resources Administration.

American Hospital Association (1979). *Hospital Statistics 1978.* Chicago, Ill.: AHA.

BATTISTELLA, R., and EASTAUGH, S. (1980). "Hospital Cost Containment," *Proceedings of the Academy of Political Science* 33:4 (Winter), 192–205.

BAUER, K. G. (1977). "Hospital Rate Setting—This Way to Salvation?" *Milbank Memorial Fund Quarterly* 55:1 (Winter), 117–158.

BERNSTEIN, M. (1955). *Regulating Business by Independent Commissions.* Princeton: Princeton University Press.

BILES, B., SCHRAMM, C., and ATKINSON, G. (1980). "Hospital Cost Inflation Under Rate-Setting Programs," *New England Journal of Medicine* 303:12 (September 18), 664–667.

COHEN, H. S. (1975). "Regulatory Politics and American Medicine," *American Behavioral Scientist* 19:1 (September/October), 122–136.

Congressional Budget Office (1979). "The Hospital Cost Containment Act of 1978," Staff Report (May). Washington, D.C.: U.S. Government Printing Office.

EASTAUGH, S. R. (1980). "Organizational Determinants of Surgical Lengths of Stay," *Inquiry* 17:2 (Spring), 85–96.

EASTAUGH, S. R. (1979). "President's Hospital Cost Containment Proposal," Subcommittee on Health Hearings, Committee on Ways and Means, 96th U.S. Congress, First Session, April 2, 1979, Part 2, Serial 96-19. Washington, D.C.: U.S. Government Printing Office, 396–418.

ENTHOVEN, A. (1980). *Health Plan.* Reading, Mass.: Addison-Wesley.

General Accounting Office (1980). "Unreliability of the American Health Planning Association's Savings Estimate for the Health Planning Program," GAO Report HRD-80-49. Washington, D.C.: U.S. Government Printing Office.

GREER, A. (1980). "Medical Technology and Professional Dominance Theory." University of Wisconsin–Milwaukee: Urban Research Center Reports.

HAVIGHURST, C. (1980). "Antitrust Enforcement in the Medical Services Industry:

What Does It All Mean?" *Milbank Memorial Fund Quarterly* 58:1 (Winter), 89–124.

HELLINGER, F. J. (1976). "The Effect of Certificate-of-Need Legislation on Hospital Investment," *Inquiry* 13:6 (June), 187–193.

HILTON, G. W. (1972). "The Basic Behavior of Regulatory Commissions," *American Economic Review* 62:2 (May), 47–54.

Hospital Association of New York State (1981). "Ninth Annual Fiscal Pressures Survey, 1979" (March). Albany, New York.

Institute of Medicine (1980). *Health Planning in the United States: Issues for Guideline Development*. Washington, D.C.: National Academy of Sciences.

Institute of Medicine (1981). *Health Policy in the United States: Selected Policy Issues*, vol. 1. Washington, D.C.: National Academy of Sciences.

KAHN, A. (1971). *The Economics of Regulation: Principles and Institutions*, volume II, "Institutional Issues." New York: Wiley.

KASSIRER, J., and PAUKER, S. (1978). "Should Diagnostic Testing Be Regulated?" *New England Journal of Medicine* 299:17 (October), 947–949.

KINZER, D. (1977). *Health Controls Out of Control: Warning to the Nation from Massachusetts*. Chicago, Ill.: Teach'em.

LEE, L. (1980). "A Theory of Just Regulation," *American Economic Review* 70:5 (December), 848–862.

Lewin and Associates, Inc. (1975). *Evaluation of the Efficiency and Effectiveness of the Section 1122 Review Process*. Washington, D.C.: Lewin and Associates.

MARMOR, T. R., and MORONE, J. A. (1980). "Representing Consumer Interests: Imbalanced Markets, Health Planning and the HSAs," *Milbank Memorial Fund Quarterly* 58:1 (Winter), 125–165.

McCLURE, W., and KLIGMAN, L. (1979). "Conversion and Other Policy Options to Reduce Excess Hospital Capacity," DHEW, Report 16 (September), Bureau of Health Planning Information Series (HRA) 79-14044.

MULLER, C., WORTHINGTON, P., and ALLEN, G. (1975). "Capital Expenditures and the Availability of Funds," *International Journal of Health Services* 5:1 (Winter), 143–157.

NATHAN, R. P., and DOMMEL, P. R. (1978). "Federal-Local Relations Under Block Grants," *Political Science Quarterly* 93:3 (Fall), 421–442.

PELTZMAN, S. (1976). "Toward a More General Theory of Regulation," *Journal of Law and Economics* 19:3 (August), 211–248.

POSNER, R. A. (1975). "The Social Costs of Monopoly and Regulation," *Journal of Political Economy* 83:4 (August), 807–827.

SALKEVER, D. S., and BICE, T. W. (1976). "The Impact of Certificate-of-Need Controls on Hospital Investment," *Milbank Memorial Fund Quarterly*, 54:2 (Spring), 195–214.

SLOAN, F. A., and STEINWALD, B. (1980). "Effects of Regulation on Hospital Costs and Input Use," *Journal of Law and Economics* 23:1 (April), 81–109.

STIGLER, G. J. (1971). "The Theory of Economic Regulation," *Bell Journal of Economics and Management Science* 2:1 (Spring), 3–21.

TRUMAN, D. R. (1951). *The Government Process: Political Interests and Public Opinion*. New York: Alfred Knopf.

Part Three

INSTITUTIONAL COST AND FINANCIAL MANAGEMENT ISSUES

Chapter 9

LIMITS TO DEBT FINANCING

> *Debt is a bottomless sea.*
>
> —THOMAS CARLYLE

> *In many situations providers may have reached maximum debt capacity which implies that the next phase may be rapid aging and deterioration of present health facilities in this country. It seems imperative that a more equitable system of capital cost reimbursement be adopted.*
>
> —WILLIAM O. CLEVERLEY

A new era of total revenue controls and decreasing numbers of hospital beds does not preclude the need to allow hospital capital to keep pace with inflation and meet the demand for more tests and procedures per day of care. Debt financing has recently become the hospital's major source of funds for the purchase of new capital. A clear danger of further government regulation of hospital revenues is the possibility that some hospitals will be unable to maintain a reasonable income margin. To insure against this, the base values for calculating annual revenue ceilings should allow for a small but significant profit margin. Three equations are derived in this chapter to measure the impact that private-sector financing authorities could have on hospital growth as a function of various suggested financial ratio ceiling requirements. After a sensitivity analysis, it is concluded that a 3 percent operating margin would be enough to reduce the case study hospital's dependence on debt. The definition of an adequate operating margin will vary among different size hospitals and ownership arrangements. However, the average hospital will require at least a 3 percent margin. Reimbursement formulas fixed in this manner would not only diminish the incentives for excessive reliance on debt financing but also allow new capital to be largely equity-financed.

Shift from Equity to Debt Financing

In recent years we have seen an explosion in the use of debt financing by hospitals to help support and expand their operations. Later in this chapter we will identify the reasons for an explosion in debt, the constraints on future increases in the debt ratio, and the implications of debt ratios for hospitals in a state of expansion or decline. In addition, the often neglected reimbursement issue concerning definition of an adequate rate of return on equity to assure sufficient private market financing of hospital capital needs will be discussed.

Two basic policy initiatives by the federal government fueled the current trend toward bonded indebtedness. First, Medicare and Medicaid substantially reduced the risk involved with debt financing by reimbursing 100 percent of interest and allowing full amortization of bonded indebtedness. Second, the Nixon Administration, acting in the spirit of what they termed "off-budget financing," encouraged investment banking firms and local government to create tax-exempt financing authorities to issue tax-exempt hospital bonds in forty-two states in the period 1970–1973. Tax-exempt bonds offered health facilities the advantages of longer payback periods, no down-payment or equity requirements,* and lower interest rates relative to taxable bonds.

Tax-exempt bonds as a percentage of hospital debt offerings increased from less than 10 percent in 1970 to 68 percent in 1974 to 81 percent in 1979 (Table 9.1). The 1980 Congressional Budget Office Report entitled "Tax Subsidies for Medical Care" suggested either eliminating the tax-exempt status of hospital bonds or containing the rate of issue of tax-exempt bonds by requiring that they be declared the general obligation issue of the state or local government unit issuing them. Placing hospital bonds under general obligation status would force hospitals to compete for capital with schools and public projects on a equal basis. Currently state and local government units have no financial responsibilities for hospital bond issues, con-

---

* Frequently the par value of a hospital bond issue accounts for over 99 percent of the total project cost.

Table 9.1 Summary of Debt Financing Trends for Hospitals, 1974–1979 (thousands of dollars)

Year	A-1 Total Funding for Hospital Construction (thousands)[1]	A-2 Number of Hospitals Reporting A-1	A-3 Total Debt from A-1 (thousands)	B-1 Total Debt Offerings in Hospitals (thousands)	B-2 Tax-Exempt Hospital Bond Offerings (thousands)	B-3 Tax-Exempt Offerings as a Percentage of B-1
1974	$3,231	899	$1,873	$2,215	$1,506	68%
1975	3,064	798	1,740	2,728	1,959	72
1976	4,475	916	2,587	3,940	2,726	69
1977	3,729	817	2,331	6,312[2]	4,734	75
1978	3,318	677	2,031	4,226	3,123	74
1979	4,345	739	2,657	4,306	3,471	81

SOURCES: Column A—American Hospital Association, Survey of Sources of Funding for Hospital Construction (next available survey year, 1981). Column B—Kidder-Peabody & Company, Inc. (1980).

[1] Due to underreporting, this is probably an underestimate that should be inflated 50 percent. Even though the A.H.A. figure includes construction costs plus some new equipment, plus refinancing, plus acquisition of land and architect fees, the Commerce Department figures for only hospital construction costs are $800 million higher in both 1977 and 1978. Commerce Department, *Construction Reporting: Value of New Construction Put in Place*, June 1979, Table F-1, U.S. Government Printing Office, Washington, D.C. The percentage of the funds in column A-1 from tax-exempt bonds increased from 28 percent in 1974 to 56 percent in 1979.

[2] 1977 was a record setter because of a four-fold increase in the number of advance refundings in that year. Hospitals took advantage of the lower interest rates of 1977 because the rates were substantially lower than those of the recent past or projected future.

sequently, they have no direct interest in limiting them. However, the marketplace for general obligation bond issues would undoubtedly reduce the ability of hospitals to borrow. Some analysts have argued that the relative ease of borrowing in the hospital industry has exacerbated the shortfall of capital available to other public sector building projects.

Many factors underlie the shift from equity to debt financing. The most important factor is the shift from cost-plus to simple cost reimbursement. This has created a shortfall in both net income and working capital, forcing hospitals to seek funds externally. The Hill-Burton program, which provided federal funds for the construction of new beds, has been eliminated. Philanthropic contributions as a percentage of total contributions have declined. In 1968 philanthropy accounted for 21.2 percent of capital funds. By 1976 philanthropy accounted for just 7.5 percent of the funding for new projects (Lightle, 1978). One should also point out that states with hospital rate regulatory programs eroded the incentives to seek philanthropy by requiring hospitals to spend a fraction of such unrestricted funds on bad debts and charity care. Finally, new technologies and equipment obsolescence have put a strain on larger hospitals in particular to come up with the funds to maintain state-of-the-art technology. This drain on funds is frequently overlooked, yet the rapid turnover in new technologies has proven to be a major cause of increasing hospital costs. Gaus and Cooper (1976) estimate that close to 50 percent of the increase in health costs from 1967 to 1975 was due to new technologies.

The approach taken in this chapter will be to suggest why we might stimulate equity financing, rather than simply reduce the availability of debt options. Government and third-party insurance carriers have resisted the explicit recognition of an operating margin that would sufficiently cover capital replacement and the technological updating of equipment. At the present time, interest on debt is an allowable cost. Hospitals that fund new equipment with debt find the actual cost of purchase to be much lower than the purchase price. To quickly see why, consider the following simplified example of a hypothetical hospital named ABC. Hospital ABC is anticipating the purchase of a new piece of capital equipment. It can fund the purchase through debt or internally generated funds. The financial officer considering these two alternatives faces the following cash flows. Hospital ABC can debt finance the equipment in 1981 through a 20-year bond issue paying interest of 10 percent per annum with repayment at maturity.

Three quarters of hospital ABC's revenues are paid by cost payers who reimburse for all interest expense. Therefore, 75 percent of interest payments will be reimbursed as allowable costs, and we will assume this percentage remains constant throughout the time period (1981–2001). The appropriate discount rate for computing the net present value of the cash flow is 10 percent, that is, the cost of borrowing. The effective cost of the debt-financed purchase to the hospital in 1981 is $36,148 (the $36,148 is composed of the net present value of the 25 percent unreimbursed interest payments equal to $21,284, plus the debt repayment of $100,000 in the year 2001, which has a net present value of $14,864). The effective cost of the internally funded purchase alternative in 1981 is $100,000. In summary, the time value of money and current full reimbursement for interest expense create powerful incentives for hospitals to fund new capital acquisitions with debt.

For some southern and western hospital markets, the incentive to debt finance is not as strong because only 50 percent of their patients pay costs, for example, half their patients are charge payers (self-pay) or represented by third parties that pay charges (commercial insurance companies, some Blue Cross and Medicare plans). If we assume that only 50 percent of the patient days are covered by cost payers, the effective cost of the debt-financed purchase in 1981 is $57,432. Consequently, it is still better to debt finance than equity finance the $100,000, but the differential has been reduced to $42,568. Although there are other cash flows involved in the capital purchase decision, such as reimbursement for depreciation, these cash flows would be the same for debt or internal fund financing alternatives, and thus are not relevant in the above comparisons.

Reasons for the Increase in Debt Financing

Hospital administrators are not entirely to blame for the critical leverage problems facing their hospitals. Administrators had been blessed with large external sources of funds for many years. The abandonment of government programs such as Hill-Burton, the rise of cost-reimbursement, and the dramatic drop in philanthropy have left hospitals groping for new capital sources. Expansion and growth have continued at a rapid pace despite the presence of forces that would dictate against growth.

Many economists (Lee, 1971; Harris, 1977) have concluded that hospitals compete for prestige in such an aggressive fashion that there is great pressure on hospital management to maintain state-of-the-art technology. The continued increase in demand for more tests and procedures per day of hospital care has placed additional pressure on hospitals to grow in order to meet the demand, arguments that the increased demand is due to increased hospital growth notwithstanding. The number of hospital beds may decrease, as suggested by the Institute of Medicine (1976), by as much as 10 percent over the 1980s, but hospital capital stock seems destined to continue to grow to meet the ever-expanding vista of new technology. Society seems unlikely to heed the warnings of Fuchs (1974a) and Wildavsky (1977) and question whether better health is purchasable through more and better technology. Politicians are concerned that a maldistributed or inadequate supply of capital can reduce public accessibility to necessary services.

A final explanation for this continuing growth trend lies with a new economic theory called the theory of rational expectations. The theory, as outlined in Chapter 8, states that individuals' behaviors take into account their own expectations of how outsiders, including the government, will behave. For instance, hospital administrators, in municipal hospitals in particular, cannot believe that the government would permit their hospitals to go bankrupt. If necessary their hospitals could become some sort of wards of the state. This is already happening in some cities. The marketplace restrictions to growth imposed on highly levered hospitals may fail if administrators believe that local governments will save their hospitals from default and if the local governments continue to do just that.

Marketing the Debt

Financing authorities organized by state governments have greatly aided hospitals in issuing tax-free debt. The need for a debt service reserve fund has been eliminated in many cases. These securities typically offer high yields and have proven to be very attractive to fire and casualty companies, banks, and mutual funds. The federal government National Mortgage Association has similarly enabled hospitals to issue debt at reduced interest costs by reducing the riskiness of the security.

There are now an increasing number of private security brokers offering hospital securities. They have also helped hospitals to better tailor their debt to the needs of both the hospital and the lender. If the issue is large enough ($10 million or more) it will attract secondary market interest, which increases its liquidity and lowers its cost enough to make it competitive with other high-volume tax-exempt bonds (such as municipal bonds). The increased demand for debt financing has been matched by an enlarged infrastructure for the issuing of that debt. The result is a growth in debt financing that is continuing into the 1980s.

Financial Constraints on Hospitals Issuing Debt

As a hospital becomes highly levered it becomes increasingly susceptible to default. To protect themselves, lenders look at many financial indicators to determine the riskiness of a debt issue. Among these indicators are ratios such as debt to total capital, debt to total plant and equipment, and the debt service coverage ratio. A bond's rating reflects its riskiness and determines the interest rate which the borrower will have to pay (the higher the rating, the safer the investment and the lower the interest rate), is determined in large part by ratios such as these. Table 9.2 shows clearly how a bond rating is reflected by two of these ratios.

Increasingly, hospitals find lenders placing restrictions on hospital finances to insure against the possibility of default. Constraints are often placed on financial ratios such as those mentioned above. Even if the constraints are not explicit in the loan agreement, hospitals find that if their leverage position deteriorates the cost of new debt increases. Eventually lenders will refuse to purchase any debt as the investment becomes too risky.

Hospitals must maintain their financial stability, as reflected in their leverage and coverage ratios, if they are to continue to finance growth through debt. However, J. B. Silvers (1975) has shown that if other sources of capital remain scarce, maintaining ceilings on financial ratios can severely limit hospitals in their ability to grow. Yet, such ceilings may be the only way to insure the solvency of the hospitals.

**Table 9.2   Selected   Comparative   Statistics   for   1977–1979   Hospital   Revenue
Bond Issues Over $5 Million**

Constraint	*BBB/BBB+*	*A−*	*A*	*A+*	*AA−/AA*
Coverage of Maximum Debt Service	1.88×	1.87×	2.13×	2.70×	3.40×
Average Occupancy Rate (percent)	69.1	78.5	78.9	81.8	82.3
Average Number of Beds	150	202	286	448	831
Percentage of the Total Number of Hospital Bond Issues	13	30	23	23	8
Average Long-Term Debt to Total Capitalization (percent)	67.4	55.2	54.9	46.0	41.5
Operating Income (Net Income as a % of Gross Revenues)	5.4	4.4	4.6	4.7	4.9
Projected Future Operating Margin in the Feasibility Study (percent)	2.8	2.8	2.9	3.0	3.9
Market Acceptance Index[1]	1.26	1.22	1.17	1.14	1.08

SOURCE: Kidder-Peabody & Company, The Health Finance Group, Public Report: *Review of Health-Care Finance*, New York, 1980.

[1] Net interest cost of the hospital bond issue divided by the Bond Buyer's Index at the time of the bond issue; e.g., the lower the issue, the better the market acceptance of the issue.

Once a hospital has reached the limit of one of the constraints, it is possible to determine the maximum growth rate a hospital can maintain and still be within the constraint. This has been done before under some very limiting assumptions, but one can actually derive equations to solve for the maximum growth rate under more relaxed assumptions. We do assume that net income may be used to help meet capital requirements in the year it is earned. Additionally, we assume straight line relationships between revenue and the capital needed to generate that revenue and between net income and revenue. Under these two assumptions, it will be shown that in order to maintain a reasonable rate of capital expansion hospitals must rely on external sources of funds. The extent of this reliance on debt is determined largely by the hospital's ability to generate profits internally. The sensitivity of three key financial ratios to net income margin will be demonstrated in the next section.

How Financial Ratios May Restrict Hospital Growth

To demonstrate how a ceiling on the ratio of debt to total capital can restrict growth, consider the case of County General Hospital (CGH) currently operating with a debt/total capital ratio ceiling of 50 percent. CGH has a net income margin of 2 percent of revenues and requires $1.15 of capital investment (plant and equipment) and working capital to support each dollar of revenue. Under these conditions the hospital is constrained in the next year to a maximum growth rate in real dollar terms of 3.6 percent.

To see that this is so, let us say that CGH generates $1,000,000 in total revenues this year. Next year the hospital will generate total revenues of $1,036,000 (see Figure 9.1). Net income will be $20,720, which can be matched by $20,720 in new debt, maintaining the 50 percent debt/total capital ratio. The sum, $41,440 is exactly equal to (except for rounding off the growth rate) the additional working capital and capital investment required to generate the $36,000 of additional revenue. At higher growth rates the capital requirements exceed the total funds that can be obtained from debt and equity. The hospital would have to become more highly levered (issue more debt) to maintain a higher growth rate. At lower growth rates, the required new capital can be generated without reaching the debt financing limit.

A formal equation can be derived to calculate the maximum growth rate for any debt/total capital ratio. This equation can be used to see the effects each variable has on the growth rate.

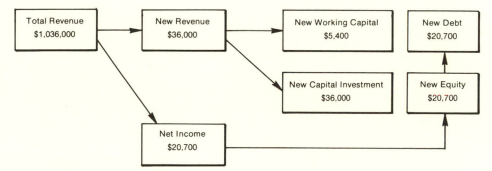

Figure 9.1 Capital Growth Under the Debt/Total Capital Restriction.

Table 9.3   Maximum Growth Rates Under Debt/Total Capital Restriction

	Net Income Margin				
Debt/Total Capital	*0%*	*1%*	*2%*	*3%*	*4%*
0.50	0	2	4	6	8
0.67	0	3	6	9	12
0.70	0	3	7	10	13
0.75	0	4	8	12	16
0.80	0	5	10	15	21
0.90	0	9	21	35	53

$$G = \text{maximum growth rate}$$
$$CI = \text{\$ of capital investment required to support \$1 of revenues}$$
$$WC = \text{\$ of working capital required to support \$1 of revenues}$$
$$X = \frac{\text{debt/total capital}}{1 - \text{debt/total capital}}$$
$$= \text{maximum debt/equity ratio}$$
$$M = \text{net income margin}$$
$$\text{funds generated by growth} = \text{funds required to support growth}$$
$$(1 + X)(M + G)(M) = (CI + WC)G$$
$$G = \frac{(X + 1)(M)}{(CI + WC) - M - (X)(M)}$$

Table 9.3 presents the maximum allowable growth rates for various values of debt/total capital and *M*. *CI* + *WC* is assumed to equal 1.15 for the purposes of these calculations. Higher values of *CI* and *WC* would result in lower maximum growth rates.

Debt/Plant Ratio

This second constraint limits hospital growth in much the same way as the first constraint. If CGH was at its debt/plant limit of 0.67 it would be restricted to a maximum growth of 4.3 percent next year. This can be seen in Figure 9.2. Here, CGH generates $43,000 in new revenues and requires $43,000 in new plant and equipment and $6,450 in new working capital to support this growth—a total cash requirement of $49,450. Net income of $20,860 is generated during the year, leaving the debt requirement at $28,590. This maintains exactly the 0.67 debt/plant ratio.

If the growth rate exceeded 4.3 percent, the additional debt re-

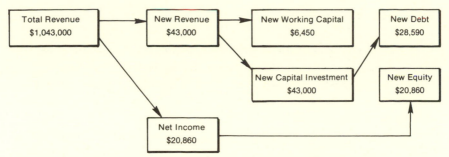

Figure 9.2 Hospital Growth Under the Debt/Plant Restriction.

quired to support operations would exceed 0.67 times the additional plant and equipment. A lower growth rate would reduce the debt requirement below the maximum allowable level. Again, we can derive an equation to determine the maximum growth rate for a hospital that has reached the limit of its debt/plant constraint.

$$G = \text{maximum growth rate}$$
$$CI = \text{\$ of capital investment required to support \$1 of revenue}$$
$$WC = \text{\$ of working capital required to support \$1 of revenue}$$
$$X = \text{maximum allowable debt/plant ratio}$$
$$M = \text{net income margin}$$
$$\text{funds generated by growth} = \text{funds required to support growth}$$
$$(CI)(X)(G) + M(1 + G) = (CI + WC)G$$

$$G = \frac{M}{(CI + WC) - (CI)(X) - M}$$

Table 9.4 presents the maximum growth rates for various values of X and M. $CI + WC$ is assumed to equal 1.15.

Table 9.4 Maximum Growth Rates Under Debt/Plant Restriction

Level of Constraint: Debt/Total	Net Income Margin				
	0%	1%	2%	3%	4%
0.67	0	2	4	7	9
0.70	0	2	5	7	10
0.75	0	3	5	8	11
0.80	0	3	5	8	13
0.90	0	4	9	14	19

Debt Service Coverage

It is reasonable to expect a lender to want some guarantee that a hospital will generate enough income during the year to repay principal and interest. The ability to repay principal and interest is reflected in the debt service coverage ratio. This is the ratio of the cash flow available to repay debt to the required debt payments. Specifically, the debt service coverage ratio equals:

$$\frac{\text{Net Income} + \text{Depreciation} + \text{Interest}}{\text{Interest} + \text{Principal Payments}}$$

Depreciation is added because it is a non-cash charge on the income statement.

Typically this ratio is required to be at least 1.0 to 1.5 with higher coverage ratios being more restrictive to the use of debt. Suppose CGH has a required margin of 1.50. Depreciable life on new capital investments at CGH averages twenty years and any new debt would be paid back in equal principal payments over twenty years. If the current interest rate on debt is 10 percent, then it can be shown that the maximum allowable growth rate is just under 3.4 percent.

In this case, CGH would generate $34,000 in new revenues. This growth would require additional plant and equipment of $34,000, to be depreciated over twenty years at $1,700 per year. Additional working capital of $5,000 is needed as well. Net income for next year would be $20,680. Additional debt of $18,420 is required to support operations. The debt will be paid back in annual installments of $921. The first year's interest due is $1,842 and the total interest plus principal due in the first year is $2,763. We can now see that the coverage ratio will be maintained at 1.5.

Additional net income is $680. Depreciation is $1,700. Interest is $1,842. The sum is $4,222 which, except for rounding errors, is exactly 1.5 times the required interest and principal payments. Table 9.5 summarizes these figures. Again, faster growth would

Table 9.5   How County General Hospital Meets Its Debt Service Coverage Ratio

Cash Inflow	=	1.5 × Required Payments	
Additional Net Income	$ 680	Principal $ 920	
Additional Depreciation	1,700	Interest $1,842	
			$2,762
Interest	1,842		
	$4,222 = 1.5 × $2,762		

require additional debt and CGH would be unable to maintain its coverage ratio.

Deriving an equation to determine the maximum growth rate under various situations is a simple task. The final equation is presented below.

G = maximum allowable growth rate
CI = $ of capital investment required to support $1 of revenue
WC = $ of working capital required to support $1 of revenue
C = required coverage ratio
I = rate of interest on debt
RP = repayment period of principal
M = net income margin
DL = depreciable life of new plant and equipment
$G = [(C*M)/RP + (C*I*M) - (I*M)]/[((WC + CI)*C)/RP + ((WC + CI)*C*I) - M - (CI/DL) - ((WC + CI)*I)]$

Table 9.6 presents the maximum growth rates for coverage ratios of 1.25 and 1.5. As the coverage ratio approaches 1 the maximum allowable growth rate approaches infinity.

For the purposes of calculations for Table 9.7, working capital and capital investment needs are assumed to be $1.15 for each dollar of revenue. The repayment period on new debt is thirty years and the average depreciable life of new capital investment is twenty-five years. These are typical figures for most hospitals, although depreciable life in proprietary hospitals tends to be a bit shorter (twenty-three years) and depreciable life in voluntary hospitals tends to be longer (twenty-seven years).*

Table 9.6   Maximum Growth Rates Under Debt Service Constraint

Prevailing Interest Rates	1.25 Coverage Net Income Margin				1.50 Coverage Net Income Margin			
	0%	1%	2%	3%	0%	1%	2%	3%
6%	0%/yr	3%/yr	10%/yr	93%/yr	0%/yr	2%/yr	4%/yr	8%/yr
8%	0	2	7	24	0	1	3	7
10%	0	2	6	15	0	1	3	6
12%	0	2	5	11	0	1	3	5
14%	0	2	4	9	0	1	3	5
16%	0	2	4	8	0	1	3	5

* Unpublished data provided by the Capital Finance Division of the American Hospital Association.

Table 9.7   Maximum Growth for Different Capital Investment Requirements

CI	Maximum Growth
0.8	12%/year
0.9	10
1.0	8
1.1	7
1.2	6

Since interest is an allowable expense for cost-based reimbursement, the coverage ratio as normally calculated does not accurately reflect a hospital's ability to repay its debt. The figures used to calculate the coverage ratio should be the unreimbursable portion of the interest expense. Assume CGH has cash flows (which includes interest *expense*) of $20,000 and interest and principle payments of $15,000 or a coverage ratio of 1.33. If 50 percent of CGH's $5,000 in interest expense is reimbursed (because 50 percent of CGH's volume is reimbursed on a cost basis), then these figures should be adjusted to $17,500 [$20,000 − 0.5 (5,000)] in cash inflow and $12,500 [$15,000 − 0.5 (5,000)] in required debt service. The coverage ratio increases to 1.40. To calculate a maximum growth rate one can simply use I' instead of I in the given equation, where $I' = I \times$ (percentage volume not cost-based).

Under typical conditions, a hospital that has reached its debt ceiling and has a small net income margin will often be limited to an annual growth rate of 4 percent or less. For hospitals with a high percentage of revenues coming from cost-based sources the net income margin is often 1 percent or less. In the future these hospitals will find it increasingly difficult to generate new funds from any source.

Hospitals that are not presently near their debt capacity may find their leverage positions weakening quickly as growth continues unabated. For example, if CGH currently has a debt to total capital ratio of 0.5, annual revenue growth of 10 percent per year, and a net income margin of 2 percent, the debt to total capital ratio would increase to 0.67 in just nine years. If the debt/plant ratio is currently 0.5, then under these conditions this ratio would increase to 0.67 in just six years.

Sensitivity Analysis

The growth rates presented in Tables 9.3, 9.4, and 9.6 are sensitive to changes in each of the variables used to derive the rates. Tables 9.7–9.10 indicate how small changes in these variables can affect the maximum growth rate under the debt service coverage constraint, which is the constraint most sensitive to small changes in a hospital's finances. Unless otherwise indicated, the variables will be assumed to have the following values:

$$CI = \text{capital investment} = 1.00$$
$$WC = \text{working capital} = 0.15$$
$$DL = \text{depreciable life} = 25 \text{ years}$$
$$RP = \text{repayment period} = 30 \text{ years}$$
$$I = \text{interest rate} = 0.10$$
$$M = \text{net income margin} = 0.02$$
$$C = \text{required coverage ratio} = 1.25$$

The results in Tables 9.7 and 9.8 indicate that small changes in the capital investment and working capital requirements can lead to

Table 9.8   Maximum Growth for Different Working Capital Requirements

WC	Maximum Growth
0.10	10%/year
0.15	8
0.20	7
0.25	6

Table 9.9   Maximum Growth for Different Depreciable Lives of New Assets

DL	Maximum Growth
20 years	20%/year
23	10
25	8
27	6

Table 9.10   Maximum Growth for Different Repayment Periods of Debt

RP	Maximum Growth
20 years	4%/year
23	5
27	7
30	8

pronounced changes in the constraint on growth. Increasing efficiency through better working capital management and general productivity increases can greatly reduce a hospital's dependence on
debt.

Tables 9.9 and 9.10 demonstrate that long repayment periods for
debt issues and a short depreciable life for new assets will place the
least short-term financial strain on the institution. However, over
the life of the debt these conditions may be more restrictive than
typical conditions would be.

Philanthropic donations can improve a hospital's leverage position
slightly. A hospital that receives enough donations to fund 10 percent of total capital expansion may increase its maximum annual
growth rate by as much as a full percentage point or more, depending on the other variables.

Finally, these conditions assume level principal payments. If loans
are paid back through level debt service (principal plus interest)
instead, then the loan would prove less constrictive to growth in the
first few years but would be more constrictive in the last few years of
the debt. This is due to the different timing of the cash flows associated with each method of repayment.

Feasibility Studies

Many analysts claim that the hospital sector has reached the limits of
its debt capacity, and will reach a point in the early 1980s when it is
unable to generate enough capital to meet demand (Grimmelman,
1980). However, such analysis ignores the subtle difference between
sufficient resources to meet capital maintenance and sufficient resources to meet the physicians' goal of capital improvement. In other
words, a national policy for cost containment might involve limiting
the ability of hospitals to expand or improve their capital position
and perhaps constrain their ability to maintain the high current
levels of fixed capital assets. A number of studies in the United
States (Fuchs, 1974b) and England (Cullis *et al.*, 1979) have argued
that erosion of hospital capital will have negligible effect on quality,
availability of non-elective care, and health status indices of the
population. If hospitals do not cut back on their capital demands in
the 1980s, they may face financial disasters if the Health Systems
Agency that approved their ten-year depreciable investment in 1980
decides that the capital asset is inappropriate and not eligible for

reimbursement in 1984. Proponents of cost containment cannot hope that prohibitively expensive interest rates will curtail costs when interest expense remains a 100 percent reimbursable item. However, rising interest rates will have some downward effect on the supply of loans available to the overregulated non-profit hospital sector if we can trust the recent congressional testimony of the investment banking community. The issue of the credit worthiness of the hospital sector will recur frequently during the 1980s.

Federal issuing agencies, institutional lenders, and bond rating agencies must evaluate the credit worthiness of the institution through quantitative measures (financial ratio analysis) and qualitative (such as community support volunteers) criteria. The obvious objective of the credit analysis is to establish whether the borrower can generate sufficient cash flows to service its debt requirements and meet other financial obligations. As President Nixon contracted the Hill-Burton program and encouraged private borrowing, the hospital feasibility study developed as the document to assess credit worthiness. Such studies were first used in the mid-1970s by state and municipal authorities monitoring bond issues.

The early feasibility studies were technically unsophisticated and offered only a few key financial ratios concerning the ability of a hospital to retire debt. The reports prepared by consultants in the 1978–1981 period offered a more comprehensive economic and financial forecast. Good feasibility reports focus on the cash-generating capacity of the hospital and estimate the adequacy of cash flows in meeting a hospital's stated financial obligations. Underwriters utilize the information to evaluate the proposed financing structure, to review the desirability of certain indenture terms, and to evaluate the appropriateness of the amount to be borrowed. Rating agencies such as Standard and Poor's or Moody's use feasibility reports in the evaluation of credit worthiness, and designate ratings that represent an assessment of the perceived quality and risk of a proposed bond issue.

The most important element of a feasibility study is the financial ratio analysis section. Many ratio analysis comparisons among hospitals have been performed. Cleverly and Nilsen (1980) and Caruana and McHugh (1980) categorized ratios into the following areas: liquidity, receivables, capital asset and equity ratios, operating ratios, and a hospital viability index. One should note that any single ratio is insufficient to assess the financial condition of an institution. At the very minimum it is necessary to review a group of ratios to make any sort of a reliable forecast of financial position and credit standing. Hospitals would be well advised to go beyond this single variable approach, whereby they consider changes in one ratio over time or relative to other hospitals. The superior alternative is to simultaneously consider the patterns in changes of a number of ratios over time. This approach has been labeled a multi-discriminant analysis methodology by Altman (1977). This method of multi-discriminant profile analysis reduces a number of problems of misclassification encountered in simple comparisons of single ratios.

Multi-Hospital Systems and Leasing Alternatives

Health economists have long complained about the lack of competition and the lack of an exit phenomenon for inefficient hospitals (Enthoven, 1980). The dual scourge of a limited payer definition of allowable costs and limited debt capacity might force some hospitals to exit into bankruptcy. The problems with this unplanned "solution" is that the beds might not close in the overbedded areas, and the private money markets that now fuel three-quarters of hospital capital projects might severely contract the availability of funds. The investment banking community frequently testified before Congress in 1979 and 1980 that they consider hospitals too much of an over-regulated credit risk to continue funding the present high debt capacity levels unless the federal government will be the receiver of each bankrupt facility and accept responsibility as the lender of last resort.

There are ways for hospitals to cope with the future limits on the availability of capital. Two frequently utilized strategies are sharing and leasing. The multi-hospital systems approach to health services management is potentially an effective structure if economies of scale can be captured by pooling financial resources and decreasing the duplication of services and facilities. In addition, multi-hospital systems make it feasible to hire more sophisticated management and offer an atmosphere conducive to long-range planning. These aspects of multi-institutional systems combine to raise credit ratings, decrease interest costs, and thus make capital financing less expensive and more feasible. The competitive financial advantages of multi-institutional systems in the 1980s may contribute more to the regionalization of health care than Health Systems Agencies.

Most analysts agree that multi-hospital systems will control 50 percent of the hospital beds by 1985 (Brown and McCool, 1980). Presently, more than 75 percent of all hospitals have entered into agreements whereby the costs of one or more pieces of equipment and the revenues generated are shared by two or more institutions (Rice, 1979). As new technologies continue to appear and hospitals are less able to fund them alone we can expect to see many more such sharing agreements. However, the capital financing repercussions of this trend are hard to predict. If most of the growth continues among investor-owned multi-hospital systems, the proprietary incentive often favors buying and equity financing. However, if most of the growth in the 1980s is in non-profit systems, leasing might become a more prevalent capital financing option.

Leasing of equipment can reduce the immediate drain on funds associated with a major purchase. Often overall costs are even reduced as the hospital takes advantage of the economies realized by the leasing firm (Guy, 1976). Current tax law encourages leasing by third parties to non-profit organizations in the following way. A vendor sells capital equipment to a proprietary intermediary. The intermediary gets the benefit of the investment tax credit and accelerated depreciation and is able to lease to the non-profit organization at a reduced price. The non-profit organization benefits from this reduced price, whereas it would reap no benefit from buying the equipment itself, as the investment tax credit is worthless to an organization that does not pay taxes. In the case of hospitals, leasing provides additional advantages in the form of: (1) a hedge against technological obsolescence; (2) an alternative source of funding when debt or equity funding is unavailable; (3) faster reimbursement; (4) better service. The financial aspects of leases will be discussed in Chapter 10, as well as the comparative advantages and disadvantages of leasing over purchasing.

Ironically, tax law has discouraged the formation of potentially cost-saving multi-hospital systems. Section 502 of the Internal Revenue Code makes it difficult for a shared service organization to qualify as a non-profit institution (Walker and Berry, 1980). According to the Code, an organization generating profit in a business or trade may not qualify for tax-exempt status on the grounds that all of its profits are returned to organizations that are exempt from tax. Section 501(e) was subsequently intended to provide exemption for cooperative hospital systems; however, the elaborate system of allocating net profits through paper dividends works to the disadvantage of the hospitals' reimbursement position.

Policy Implications

Hospitals turned to debt financing because it was cheap and because other sources of funding had disappeared. As hospitals become more and more highly levered new debt issues will be perceived as being more and more risky. Interest rates will increase, increasing the cost of debt. Much of this increase will be passed along to consumers through reimbursement mechanisms, but hospitals will have to shoulder a lot of the burden themselves.

Hospitals that have small net income margins must become highly levered in order to maintain growth rates above 4 or 5 percent annually. Yet in recent years hospitals have been growing at rates in excess of 10 percent annually (American Hospital Association, 1980). Hospitals that have been unable to generate funds internally have brought themselves to the brink of default. This problem has been most acute in New York City, and the New York experience may foreshadow the problems many more hospitals will have to face during the 1980s.

Interest on debt and foregone interest on expended equity must be treated in the same fashion when being recognized as allowable or non-allowable costs. It would be unwise to suddenly disallow all interest costs, as this is a large expense for many hospitals. However, disallowing interest costs on new debt would serve to reduce overall growth and especially to reduce the use of debt.

Simple cost reimbursement forces hospitals to operate at a break-even level unless they can increase charges to self-payers. Hospitals that rely heavily on cost-reimbursed patients must operate at net income margins of 1 percent or less. Even a small increase in profit margin above 1 percent can greatly reduce a hospital's dependence on debt. Indeed, administrators of the New York City hospitals that have gone bankrupt blame Medicaid and Blue Cross rates for their financial woes.

The Congress has recently considered a number of revenue cap proposals for the hospital industry. President Carter proposed a revenue cap allowing for a maximum annual growth rate of 9.7 percent.* A similar revenue ceiling of 10.9 percent was a fundamental part of Senator Kennedy's Cost Control Proposal (S.570, 1979). A clear danger in the proposed ceilings is the possibility that some hospitals will be unable to maintain a reasonable income margin. To

---

* The Carter proposal also included a nationwide cap on capital expenditures equal to approximately half the current level of capital spending.

insure against this, the base values for calculating annual revenue ceilings should allow for a small but significant profit margin. We have seen that a 3 percent margin would be enough to reduce the case study hospitals' dependence on debt. Ceilings fixed in this manner would not only remove the incentives for excessive growth but also would allow that growth to be largely equity-financed. The three important financial ratios considered herein do not define all conditions necessary to determine the correct operating margin for assuring the hospital sector of adequate private market financing. For example, the definition of an adequate operating margin will vary among hospitals as a function of size and ownership. It could be argued that the 3 percent operating margin suggested for the 200-bed case study hospital is niggardly for a 1,000-bed university medical center. Obviously, differences among hospitals do affect their capital needs and, consequently, the "correct" operating margins sufficient to freeze or reduce the amount of capital that is debt financed.

In drawing comparisons between the degree of regulatory involvement in the hospital industry and public utilities, one encounters two important differences. First, the degree of regulatory involvement in hospitals is less rigid, more variable across state lines and Blue Cross catchment areas, and is handled in an illogical fashion that can best be described as muddling through. Consequently, the hospital sector has the benefit of being less regulated than most public utilities. Second, the *ad hoc* swings in the reimbursement rules have prevented many hospitals from preserving their capital purchasing power to anywhere near the degree that public utilities are allowed in order to assure future operations. In summary, hospitals have not received the same basic treatment that we accord to other highly regulated utility industries. The industry should improve financial management techniques and the government should allow reimbursement of a capital maintenance factor or incorporate price-level depreciation. These issues will be discussed in further depth in the next chapter. The dependence on debt financing will increase if the third-party payers continue to prevent an adequate return on equity, fail to adjust depreciation schedules in line with inflation, and pay for only a miserly share of bad-debt cases.

Conclusions

For many hospitals the capital crisis is already here. For others, debt ceilings are just a few years away. These hospitals can improve their financial positions somewhat through sharing of equipment, leasing instead of buying outright, and general improvements in efficiency. The ultimate solution, however, rests on returning to a reimbursement system that recognizes reasonable growth as a legitimate cost of operating a hospital and provides a large enough income margin for hospitals to grow without an excessive dependence on debt financing.

The lack of a reimbursement multiplier to allow purchasing power of the fund balances to keep pace with inflation has always been a research problem in hospital cost accounting. From the limited sensitivity analysis, it has been suggested that a maintenance factor for capital replacement would require at least a 3 percent operating margin. In addition to the simple replacement concept of capital maintenance, society may wish to consider adding on a technological maintenance factor to assure that the hospital has funds for updating capital to keep pace with peer institutions. Given that medical technology is likely to be cost-increasing in the future, preservation of capital position implies both capital replacement and a capital improvement concept that keeps pace with new technology. Advocates of negative growth in the hospital industry may fight any reimbursement formula that explicitly recognizes the need to update hospital capital, but the institutional manager can ill afford to count on hopes for a resurrected Hill-Burton program to finance new technology and plant modernization.

References

ALTMAN, E. (1978). "Financial Ratios, Discriminant Analysis, and the Prediction of Corporate Bankruptcy," *Journal of Finance* 23:4 (September), 589–607.

American Hospital Association (1980). *Hospital Statistics 1979*. Chicago, Ill.: AHA.

BROWN, M., and MCCOOL, B. (1980). *Multihospital Systems*. Germantown, Md.: Aspen Systems.

CARUANA, R., and MCHUGH, T. (1980). "Comparing Ratios Shows Fiscal Trends," *Hospital Financial Management* 10:1 (January), 12–28.

CLEVERLEY, W., and NILSEN, K. (1980). "Assessing Financial Position with 29 Key Ratios," *Hospital Financial Management* 10:1 (January), 30–36.

Council of Economic Advisers (1980). *Economic Report of the President 1980*, including data from the American Hospital Association Annual Survey. Washington, D.C.: U.S. Government Printing Office.

CRAIG, J. (1978). "The Urban Fiscal Crisis in the United States, National Health Insurance and Municipal Hospitals," *International Journal of Health Services* 8:2 (Spring), 329–345.

CULLIS, J. G., FORSTER, D. P., and FROST, C. E. (1979). "Demand for Inpatient Treatment: Some Recent Evidence," *Applied Economics* 12:2 (December), 43–60.

ENTHOVEN, A. C. (1980). *Health Plan.* Reading, Mass.: Addison-Wesley.

FUCHS, V. (1974a). *Who Shall Live?* New York: Basic Books.

FUCHS, V. (1974b). "Some Economic Aspects of Mortality in Developing Countries," in M. Perlman (ed.), *The Economics of Health and Medical Care.* London: Macmillan.

GAUS, C., and COOPER, B. (1976). "Technology and Medicare: Alternatives for Change," Proceedings of the November 19–20 Conference on Health Care Technology and Quality of Care, Boston University Health Policy Center.

GRIMMELMAN, F. (1980). "Borrowing for Capital: Will It Empty Your Pockets?" *Hospital Financial Management* 6:12 (December), 19–25.

GUY, A. (1976). "Six Leasing Considerations," *Hospital Financial Management* 6:6 (June), 40–46.

HARRIS, J. (1977). "The Internal Organization of Hospitals: Some Economic Implications," *Bell Journal of Economics* 8:2 (Autumn), 467–482.

HEE, D., and HOWIE, C. (1980). "First-half Financing Up Despite High Interest Rates," *Hospital Financial Management* 10:11 (November), 28–37.

Institute of Medicine, National Academy of Sciences (1976). *Controlling the Supply of Hospital Beds.* Washington, D.C.: National Academy of Sciences.

Kidder-Peabody & Company, The Health Finance Group (1980). Public report: *Review of Health-Care Finance.* New York.

LEE, M. (1971). "A Conspicious Production Theory of Hospital Behavior," *The Southern Economic Journal* 20:7 (July), 48–61.

LIGHTLE, M. (1981). "Changes in The Sources of Capital," *Hospital Financial Management* 11:2 (February), 42–47.

LIGHTLE, M. (1980), "1970's See New Approaches to Capital Financing for Hospitals," *Hospitals,* 52:14 (July) 135–141.

MULLNER, R. (1980), "Hospital Trends in Construction Financing, Costs," *Hospitals* 54:11 (June) 59–62.

MULLNER, R., MATHEWS D., BYRE, C., and KUBAL, J. (1981). "Construction in U.S. Hospitals 1979: Costs and Sources of Funds," *Hospitals* 55:9 (May 1), 60–66.

RICE, J. (1979). "Voluntary, For-Profit Chains Differ on Shared Service, Consulting Strategies," *Modern Health Care* 16:5 (May), 72–76.

SILVERS, J. B. (1975). "How Do the Limits to Debt Financing Affect your Hospital's Financial Status?" *Hospital Financial Management* 5:2 (February), 32–41.

United States Congress, Office of Technology Assessment. (1980). *The Cost-Effectiveness of Medical Technologies,* Volume 2, "Methodology and Literature Review." Washington, D.C.: U.S. Government Printing Office.

WALKER, S., and BERRY, R. (1980). "Hospitals are Caught in the Regulatory Cross-ruff," *Hospitals* 53:12 (June), 74–76.

WILDAVSKY, A. (1977). "Doing Better and Feeling Worse: The Political Pathology of Health Policy," *Daedalus* 106:1 (Winter), 105–124.

Chapter 10

EVALUATION OF FINANCING ALTERNATIVES

We do not render service in order to collect money, but we must collect money in order to render service.

—Dr. Marcus Welby

Finance is somehow both the implicit culprit and the expected savior of an industry rapidly approaching bankruptcy. The health field, in large part, has been managed by professionals who often had a clear view of part of their external and internal environment without being able to relate these to financial realities.

—J. B. Silvers

Hospitals have an excessive reliance on debt relative to other sectors of the economy. Public utilities borrow on the average about 50 percent of total capitalizataion, and manufacturing firms about 30 percent. Hospital debt loads currently are in the 70–80 percent range. According to Kidder-Peabody and Company (1980), total debt offerings in the hospital industry increased from 2.2 billion dollars in 1974 to 12 billion in 1979. As sources of philanthropy and free Hill-Burton funds dramatically declined in the mid–1970s, one out of six hospitals planning a capital expansion or modernization were forced into the private debt markets.

This trend toward heavier debt financing has been encouraged by reimbursement formulas that include interest on debt as an allowable cost. Currently, Medicare, most Medicaid plans, and two thirds of the Blue Cross plans reimburse capital costs on the basis of historical cost depreciation. Most third-party payers have followed the lead of Medicare, which covers both depreciation on prior-approved capital expenditures and interest expense. However, debt principal payments, capital expenditures on replacement and expansion, and working capital are not reimbursable costs. This creates an incentive for hospitals to use debt financing rather than equity financing for major purchases, in order to preserve or minimize the erosion of their capital asset base.

The eight most frequently utilized debt instruments are: publicly sold tax-exempt revenue bonds; direct placement Farmers Home Administration (FHA) insured mortgage notes guaranteed by the Government National Mortgage Association (GNMA); direct placement of mortgage notes insured through FHA, Section 242; private placement of tax-exempt bonds; publicly sold mortgage notes; publicly sold (unsecured) direct obligation notes; private placement of mortgage notes; private placement of direct obligation notes. The particular benefits and costs of each debt method has been reviewed elsewhere (Berman and Weeks, 1979). For our purposes it is important to note at this juncture that the hospital industry might increasingly rely on leasing opportunities if the upper limits of debt capacity have been reached.

The Advantages of Leasing

The rapid development of new medical products in combination with consumer demands for more comprehensive insurance to cover the ever-expanding vista of medical technology has pressured hospital administrators to replace their equipment more frequently and at a higher cost. Most corporate financial analysts are shocked to learn that hospitals lease less than 10 percent of their capital equipment. Given the non-profit nature of more than 90 percent of the hospital industry, there are no tax incentives to discourage leasing and favor purchasing (see Chapter 9). The rule of thumb is that a non-profit firm should lease all or most of its equipment. The resistance of hospital administrators to considering new financing options or performing net present value (NPV) analysis is especially appalling given the high rate of medical technological obsolescence. For example, only 8 percent of a 1973 sample of large complex hospitals calculated the NPV of a project (Williams and Rakich, 1973).

The main advantage of lease financing is that it allows the health institution to be more flexible with regard to rapid technological changes in hospital equipment. The facility can lease equipment for the duration of the equipment's useful life, which is frequently less than the item's physical life. The possibility that the cost of future obsolescence will be built into the contract price is partly offset by the higher residual value the equipment may have for the leasing company, which has greater access to national resale markets.

Leasing is also attractive to the smart health facility administrator because of flexibility in financing. There is no requirement for a large initial payment. Moreover, even if the project is debt financed with low annual payments, the debt contract frequently involves restrictive clauses on future borrowing. Lease financing establishes a new line of credit that is useful as a supplemental financing source in times of high interest rates and limited borrowing opportunities. For example, leasing companies expanded following President Carter's May 1980 Executive Memorandum to all federal agencies asked for a moratorium on hospital bed construction and capital project financing in areas with more than 4.0 beds per thousand (the current national average is 4.5).

One indirect advantage of leasing is that the administrator may apply leverage on the leasing company, through future lease payment options, to force the lessee to provide better maintenance service. For example, hospital labs with leased equipment tend to have lower down-time and lower maintenance and repair costs.

Another advantage of leases is the treatment of lease costs by third-party payers.* By leasing, the hospital can utilize the services of the asset and be reimbursed for the periodic lease payments. When equipment is bought outright, straight-line depreciation is normally required. Thus, the early large cash inflows associated with reimbursement for accelerated depreciation are not realized. This is important in view of the increasingly high time value of money. Moreover, no third-party payers' reimbursement policies include full price adjustments for inflation over the economic life of the equipment. These negative effects of third-party reimbursement can be avoided when a true lease is used for financing.

There is one other potential reason why leasing may be financially

---

* Some state rate regulators in Massachusetts and New Jersey have argued that leasing should be discouraged, so as to force hospitals that have purchased equipment that became prematurely obsolete to suffer the full costs of their actions.

superior to buying. It is currently a moot point to argue whether tax concerns have favored lease or buy decisions. Some analysts argue that the for-profit lessor benefits from the ability to utilize accelerated depreciation and the investment tax credit (not available to non-profit institutions), and consequently passes on partial benefits (in the form of slightly lower lease payments) of this asymmetry in the tax treatment to the lessee's. On the other hand, some analysts have argued that the lessor simply charges an amount equal in present value terms to the cost of buying the equipment plus whatever taxes must be paid. This last scenario suggests that it would be financially advantageous for a tax-exempt lessee to buy rather than lease (and pay the lessor's taxes). There is clearly a need for future research to determine which of the two viewpoints is correct. Our intuition suggests that the former scenario may occur more frequently, especially in urban markets that have many competing medical leasing companies.

Capital Leases and Operating Leases

There are two types of leases from the standpoint of the lessee: operating leases and capital leases. A capital lease is viewed as a purchase agreement whereby the risks and benefits of ownership of the asset are transferred to the lessee. This type of lease is not cancellable and is fully amortized so the asset, and related debt, must be recorded on the balance sheet.

Under an operating lease, the risks and benefits of ownership are not transferred to the lessee and the payments under the lease contract are not sufficient to purchase the leased equipment. Thus an operating lease is not fully amortized and does not affect the balance sheet. Operating leases usually contain a cancellation clause and may call for the lessor to maintain and service the equipment.

Two organizations have attempted to classify leases according to whether the contract entered into is viewed as more of a purchase agreement or an actual lease/rental type of agreement. The relatively new FASB (Financial Accounting Standards Board) rule 13 distinguishes between a *capital* lease, which is a purchase agreement, and an *operating* lease, which is a rental agreement. On the other hand, the IRS uses the term *financial* lease to signify a purchase, and *true* lease to signify a lease agreement. However, be-

Exhibit 10.1

FASB Criteria for a Capital Lease (Financial Accounting Standard 13)

  i. Ownership is transferred to the lessee by the end of the lease term.

 ii. The lease contains a bargain purchase option.

iii. The lease term is equal to 75% or more of the estimated economic life of the leased property.

iv. The present value at the beginning of the lease term of the minimum lease payments equals or exceeds 90% of the excess of the fair value of the leased property over any related investment tax credit retained by the lessor.

IRS Criteria for a Financial Lease (Rule 55-540)

  i. The lessee will acquire title upon payment of a stated amount of "rentals" under the contract, i.e., portions of periodic payments are used to establish an equity position to be acquired by the lessee.

 ii. The "rental" payments materially exceed the current fair rental value, which indicates that the payments include an element other than compensation for the use of property.

iii. The total amount which the lessee is required to pay for a relatively short period of use constitutes an inordinately large proportion of the total sum required to be paid to secure transfer of title.

iv. Some portion of the periodic payment is specifically designated as interest or is otherwise readily recognizable as the equivalent of interest.

 v. The property may be acquired under a purchase option at a price which is nominal in relation to the value of the property at the time when the option may be exercised, as determined at the time of entering into the original agreement, or which is a relatively small amount when compared with the total payments which are required to be made.

---

cause the FASB is more stringent in their criteria, it is possible for a *capital* lease by FASB standards to be classified as a *true* lease by the IRS (Exhibit 10.1). This inconsistency on the part of the two agencies has led to some confusion in reimbursement by cost-based third-party payers.

The FASB standards must be used for financial statement reporting purposes. However, for third-party reimbursement purposes (Blue Cross and Medicare) the IRS standards are usually applied. If a contract qualifies as a true lease, the rental payments may be expensed on a periodic basis. If the contract is considered to be a purchase agreement (or conditional sale), the allowable expenses are interest and depreciation, as period costs.

Reimbursement

Current reimbursement policy among third-party payers favors true leases over capital leases if revenue maximization is the objective. The capital lease is treated in a fashion similar to debt, with allowable costs being determined for depreciation and interest in a fashion that may not reflect the full costs of the contract.

Medicare and most third-party reimbursement schemes create a disincentive for capital leasing by not allowing the depreciation of an asset below its estimated salvage value, and limiting historical cost to the lower of fair market value or purchase at the current cost of replacement (adjusted only by straight-line depreciation and pro-rated over the useful life of the asset). On the other hand, a contract defined as a true lease allows full reimbursement of both operating costs and the entire lease payment. Consequently, true leases give full reimbursement for the current costs of ownership. As a rule, most third-party payers follow the lead of Medicare in creating incentives that favor leasing over purchase. If the machine is purchased with either debt or equity capital, third-party payers reimburse a hospital for depreciation and operating costs. When the machine is financed by debt, hospitals are additionally reimbursed for interest. Depreciation is usually done by the straight-line method, although Medicare and most Medicaid plans will allow a financially troubled hospital to use a declining-balance method of determining depreciation as long as it does not exceed 150 percent of the straight-line method. For most movable scientific equipment, the life of the asset as established by the American Hospital Association is assessed as eight to ten years.

An unanticipated consequence of FASB rule 13 was that hospitals were subsequently required to submit leases with discounted (at 10 percent) present values of over $100,000 to the Certificate-of-Need and Section 1122 review process (Horwitz, 1979). If the institution fails to receive dual regulatory approval for the equipment, the hospital loses the reimbursement for imputed depreciation and interest expenses for the capital lease. Moreover, Medicare has "an unnecessary borrowing" provision which, if applied to include capital leases in the 1980s, could require that the hospital use all unrestricted liquid assets, including future capital expansion funds, to reduce the amount of the debt lease.

Fortunately for the hospital industry, most third-party payers and

Medicaid plans have been slow to adopt the four FASB criteria. Consequently, if the lease is defined as a true lease in the reimbursement contracts, the total rental payment is fully expensed on a period basis, even if the lease is classified as a capital lease for FASB reporting purposes. However, the FASB criteria are being adopted, and interpreted in a less flexible fashion, by third-party payers concerned with cost containment. What previously passed as a true lease contract allowing for transfer of ownership title at a nominal fee, in violation of FASB criteria two, is increasingly being appropriately labeled as a variant of the capital lease known as a conditional sales contract or financial lease. If an institution selects a capital lease, they should require the lessor to explicitly document the interest charges implicit in the lease. The hospital would then have a point of defense against the third-party payer that attempts to impute unfairly low interest costs.

Potential Changes in Reimbursement Incentives

Cleverley (1979) has suggested two interesting alternatives to the currently popular method of treating depreciation. The first alternative Cleverley suggests is a form of replacement cost depreciation (RCD) with debt financing adjustment. In the case of RCD, debt financing adjustment, it is assumed that third-party payers will reimburse totally for the debt service costs, both principal and interest. In addition, replacement cost depreciation will be reimbursed, but not totally. The amount of allowed reimbursement will equal replacement cost depreciation times the desired proportion of equity financing, for example, a target proportion of 0.20 in each of the ten years. This would stimulate containment of total capital financing costs, since debt would be used to supplement somewhat lower levels of reimbursement. The use of a given proportion of debt is desirable because the non-profit hospitals can take advantage of the availability of lower tax-exempt interest rates. Moreover, the hospital can adjust the desired equity financing ratio to suit its financial needs. In the example provided by Cleverley, the target proportion of 0.20 over ten years resulted in an effective 0.016 decline in the proportion at the end of the period. This decline occurred because the inflation rate was 2 percent higher than the presumed investment income rate. Thus, one disadvantage of this RCD alternative is that if surplus reimbursement funds cannot be invested at a rate of return greater than or equal to the inflation rate, the targeted equity ratio would have to be continually increased to achieve the desired target ratio.

The second practical alternative suggested by Cleverley is an annuity deposit. Under this method, the amount of equity financing necessary to purchase replacement equipment can be accumulated over the life of the present asset. This would allow for replacement of equipment while minimizing financial incentives for over-capitalization. A third alternative is to allow a capital maintenance factor in the reimbursement formulas, that is, a fixed percentage levied against all patients to finance the maintenance of equivalent state-of-the-art equipment and plant assets. This percentage surcharge might range from 3 to 5 percent.

One infrequently mentioned advantage of total replacement cost depreciation, or price-level depreciation, is that it reduces the long-term cost of services to the public. In basic economic terms, future capital funds are best held in the hands of the institution that can earn a higher rate of return on the investment over time. The average hospital, because it is a large, non-profit firm, can earn a rate of return on its investments that is typically more than 4 percentage points higher than the average individual, whom we shall call John Q. Public. To make this point clear, let us consider the hypothetical example of a hospital that must replace a piece of equipment in the diagnostic radiology department in five years. The original equipment costs $500,000 in year zero (1980). The equivalent state-of-the-art replacement appreciates in value at the rate of 15 percent per year, and will cost $1,006 thousand ($1.006 million) in 1985. At the end of the time period the hospital can finance the new equipment in one of two ways: (1) historical cost depreciation of $100,000 per year for five years with a bonus to make up the difference from the rate setters in year 5 (this bonus is called the Planned Capital Service Component in some states), or (2) allow price-level depreciation (with cash inflows of $115,000, $132,000, $152,000, $175,000, and $201,000 for the five years, to net, after adding in the accumulated interest at 12 percent per year from the depreciation fund, a total of $1,006 thousand).

In the first case the control over the equity of the institution is effectively out of the hands of the trustees and vested under the control of the rate commission. If the hospital receives $100,000 each year for five years and earns 12 percent annual interest on those funds, they will accrue $635,285 at the end of the period (1985). The

differential between replacement costs and accumulated depreciation funds ($370,715) will have to be paid by the consumers in the
form of increased rates. If the public had to budget for that difference over the same five-year period, earning 8 percent per
annum on the funds, John Q. Public would collectively have to save
$63,191 per year for five years to finance the $370,715. However, if
hospitals were reimbursed on the basis of price-level depreciation,
they could invest the funds at 12 percent interest, and need save
only $58,354 per year for the five years to achieve the $370,715 at
the end of 1985. Consequently, it is $31,002 less expensive (future
value of savings in 1986, discounted at 12 percent) in the long run for
consumers to keep the funds in the hands of the hospital, rather than
under-reimburse the hospital and pay out the bonus differential
($370,715) in year 5.

Some cynics argue that politicians support rate setting commissions because they do apparently save money in the short term,
irrespective of whether they are perhaps inflationary in the long run.
Supporters of rate regulation and planning argue that society could
save money in the long run if they could only force some hospitals
not to purchase replacement equipment. The econometric results
reported in Chapter 8 indicate that planners have not been successful in curtailing the hospital sectors annual growth in assets. Consequently, one might advocate cost containment and still question
the wisdom of a regulatory system that treats hospital management
like a beggar with a tin cup, where the government rate commission
has the right to determine how full the cup should be. Allowing the
hospital a return on equity capital is more efficient than letting the
government arbitrarily decide how much each hospital deserves and
when it should receive the funds.

Blue Cross plans in six states and one state rate commission currently recognize some form of price-level depreciation. There is an
irony that the one state government (New Jersey) that is progressive
concerning the need for inflation-adjusted depreciation has become
equally regressive in disallowing reimbursement for future lease
contracts. Price-level depreciation is currently being implemented
as part of the New Jersey DRG experiment. Major equipment acquired since 1970 is adjusted to 1979 base year prices, and then
successively inflated annually according to national price increases.
Each New Jersey hospital is allowed a sinking fund for accumulating
annually 10 percent of the price level depreciable value of the
equipment. The New Jersey rate experiment explicitly discourages

both leasing and borrowing in future capital decisions. Future lease contracts in New Jersey will not be reimbursed by cost payers in 1981–1982. Fortunately, the climate for reimbursement of leases is much better in other states.

The Financial Cost of Leasing

Leases are not always a cost-beneficial mode of capital financing. One common misconception about leasing is that it conserves capital. For example, the lease payments are frequently larger than the combined principal and interest payments on debt necessary to buy equipment, especially in Southern states where leasing companies have a natural monopoly. Henry and Roenfeldt (1978) report that the majority of hospital financial managers did not know how to correctly determine the charges associated with leasing. Lack of financial expertise did not inhibit the estimated doubling in assets leased by the hospital sector from 1975–1978 (Standard and Poors, 1978). Hospital financial managers should force leasing company representatives to break out the costs that can be expensed rather than capitalized. Such costs include service arrangements, shipping and installation charges, training, and supply fees.

Another common misconception among hospital managers is that leasing has an intrinsic cash-flow timing advantage. However, some lease contracts require the institution to borrow a sum (for security purposes) in advance, which is comparable to a loan repayable in arrears in annual installments. Consequently there is no cash-flow advantage to a leasing agreement if correctly compared to a loan of equivalent interest cost and a comparable schedule for repayment. The one advantage that leasing has over purchasing is that the interest costs are typically one or two percentage points lower. Probably, the most widely held misconception concerning leasing is that it represents an undetected mode of debt financing, hidden from regulatory oversight. The hidden debt argument is at best cosmetic, and at worst a zero-sum manipulation in that neither the asset, nor the future liability for the lease payments, appear on the balance sheet.

Another unanticipated side effect of defining true leases as capital leases is that a number of the financial ratios used to assess the credit worthiness of the facility deteriorate. If the debt ratio or interest coverage ratio diminishes, then the hospital's bond rating deteriorates, causing the public to pay for incrementally higher interest rates on future capital purchases. We have reviewed the subject of credit ratings and the limits of debt financing in Chapter 9.

Claims by lessors that leasing rates are lower than borrowing rates are not always valid. For example, miscellaneous leasing charges can significantly increase the effective interest rate over the quoted rate for the term of the lease. Leases often include hidden charges such as late payment penalties. The calculated salvage value of the asset also affects the effective interest rate. This means that careful analysis of the net present cost (NPC) of a lease must be carried out to find the effective rate of interest, in order to compare this mode of financing with other alternatives.

Net Present Cost Analysis of Leasing, Debt Financing, and Equity Financing Alternatives

There are no simple rules to suggest one form of financing is uniformly superior to another. For example, leases are purported to transfer the risk of medical equipment obsolescence to the leasing firm. However, the hospital could carry 110 percent (or 90 percent) of the risk in the form of higher (or lower) than "fair" lease payment terms. One cannot adopt a simple decision rule, such as "purchasing is best because it adds to the hospital's asset base on the balance sheet." Capital leases also add to the asset base, and the asset base is not critical by itself (that is, increases in assets are offset by increases in long-term debt on the same balance sheet).

In the following example, we consider four modes of financing a $100,000 blood analyzer. We assume that the hospital's objective function is to minimize the net present cost to the institution. One way to do this, although not the only way, is by selecting the method of financing that maximizes reimbursement from third-party payers. One could also minimize net present cost (NPC) by selecting the alternative that has a lower present cost because it had a lower initial cost, whether or not it had higher reimbursement. The net present cost estimates that we derive are sensitive to discount rates, interest rates, the time span of the lease or loan, the size of the down payment, the percentage of cost-based reimbursement, and the estimated salvage value.

In considering the cash flows for the four financing options in Tables 10.1 and 10.2, we have assumed that the hospital uses straight-line depreciation. The blood analyzer is assumed to have a

Table 10.1   Net Present Cost Calculations with an 8 Percent Discount Rate

	A *True* *Lease*[1]	B *Debt* *Financing*[2]	C *Capital* *Lease*[3]	D *Equity* *Financing*
1. Principal Payments	—	73,680	—	—
2. Interest Payments	—	49,348	—	—
3. Maintenance (at $2000/yr.)	—	7,985	7,985	7,985
4. True Lease Payments	112,115	—	—	—
5. Capital Lease Payments	—	—	108,496	—
6. Cash Purchase	—	—	—	100,000
Net Outlay	112,115	131,013	116,481	107,985
7. Reimbursement for Depreciation (years 1–5)[4]	—	22,459	22,459	22,459
8. Capital Asset[5] Write-off ($50,000)[6]	—	19,141	19,141	19,141
9. Reimbursement for Maintenance (at 75%)	—	5,989	5,989	5,989
10. Reimbursement for Interest (at 75%)	—	37,011	16,566	—
11. Reimbursement of True Lease (at 75%)	84,086	—	—	—
Net Reimbursement	84,086	84,600	64,155	47,587
12. NPC without Salvage Value	28,029	46,413	52,326	60,396
Ranking	1	2	3	4
13. Salvage Value ($25,000)	—	17,015	17,015	17,015
14. NPC with Salvage Value	28,029	29,398	35,311	43,381
Ranking	1	2	3	4

[1] $26,000 per year for five years (includes maintenance, service, and insurance). The FASB term is operating lease.
[2] 15 percent interest and 20 percent down-payment.
[3] 13 percent interest, five equal payments of $25,160.58 per year. The IRS term is financial lease.
[4] ($75,000 ÷ 5) × 0.75 = $5,625 per year for 5 years.
[5] The asset is not fully depreciated at the time at which the useful life of the asset expires, so the remaining value of the asset must be written off.
[6] $7,500 × 5 × 0.75 = $28,125.

useful life of five years and a book life of ten years. The debt financing option calls for a $20,000 down payment, payments on principal of $8,000 per year for ten years, and an interest rate of 15 percent.

In the case of both the capital and true (operating) leases, the lease contract is for a period of five years. The payment is at the beginning of the year for both leases. An interest rate of 13 percent is implicit

Table 10.2   Net Present Cost Calculations with a 12 Percent Discount Rate

	A *True* *Lease*[1]	B *Debt* *Financing*[2]	C *Capital* *Lease*[3]	D *Equity* *Financing*
1. Principal Payments	—	65,202	—	—
2. Interest Payments	—	43,496	—	—
3. Maintenance (at $2000/yr.)	—	7,209	7,209	7,209
4. True Lease Payments	104,971	—	—	—
5. Capital Lease Payments	—	—	101,582	—
6. Cash Purchase	—	—	—	100,000
Net Outlay	104,971	115,907	108,791	107,209
7. Reimbursement for Depreciation (years 1–5)[4]	—	20,277	20,277	20,277
8. Capital Asset Write-off ($50,000)[5]	—	15,959	15,959	15,959
9. Reimbursement for Maintenance (at 75%)	—	5,407	5,407	5,407
10. Reimbursement for Interest (at 75%)	—	32,622	15,425	—
11. Reimbursement of True Lease (at 75%)	78,728	—	—	—
Net Reimbursement	78,728	74,265	57,068	41,643
12. NPC without Salvage Value	26,243	41,642	51,723	65,566
Ranking	1	2	3	4
13. Salvage Value ($25,000)	—	14,186	14,186	14,186
14. NPC with Salvage Value	26,243	27,456	37,537	51,380
Ranking	1	2	3	4

[1] $26,000 per year for five years (includes maintenance, service, and insurance).
[2] 15 percent interest and 20 percent down-payment.
[3] 13 percent interest, five equal payments of $25,160.58 per year.
[4] ($75,000 ÷ 5) × 0.75 = $5,625 per year for 5 years.
[5] $7,500 × 5 × 0.75 = $28,125.

in the capital lease and the bargain purchase option (nominal $1) is exercised.

The reimbursement rate for the following example is taken as 75 percent; 75 percent of patients are cost-payers covering three-quarters of allowable costs. This reimbursement rate is assumed to be constant over the ten-year period. A 75 percent reimbursement rate is considered appropriate, as the fraction of charge-based payers has declined from 50 percent to 25 percent for the typical American hospital in the last decade.

Given these assumptions, the true lease* is the best alternative given a discount rate of either 8 percent or 12 percent, and with or without salvage value. However, it is important to remember that the choice of alternative is sensitive to the assumptions that were made at the beginning. For example, debt financing can be brought into parity with the true lease option if the interest charge were to decrease relative to the discount rate by more than 2–3 percentage points. Likewise, debt would be the preferred option if the salvage value were to increase to more than $28,000 or 28 percent, or if the down payment were 10 percent or less given a 25 percent salvage value. In addition, the time span of the loan or lease and the reimbursement rate will each affect the choice of financing method.

In this example capital leases were assumed to have a 13 percent interest rate; however, such leases are not competitive with true leases or debt financing even if the interest rate is dropped substantially. Capital leases are basically debt financing with a higher down payment (in this example). Thus capital leases are intermediate between equity and debt financing, because as the down payment increases, reimbursement for interest decreases. Why then do so many hospitals currently hold capital leases? Their popularity is largely due to clever marketing efforts on the part of leasing companies who are able to obscure the actual cost of the lease by quoting low interest rates and then adding on miscellaneous charges. It may also be that hospitals that cannot obtain debt financing go instead with a capital lease. Prior to the adoption of FAS 13 in 1977, hospitals had the cosmetic advantage that the debt incurred through a capital lease did not affect their financial ratios; however, this is no longer the case.

A number of factors have been ignored in this simple analysis. The really crucial decision might not be how to finance the $100,000 blood analyzer, but rather: "Shall we purchase the new blood analyzer under any conditions?" The answer to this question is normally "yes" if the net present value is greater than zero, or if the net present cost is less than zero. In the example above, any income streams associated with the purchase of the blood analyzer have not been considered, other than the cash inflows associated with 75 percent cost-based reimbursement. If such income is considered, a

---

* Discounted at the incremental borrowing rate of 15 percent, the true lease meets the requirements of having a net present value of less than 90 percent of the fair value of the equipment if $2666 per year is allocated for maintenance, insurance, and service (as required under FAS 13).

net present cost of less than zero is required if a decision to purchase the machine is to be made on purely financial grounds.

The choice of discount rate is critical in determining the net present cost or net present value of a proposal. There are two factors to consider when determining the appropriate discount rate: the cost of funds and the yield from alternative uses of the funds. The correct figure to use depends on where the money is coming from. If equity is being spent (anything that is not debt), then the appropriate discount rate is the return from the best alternative use of the funds (including depositing the money in a bank). If the money is obtained via a debt issue, then the appropriate discount rate for evaluating a specific project is the borrowing rate or the rate of return for the best alternative use of funds, whichever is higher. If the rate of return for the best alternative project and the rate of return on the proposed project both exceed the borrowing rate, then both projects should be completed if enough money can be borrowed (otherwise do the one with the higher NPV).

Miller (1979) argues that a complete financial analysis should include a multivariate sensitivity analysis for a range of interest rates, purchase functions, lease cost functions, salvage values, and discount rates. Burns and Bindon (1980) have pointed out the potential for linear programming applications in buy–lease decisions. However, these models are severely limited by our ability to estimate discount rates and the age at which obsolescence will occur.

The trend toward heavier debt financing may be replaced by a trend toward leasing options in the 1980s. The decision to lease rather than buy-borrow should be analyzed in each individual case. We have reviewed the important net present cost analysis assumptions that must be made explicitly. We shall now consider two highly specialized management topics: financial ratio analysis for medical school policy makers (Chapter 11), and cost and utilization studies of teaching hospitals (Chapter 12).

References

BERMAN, H., and WEEKS, L. (1979). *The Financial Management Hospitals*, fourth edition. Ann Arbor, Mich.: Health Administration Press.

BURNS, J., and BINDON, K. (1980). "Evaluating Leases With Linear Programming," *Management Accounting* 61:8 (February), 48–53.

CLEVERLEY, W. (1979). "Reimbursement for Capital Costs," *Topics in Health Care Financing* 6:1 (Fall), 127–139.

DANDION, J., and WEIL, R. (1975). "Inflation Accounting: What Will General Price Level Adjusted Income Statements Show?" *Financial Analysts Journal* 15:1 (January-February), 30–38.

Financial Accountings Standards Board (1979). *Professional Standards: Accounting*, Volume 3. Chicago, Ill.: Commerce Clearing House.

GRIMMELMAN, F. (1980). "Borrowing for Capital: Will It Empty Your Pockets?" *Hospital Financial Management* 6:12 (December), 19–25.

HENRY, J., and ROENFELDT, R. (1978). "Cost Analysis of Leasing Hospital Equipment," *Inquiry* 15:1 (March), 33–42.

HORVITZ, R. (1979). "Accounting Management Impact of FAS 13," *Hospital Financial Management* 9:8 (August), 16–21.

JOSKOW, P. (1980). "The Effect of Competition and Regulation on Hospital Bed Supply and the Reservation Quality of the Hospital," *Bell Journal of Economics* 11:2 (Autumn), 421–447.

Kidder-Peabody & Company, The Health Finance Group (1980). Public report: *Review of Health Care Finance*. New York.

MIDYETTE, S., and PRYOR, W. (1978). "Equipment Ownership Financing Has Advantages for Hospitals," *Hospital Financial Management* 8:3 (March), 64–69.

MILLER, J. (1979). "Hospital Equipment Leasing: The Breakdown Discount Rate," *Management Accounting* 25:3 (July), 21–25.

SIMPSON, J. (1978). "The Health Care Dilemma and Corporate Debt Capacity," *Hospital and Health Services Administration* 23:3 (Summer), 54–67.

Standard and Poor's (1978). "Evaluation of Future Hospital Capitalization," Standard and Poor's Report. New York.

SURER, J., and NEUMANN, B. (1978). "Cost of Capital," *Hospital Financial Management* 8.2 (February), 20–26.

TOOMEY, R. E., and TOOMEY, R. C. (1976). "Political Relations of Capital Formation and Capital Allocations," *Hospital and Health Services Administration* 21:2 (Spring), 11–27.

WILLIAM, J., and RAKICH, J. (1973). "Investment Evaluation in Hospitals," *Financial Management* 23:2 (Summer), 30–35.

Chapter 11

FINANCIAL CONCERNS IN MEDICAL SCHOOL MANAGEMENT

A little publicized but interesting and important trend over the past ten years has been an increasing dependence of many schools on fees for service from Medicare and Medicaid as well as private patients. Many medical schools are making an organized effort to increase this source of income to compensate for the loss of research and training grants and in some it has already become the principal source of funds.

—RONALD V. CHRISTIE

Obviously this sharp dampening of general economic growth will have far-reaching implications for all our institutions. We cannot easily deny medical care for the poor. Therefore changes in the availability of federal funds have already led to some dramatic changes in the way medical schools support themselves. To survive and to prosper in the decade to come, medical academe must adjust to a period of no growth and change imaginatively to allow progress to continue.

—DAVID E. ROGERS

As the supply of physicians per capita more than doubled between 1963 and 1979, there is no longer justification for the federal medical school capitation program. In this chapter we shall question the value of a uniform program of financial assistance to medical education and research. Medical schools have an uneven ability to compensate for declining federal capitation and research grants.

Financial-ratio analysis and cluster analysis are utilized and four adaptive responses to future financial pressures are suggested. The four potential avenues of response involve reducing faculty size, expanding faculty involvement in medical practice plans, raising tuition, and in some cases increasing state-government support. Medical schools will have to strive also for better financial management if the eighty-eight institutions revealed to be in poor financial health are to survive.

The Current Policy Context

The 1970s were a time of great stress for American medical education. Schools had to grant substantial salary increases to enable their employees to maintain purchasing power. Moreover, the certain decline of federal capitation support grants and the potential decline of future federal research grants threaten the financial health of the nation's medical schools. Private medical schools are especially vulnerable. The private medical schools and their parent universities have watched the market value of their invested assets decline. The lack of data concerning the financial state of the medical schools seriously inhibits our ability to assess the impact of policy alternatives.

The Carter Administration recommended reduction and elimination of capitation awards to medical schools. In fiscal year 1980 the schools received only $685 per student instead of the $785 per student appropriated by Congress. The liberal Kennedy Health Manpower Bill (S.2375) that was debated in the summer of 1980 provides schools with only $560, $610, and $655 per student in fiscal years 1982–1984. The federal government predicts that the enrollment expansion already achieved is sufficient to meet the national demand for physicians. It is withdrawing its previous level of support for medical education and cutting general institutional operating subsidies. Reduced funding will require some reaction on the part of the medical schools and university medical centers. Grants that induced changes in academic health centers presumably increased reliance of those institutions on the federal government. It has been said that, with grants, a cut in revenues means an equal cut in expenditures, but this does not follow. Grants pay for many of the indirect costs of running an institution. When grants are reduced or eliminated, funds must come from some other source to cover these indirect costs. Action can come in the form of changes in programs or shifts to greater reliance on alternative sources. One source is the student on whom the federal government explicitly wishes to place more of the burden of financing medical education.

Medical schools are multi-product institutions producing patient care (13.8 percent of expenditures), research (25 percent of expenditures), and instruction (60.5 percent of expenditures) (Eastaugh, 1980). Most experts agree that a decline in medical school student capitation support cannot be compensated for by a growth in funding for research activities. The Reagan Administration's proposed 1982 budget decreases biomedical and behavioral research 20–40 percent below the 1980 levels. There will not be any increases in National Institutes of Health research grants and appropriations for research projects, research centers, and biomedical research support.

The Carter Administration was unsuccessful in enacting any new desirable elective programs in 1979 and 1980 for schools of medicine to expand and maintain departments of family medicine, preventive medicine, nutrition, and gerontology. Consequently there was no test of the theory that poor financial health would force more medical schools to accept "desirable" prodding to act in these aforementioned areas. No funds will be appropriated for construction of the health professions' teaching facilities since the federal government has determined that more teaching facilities are not needed. Opponents of federal manipulation argue that the reduction in discretionary fund balances will stifle innovation and eliminate the possibility for creating new programs.

The Historic Policy Context

Behn and Sperduto (1979) have recently reviewed the growth of a medical school "entitlement ethic" since passage of the first health manpower bill in 1963. In response to the national perception of a doctor shortage, the 1965 amendments to the 1963 Health Professions Education Assistance Act required only that the school expand enrollments by 2.5 percent per annum. In the following years, Fein (1967) questioned the validity of the assumption that a doctor shortage existed regionally or nationally. However, the Congress was predisposed to respond to the 1970 Carnegie Commission assertion that the nation had a shortage of 50,000 doctors. The 1971 Health

Manpower Act replaced the basic improvement grants of the 1960s with a program of capitation grants to stimulate rapid growth in class size. The capitation grant program stipulated that small schools with less than 100 students per class expand the class by 10 students, and larger schools expand class size by 5 percent.

These financial incentives to expand class size were a smashing success story. By 1968 the nation had already exceeded the American Medical Association's declared appropriate supply ratio of 154 physicians per 100,000 population (Carnegie Commission, 1970). By 1975 the national supply of physicians exceeded the Carnegie Commission's (1973) most optimistic projection of 171.3 physicians per 100,000 population for 1982. In renewing the capitation program in 1976, the Congress expressed concern over the doctor surplus in the preamble, and concluded that the nation had a maldistribution, but not a shortage, of physicians. Stevens (1971) and Reinhardt (1975) had argued that productivity, and not supply ratios, was the more salient public policy issue. Stevens went so far as to suggest that the physician supply could be reduced 12.5 percent if all U.S. physicians had the same level of productivity as physicians in the Kaiser Health Plan, or reduced 42.5 percent if U.S. physicians had Kaiser productivity and patient utilization rates.

Medical education policy was formulated in various statements to the effect that medical schools were a precious national resource in need of federal aid. From 1971 to 1980 Congress ignored the arguments of economists and accountants to terminate capitation grants. Congress followed the advice of social activists to address the specialty maldistribution problem, and the advice of medical lobbyists to perpetuate the entitlement ethic and foster increased government funding. Paradoxically, federal support had not kept pace with the inflation in medical school expenditures. From 1966 to 1976 federal research support declined from 34.1 percent of revenues to 19.6 percent, and federal grants for teaching and recovery of indirect costs declined from 18.5 percent of revenues to 17.5 percent. Social activists' concerns for the overproduction of specialists were placated by the 1976 Capitation Bill provision that specified annual national targets for percentage of filled residencies in primary care. If the targets of at least 35 percent primary care residencies by 1977, 40 percent by 1978, and 50 percent for 1979 were not met in any given year, then each school had to meet the target in succeeding years as a mandatory condition for capitation supports.

One important policy question concerns how medical schools can cope with the anticipated elimination of the capitation grant program in the early 1980s. Protecting the public interest requires that the resulting short-run financial problems of the schools be managed in ways that have the fewest adverse long-run effects on medical education. To accomplish this the schools must devote more systematic attention to financial ratio assessment. It is equally important for school administrators and federal officials to realize that different clusters or categories of medical schools must be treated differently. The uneven ability of medical schools to compensate for declining federal support cannot be overemphasized.

The objective of this chapter is to suggest potential management strategies which different types of medical schools might consider implementing in the 1980s.

Financial Ratio Analysis

Financial ratio analysis is suggested as a tool that would enable medical school deans to assess their financial position in absolute and normative terms. The appropriate ratios, calculated from data reported in balance sheets and income statements, may be used to determine an organization's profitability, liquidity (ability to meet short-term obligations), and leverage (ability to meet debt obligations). The point was made in Chapter 9 that any institution can monitor its performance by comparing financial ratios over time or by comparing its ratios against industry norms. Ratios that change significantly or are markedly different from the industry norms serve as warning signs, indicating that an evaluation of the institution's financial position is warranted (Cleverley, 1978).

Only recently has ratio analysis been utilized in the health sector. Ratios have seldom been used by hospital administrators to monitor hospital performance (Choate, 1974). Regulatory agencies may examine some key ratios when determining Certificate-of-Need (CON) eligibility. For example, one hospital may be granted a CON to purchase a CAT scanner (Computerized Axial Tomography) while a competing hospital is refused a CON because the former is highly unlevered (low debt/equity ratio) while the latter is already highly capitalized (high fixed assets/total assets ratio). Other considerations being equal, the first hospital would be better able to finance the purchase of a CAT scanner since it has yet to rely heavily on debt financing. The second hospital is already capital intensive and the high fixed assets/total assets ratio is a sign that the hospital might achieve greater efficiency with better use of short-term funds (working capital) coupled with a more labor-intensive approach to its operations.

Until now, no attempt has been made to establish national norms to facilitate ratio analysis of medical schools. At a time when many medical schools are facing fiscal crises it is important that deans and financial officers have the data base to enable them to assess their school's financial position. A comparison of ratios over time, or between schools, might prove helpful in understanding why some medical schools are being forced to erode their endowment in order to survive.

Financial Data

Financial data utilized in the ratio analysis was obtained from an Association of American Medical Colleges (AAMC) annual questionnaire. Included in the questionnaire are data items from the financial statements. These cash-flow items indicate the school's sources and uses of funds. No balance sheet information, however, is provided about fund balances, assets, and liabilities. The AAMC provided the author with data for the following ten ratios in the years 1973 and 1978, expressed in percentages:

1. *Profitability:* total revenues minus expenses as a percentage of total revenues.
2. *Tuition and fees:* total student tuition and fees, including undergraduate medical programs as well as other degree programs, as a percentage of total revenues.
3. *Restricted revenues:* current revenues that are designated to be spent for specific projects, as a percentage of total revenues. Since very little federal money is unrestricted, this classification covers virtually all federal sources of revenue.
4. *Government appropriations:* unrestricted revenues made available to the school by legislative act or local taxing authorities and restricted revenues from the same sources used for general operations.
5. *Federal appropriations:* federal revenue as a percentage of total revenues.
6. *Private gifts, grants, and contracts:* includes all unrestricted and restricted gifts from nongovernmental sources as well as

contracts for the furnishing of goods and services of an instructional, research, or public service nature, as a percentage of total revenues.

7. *Medical practice plan:* patient care reimbursement for faculty service to the medical practice plan (MPP), as a percentage of total revenues.

8. *Instruction and departmental research:* expenditures for all activities that are part of the school's instructional program, and departmental research expenditures that are not separately budgeted, as a percentage of total expenses.

9. *Sponsored research:* includes all expenditures for research activities that are externally commissioned or separately budgeted, as a percentage of total expenses.

10. *Administration and general expenditures:* includes academic and institutional support and funds for student support services, as a percentage of total expenses.

Table 11.1 presents the average values of these ten basic ratios for the years 1973 and 1978 for public and private schools.

The best indicator of the medical schools' financial problems is the sharp decline over the five year period in profitability margin, the excess of revenues over expenditures expressed in percentage terms. Public schools had a substantial income or profit margin of 3.7 percent in fiscal 1973. Private schools earned far less on each

Table 11.1   Medical School Ratios (percent)

	1973		1978	
	Public	*Private*	*Public*	*Private*
Profitability	3.7	1.2	1.2	0.7
Tuition and Fees	2.6	12.6	2.7	10.1
Restricted Revenues	42.3	54.1	33.8	47.1
Government Appropriations	47.8	10.1	43.2	7.8
Federal Appropriations, Grants, and Contracts	32.6	38.5	22.9	28.2
Private Gifts, Grants, and Contracts	7.6	11.5	5.6	9.3
Medical Practice Plan	6.8	6.9	10.3	15.5
Instruction and Departmental Research	38.3	24.3	37.9	23.7
Research	19.0	28.3	17.8	24.5
Administrative and General Expenses	11.4	11.5	13.0	12.3

dollar of revenue—just 1.2 percent. By 1978 the income margins of public and private schools had fallen precipitously, to 1.2 percent and 0.7 percent, respectively. The percentage of schools with a net margin of 2 percent or higher declined from 44 percent to 8 percent. Fewer and fewer schools, therefore, have any margin for inefficiency before they operate in the red. The conclusion from this data is that all medical schools are facing increasing fiscal pressures, but private medical schools are in far greater fiscal danger than public medical schools.

Moreover, there has been an observable decline in sponsored research support over the past five years. This may be due to a change in priorities among both big business and government. The benefits of medical research are often not realized for dozens of years. In a period of fiscal belt-tightening, medical research has been assigned a low priority.

Private schools have always relied heavily on sponsored research projects for the bulk of their revenues. These revenues pay faculty salaries and support new technologies for tertiary care medicine and basic research. The rapidly escalating costs of biomedical research leaves little room for an excess of revenues over expenditures (profit). As these sponsored programs are cut back, as they were from 1973 to 1978, and the machinery and personnel remain, the financial squeeze begins. A gap is created between funds available and funds necessary for operation of the school. This hits most private schools harder than public schools, but it is felt everywhere.

Appropriations from state and local governments, and grants and appropriations from the federal government, have also fallen off sharply over the last five years. These items accounted for 80 percent of public schools' revenues and 49 percent of private schools' revenues in 1973, but fell to just 72 percent and 36 percent, respectively, by 1978.

Filling the financial gap between funds available and funds required is a major problem for medical school deans and budget officers. The tactics used have been partially successful but often create additional problems. One tactic that has gained virtually universal acceptance is the expansion of medical practice plans (MPPs). In private schools, especially, often 20 to 30 percent of the school's revenues come from patient services rendered by the faculty. At first these MPPs were justified to the physicians as a way of keeping up to date with new techniques. Now all involved realize that these MPPs are a critical source of funds to the medical school and some schools could not survive without them.

Another issue, as yet unresolved, is whether medical researchers become better researchers and/or teachers when exposed to a few hours of clinical medicine daily. It is clear that medical school faculty now must wear three hats, the traditional ones of teacher and researcher, and now the additional one of practitioner. Salaries are not necessarily commensurate with the job responsibilities. The time available for research is reduced, and individuals interested purely in biomedical research have much to consider before agreeing to a medical school staff appointment. Thus, it is conceivable that the explosion of MPPs may adversely affect the quality of biomedical research at medical schools.

The financial figure with which the public is most familiar—tuition—has skyrocketed as well. As expenses have gone up, all medical schools have raised tuition to meet them. Much of the state appropriations to public schools are tuition subsidies. Nationwide, tuition in 1978 accounted for only 4.6 percent of school revenues and an estimated 7.6 percent of the actual cost of instruction. Some private schools have increased tuition by 25 percent per year. The medical school tuition at both Georgetown University and George Washington University, two schools that receive no appropriations from their "state" government, now equals $15,000 per year. Many other private schools are nearing five-digit tuition charges per year.

The impact of rapidly escalating tuition figures on the finances and attitudes of students is unclear. Loans are always available to students, but the thought of being $60,000 in debt upon graduation may frighten some of them away from private schools. Private schools may find that they have a student body composed of a few scholarship students from lower-class backgrounds, many students from upper-middle class backgrounds, and no one in between. Perhaps the greater danger lies in the probability that some new physicians who may otherwise have chosen family practice, or a practice in an underserved area, may opt for a specialty practice that promises a better cash return on their investment.

The Eight Types of School Clusters

Cluster analysis is a technique that groups firms or subjects together according to shared characteristics. The Department of Health, Education and Welfare (McShane, 1977) performed a cluster analysis of medical schools and devised eight clusters for 1978, grouped according to six factors. These clusters were developed from AAMC data and characterize different kinds of medical schools. These groupings were not developed on the basis of any of the financial ratios. The specific objective of this chapter is to study the shifts in financial ratios across clusters and time periods.

Schools were divided into eight clusters based on the following six shared characteristics:

1. *Emphasis on graduate medical education program.* Schools that are strong in this area have high ratios of interns and residents to undergraduates, a high proportion of faculty with M.D. degrees, and a low ratio of undergraduates to faculty. A disproportionately small number of graduates of these schools go into general practice.
2. *Size and age of school.* This factor includes the rate of growth of the school, with low growth being considered a sign of age.
3. *"Control."* Public schools rate low and private schools high on this factor. Included is the proportion of in-state students in the school.
4. *Research funding success.* This is proxied by the approval rates for grants from the National Institutes of Health.
5. *Developmental stage of school.* This is a better measure of maturity than size and age.
6. *Research emphasis.* This is the level of sponsored research activity.

The eight clusters contain schools that are roughly similar in the six aforementioned factors. Several schools were excluded from this analysis because of lack of data. Descriptions of the eight clusters are listed below:

1. Cluster 1 contains 17 public medical schools. These are all established schools with few other distinguishing characteristics. They have below-average emphasis on graduate medical programs and research, and are below average in research funding success.
2. The 8 schools in Cluster 2 are the oldest and largest medical schools. Six are public with average total enrollments of around 900 undergraduate medical students. These schools do not place much emphasis on research or graduate medical education.
3. The 16 public schools in Cluster 3 have a high degree of emphasis on research and have good research funding success. There is less emphasis on graduate medical education. They

are of moderate size with little growth, except in research funding.

4. Cluster 4 has 14 large well-established medical schools with strong education programs at all levels.
5. Cluster 5 contains the newest schools. It should be interesting to examine how their finances differ from the rest of the medical schools.
6. Relatively new public schools experiencing rapid growth are in Cluster 6. Research support is not a substantial fraction of revenues, but is rapidly growing.
7. Cluster 7 contains mainly older private schools with low emphasis on research and graduate education. These schools have the highest tuition but the lowest annual revenues.
8. The 17 schools, mostly private, in Cluster 8 have strong research and graduate medical education programs. They are smaller than average and have the highest house-staff to student ratio of any cluster. They rely on federal support more than any other cluster.

Table 11.2 presents the values of various ratios for each cluster in the years 1973 and 1978. The data presented are only for the 60 medical schools in 1978 that subscribed to the uniform financial reporting practices of the AAMC. It can be readily observed that the decline in profit margin present in all medical schools as a whole is present in most of the clusters. Only one group of schools, Cluster 2, experienced an increase in profit margin. Apparently, the inertia present in these older, larger schools gives them a unique fiscal stability. With this exception, the decline in net profit margin is a broad-based phenomenon.

The percentage of expenditures for restricted purposes, such as sponsored research programs, declined in all clusters except for Clusters 5 and 6 (the newest schools). Sponsored revenues declined in all clusters in the period from 1973–1978. This cutback in research funding is perhaps the biggest cause of medical schools' fiscal problems and it has not struck medical schools selectively.

The prestige schools (Clusters 4 and 8) do not attract much state or local money, but they still attract their share of state and federal research funds. Most of these schools continue to run in the black. The schools with the deepest trouble are the less prestigious private schools. The schools in Cluster 7 actually showed a net income loss for fiscal year 1978. Reduced government appropriations coupled with major cutbacks in sponsored programs are the chief

Table 11.2 Cluster Analysis of Medical School Finances, 1973 and 1978, for Nine Financial Ratios, Expressed in Percentages

Item	Mean 1973 Cluster Values[1]								Mean 1978 Cluster Values							
	I	II	III	IV	V	VI	VII	VIII	I	II	III	IV	V	VI	VII	VIII
Sample Response	9/17	2/8	6/14	5/14	3/4	11/12	7/17	12/17	8/17	4/8	10/16	8/14	2/5	8/13	9/19	11/17
Revenue Ratios[2]																
Profitability Ratio (percent)	1.7	0.95	1.3	1.0	8.3	10.7	0.25	2.0	0.5	1.4	0.79	1.0	0.75	2.1	−0.17	1.0
Tuition Ratio	12	11	12	10	23	6	16	9	4	6	2	5	19	2	15	6
Restricted Revenue Ratio	41	43	49	61	45	26	52	58	34	39	36	49	17	26	44	51
State Government Ratio	41	38	28	17	40	60	15	5	41	38	33	18	54	51	9	3
Federal Government Ratio	30	28	38	33	39	27	39	42	21	20	27	26	28	19	29	31
Medical Practice Plan Ratio	6	4	13	6	1	4	8	7	11	6	18	10	9	12	16	16
Expense Ratios[3]																
Instruction and Departmental Research	39	34	34	19	48	47	27	23	40	36	35	22	69	42	25	21
Sponsored Research	17	20	24	28	7	15	27	34	15	17	23	27	13	17	22	32
Administration and General Expense	Data Not Available in 1973								10	12	9	10	20	17	14	9

[1] Definitions of the 8 clusters appear in the text.
[2] Expressed as a percent of total revenues.
[3] Expressed as a percent of total expenditures.

culprits. The ability of these schools to survive in the future is uncertain.

The growth in medical practice plans (MPPs) has been dramatic in all eight clusters. MPPs have been expanded to fill the gap between educational expenses and tuition dollars; for example, observe the across-the-board reduction in percentage of revenues coming from tuition. Medical practice plans were a major source of funds in only Cluster 3 in 1973; despite the fact that this cluster contains strong public schools with good research programs, the physicians were called upon to perform a large amount of clinical work. The increasing percentage of medical school revenues derived from MPPs obviously indicates that the faculty is expected to spend more time on patient care. Alternatively, it could be that more schools within clusters are establishing school-wide MPPs, redistributing faculty designation from geographic full-time to strict full-time. The growth in MPPs has not been consistent across clusters; for example, in Cluster 8 the plans have become much more important than they have in Cluster 4. The schools in both clusters are private, prestigious schools. The main difference between them is size—the schools in Cluster 8 are small and the educational programs are de-emphasized. As MPPs grow, it will be interesting to see from where the faculty's work time in these plans is taken. In less prestigious schools which no longer can attract as much research funding, the faculty may discover that hours previously spent on research need to be dedicated to clinical work if the school is to survive.

Potential Adaptive Responses by the Schools

Even without the elimination of federal capitation grants and the reduction in research grant support, it appears probable that most schools will face difficulties in meeting increasing direct costs. Expanded graduate medical education and continuing education programs have not contributed significantly to the medical school financial picture. Rogers and Blenden (1978) have recently pointed out that the academic medical center is becoming a stressed institution that cannot find relief from any of the financial pressures it is facing. Given that hospital-rate regulators will not allow teaching hospitals to bail out medical schools, the schools have four potential avenues of response: raise tuition, increase state support, induce faculty to devote more time to reimbursable patient services in MPPs, or reduce faculty size.

The first possible response in the minds of many school administrators is to raise medical school tuition. In 1978 tuition and other student fees represented a mere 4.6 percent of school revenues. Net present value computations of the returns on investment in a medical education are in excess of the dollar returns on an education in other professions (Mennemeyer, 1978). In view of the fact that medicine is the most lucrative profession and is the only profession in which students' tuition fees are less than 7 percent of expected average future earnings, the general feeling is that medical students can absorb potential tuition increases. However, the tuition increases may exacerbate the financial burdens of poor and minority students, and the medical schools may have to resort to a policy of price discrimination in their tuition decisions. For example, the schools could pursue a policy of three-tiered tuition pricing for poor ($2,000), middle class ($6,000), and rich students ($20,000 per annum). The growing numbers of rich students willing to pay exorbitant tuitions and the existence of large pools of qualified rejected medical school applicants and students willing to undertake the expensive task of attending a foreign medical school suggest that schools can substantially raise tuition.

One potential problem of increasing the tuition burden is that newly graduated physicians may charge excessively higher fees to compensate for unmanageable debt burdens. Raising the debt burden of students exacerbates two existing problems for the medical schools. University-sponsored loans typically subsidize medical education by not requiring interest payments or repayment of principal until completion of a post-graduate residency or entrance into practice. Second, many university officials have observed that even following payment of the debt principal, the debtor is less likely to donate to the medical school than the average alumnus.

A second potential response to declining federal revenues is to ask state government for increased financial support. State subsidies are becoming important to private schools as federal subsidies decrease. However, medical school deans fear that if state governments are going to sustain the private schools, they will insist on some new conditions, for example, admissions-committee discrimination in favor of more state residents each year, and in time the state may attempt to dominate or take over the school.

Two other potential responses to declining federal financial support involve changing the composition or size of the faculty. Medical school faculties are divided into three major categories: full-time teaching and research, part-time, and geographic full-time (faculty members allowed to have private practices). One response would involve inducing faculty members to devote more time to medical practice plan activities and spend less time in research activities or independent private practice. Rather than raise revenues, a fourth response would be to decrease costs by reducing faculty size. The number of full-time clinical faculty in the United States increased over 300 percent from 1961 to 1976, according to an unpublished 1977 AAMC report on "Medical Education: Institutions, Characteristics, and Programs." The prime candidates for elimination are full-time faculty members who do not contribute substantially to the medical practice plan, and part-time faculty members who receive a school salary out of line with their limited teaching activities. Faculty members in "soft-money" areas that lack a solid base of political support in negotiating with the dean are most likely to be eliminated. Unless the federal government is willing to provide increased targeted financial support, a number of new programs and faculty may be eliminated in the areas of ghetto medicine, rural medicine, and family practice, and in cost-effective clinical decision making instruction (Hudson and Barslow, 1979). Fein and Weber (1971) indicate that innovative curriculum areas are infrequently supported by extracting a percentage of the cash flow from established departments and activities. Medical school may no longer be able to subsidize the educational activities of nursing, pharmacy, and allied health schools.

The clusters separate into three groups according to dependence on capitation grants. Clusters 2 and 6 are financially sound, highly dependent on state grants, and not in serious need of capitation grants. The second group, Clusters 1, 3, and 5, is highly dependent on federal capitation grants but has the option to appeal for more state support. All thirty-eight schools in this second group could compensate for total elimination of the capitation program by increasing tuition 20–100 percent or revenues from the medical practice plans 10–125 percent or state grants 2–27 percent. The members of Cluster 3 might be most resistant to an expansion of medical practice plans since their faculties are perceived to be above-average-quality researchers. Schools in Cluster 5 are the newest and most publicly supported institutions and consequently might find negotiations with state government for increased support to be their easiest course of action.

A third group of medical schools, Clusters 4, 7, and 8, is facing the tightest fiscal squeeze because these schools are the most dependent on capitation grants and are largely unable to increase state support if they maintain private-school status. All fifty schools in this group could compensate for total elimination of the capitation program by raising tuition 50–170 percent or by increasing revenues from medical practice plans by 40–230 percent. These schools will be in a particularly vulnerable position if the faculty is resistant to MPP expansion or if the students fight large tuition increases. The fifty schools in these three clusters would be the most likely to cut faculty size in response to the student argument that tuition is a small percentage of revenues, and the faculty is too large and overpaid. A recent study by Hall and Lindsay (1980) of sixteen medical schools over a fourteen-year period suggests that excessive increases in tuition could decrease the number and quality of medical students. The authors suggest that for each 10 percent rise in tuition, there will be a 4 percent decline in the number of qualified applicants, all other factors held constant.

Problems for the Future

The federal government has lately been pressured to bail out medical schools because they are a precious national resource. The basic dilemma faced by the medical schools is whether they can acquire increasing federal support and maintain their current degree of autonomy from government bureaucrats. Congress' problem is how to allocate resources effectively among many competing high-priority national needs in the face of limited discretionary funds. The presence of financial exigencies felt by government and the schools means that careful attention must be paid to find a solution that is cost effective. A segmented approach for different categories of schools may be better than the current uniform approach to federal financing of medical school operations.

Many adaptive response tactics have not been explored in this study. For example, increasing the number of non-M.D. graduate degrees and offering more continuing education programs could increase revenues. Most analysts assume that medical schools' primary response will be to increase revenues by raising tuition charges. But the schools should not ignore the importance of reducing costs. The earlier Carnegie Commission (1970) on Higher Education has made a number of recommendations for program changes that would lead to reduced costs, including reducing the length of time required in order to receive an M.D. degree from four years to three years, making fuller use of facilities by having year-round programs, and entering two classes each year. A number of medical schools did institute the three-year curriculum but found it unsatisfactory and have reverted to the four-year program (Beran, 1979).

The second Carnegie Commission report (1973) recommended that medical schools be organized into university health science centers responsible for coordinating the education of all health care personnel in their respective geographic areas. The Commission also recommended that these health science centers be treated as a national resource, protected and supported by the federal government. Since it appears that the federal government is not prepared to support medical schools and ensure their existence, medical schools will have to become better managers of their resources.

Most medical schools will find it difficult to preserve their financial position through the 1980s. In the 1970s the schools tended to erode their limited endowments, withdrawing funds for operations and capital projects. Many poor capital expansion and stock investment decisions were made, and there were large investments in new facilities. As the endowments began to shrink, they became increasingly harder to rebuild, and the resultant income from investments declined. Drucker (1973) was one of the first to point out that diagnosing schools as "inefficient" because they operate on the basis of a service ethic rather than a business management ethic is overly simplistic. Nevertheless, there is an obvious need for more medical school managers with business training. However, such individuals would have to be sensitive to the health service ethic so as not to put considerations for revenue maximization and cost minimization ahead of quality education. Talented management personnel might compel schools to respond to the public cry for more primary care services. However, their real challenge would be to trim the fat from tertiary care medicine without harming the basic research and development functions of medical schools.

References

American Medical Association (1978). "Medical Education in the United States, 1976–1977, Part III," *Journal of the American Medical Association* 240:26 (December), 2827–2835.

BEHN, R. D., and SPERDUTO, K. (1979). "Medical Schools and the 'Entitlement Ethic'," *Public Interest* 14:57 (Fall), 48–68.

BERAN, R. L. (1979). "The Rise and Fall of Three-Year Medical School Programs," *Journal of Medical Education* 54:3 (March), 248–249.

Carnegie Commission on Higher Education (1973). *Priorities for Action: Final Report of the Carnegie Commission on Higher Education.* Los Angeles: Maple Press.

Carnegie Commission on Higher Education (1970). *Higher Education and the Nation's Health Policies for Medical and Dental Education.* New York: McGraw-Hill.

CHOATE, G. M. (1974). *Medical Education and the State,* Fogarty International Center Proceedings No. 31, Publication NIH 76-943. Washington, D.C.: Department of Health, Education and Welfare.

CLEVERLEY, W. (1978). *Essentials of Hospital Finance.* Germantown, Md: Aspen, 53–80.

DRUCKER, P. F. (1973). "Managing the Public Service Institution," *Public Interest* 9:33 (Fall), 43–60.

EASTAUGH, S. R. (1980). "Financial Ratio Analysis and Medical School Management," *Journal of Medical Education* 55:10 (October).

FEIN, R. (1967). *The Doctor Shortage.* Washington, D.C.: Brookings Institution.

FEIN, R., and WEBER, G. I. (1971). *Financial Medical Education: An Analysis of Alternative Policies and Mechanisms.* New York: McGraw-Hill.

General Accounting Office (1978). "Federal Capitation Support and Its Role in the Operation of Medical Schools." Washington, D.C.: U.S. Government Printing Office.

HALL, T. D., and LINDSAY, C. M. (1980). "Medical Schools: Producers of What? Sellers to Whom?" *Journal of Law and Economics* 22:22 (April), 55–80.

HUDSON, J. I., and BARSLOW, J. B. (1979). "Cost Containment Education Efforts in United States Medical Schools," *Journal of Medical Education* 54:11 (November), 835–840.

Institute of Medicine, National Academy of Sciences (1974). *Cost of Education in the Health Professions.* Washington, D.C.: U.S. Government Printing Office.

KELLY, J. F. (1978). "Options for Financing Graduate Medical Education," *Journal of Medical Education* 53:1 (January), 26–32.

McSHANE, M. G. (1977). "An Empirical Classification of United States Medical Schools by Institutional Dimensions," Final Report of the Association of American Medical Colleges to the Department of Health, Education and Welfare, Publication HRA 77-55. Washington, D.C.: Health Resources Administration, Bureau of Health Manpower.

MENNEMEYER, S. (1978). "Really Great Returns to Medical Education?" *Journal of Medical Education* 13, 73–90.

PERRY, D. R., and CHALLONER, D. R. (1979). "A Rationale for Continued Federal Support of Medical Education," *New England Journal of Medicine* 300:22 (January), 66–71.

REINHARDT, V. (1975). *Physician Productivity and the Demand for Health Manpower.* Cambridge: Ballinger.

ROGERS, D. E. (1980). "On Preparing Academic Health Centers for the Very Different 1980's," *Journal of Medical Education* 55:1 (January), 1–12.

ROGERS, D. E., and BLENDON, R. J. (1978). "The Academic Medical Center: A Stressed American Institution," *New England Journal of Medicine* 298:17 (April), 940–950.

STEVENS, C. (1971). "Physicians Supply and the National Health Care Goals," *Industrial Relations* 10:5 (May), 119–144.

United States Congress, Office of Technology Assessment (1980). *Forecasts of Physician Supply and Requirements.* Washington, D.C.: U.S. Government Printing Office.

Chapter 12

COST AND UTILIZATION STUDIES IN HOSPITALS

> *Future research that explicitly recognizes variations in medical staff characteristics and organizations may be fruitful in discovering reasons underlying variations in hospital performance in response to regulation. Put another way, is "control" of medical staff a necessary condition for containment of hospital costs?*
>
> —FRANK A. SLOAN

> *In the case of a multi-product firm it is not possible to calculate the average cost of each product, only marginal costs are calculable.*
>
> —GEORGE J. STIGLER

Overutilization of hospital beds and ancillary services has been cited as the most prevalent source of inefficiency in the medical economy. A central problem in making efficiency comparisons between hospitals is the joint product nature of the institution. In the cost accounting sense, "joint product" costs are costs that are incurred when producing a group of individual products simultaneously. For example, hernia operations, pediatric days, medical students trained, and research projects completed are all products that cannot usually be separated in the production process. Little analytical work has been done in this area, with the exception of a study on joint production in ninety Veterans Administration radiology departments (Massell and Hosek, 1975).

One of the conceptual problems that economists have had, in the area of utilization in hospitals, is understanding the wide range of heterogeneous products that physicians identify in the teaching hospital setting. In teaching hospitals, physicians simultaneously produce the joint products of education, research, and patient care. Even within the category of patient care, the care "produced" is quite diverse, due to the great variance in the complexity of cases handled. Thus physicians have largely ignored medical economics studies because they do not capture the diversity of patient care within hospitals or across different hospital types. For example, the product of a hospital cannot be captured with just four figures: in-patient days, operative cases, out-patient visits, and number of residents on staff. Specifically, any efficiency comparison between hospitals must involve a perfect matching of patient characteristics and a more complete treatment of physician characteristics. The objective of this chapter is to explore ways in which economists might cooperatively work with physicians in microanalytical studies with the individual patient as the unit of analysis. Variation in cost and utilization of days of stay and tests per admission will be explained by three sets of factors: product-type (patient) characteristics, input-type hospital characteristics, and input-type physician characteristics. In addressing the patient case mix problem, this chapter begs the more difficult issue of costing out each of the components in the joint production of teaching and research.

The Policy Context

Excessive number of tests and long lengths of stay are two central issues in the public debate about rising hospital costs. The purpose of this chapter is to discover some of the factors contributing most to excessive utilization of hospital services.

There has been a dramatic growth in laboratory tests per patient episode. Scitovsky (1976) found that between 1964 and 1971, lab tests per episode increased from 25 to 33 percent for simple, well-defined diagnostic categories such as simple appendicitis and acute myocardial infarction, and increased 90–110 percent for perforated appendicitis and breast cancer cases, respectively. In a sample of 285 hospitals during the period 1968–1971, Redisch (1978) found that laboratory tests per patient day increased at an average annual rate of 9 percent. Expenditures for laboratory tests and other nonpersonnel items have the highest rate of increase of any element responsible for rising hospital costs (Rivlin, 1976).

Excessive use of tests and procedures is a source of concern not only because it is costly but because it is unnecessary. Evidence that American medicine has a high degree of unnecessary utilization has frequently appeared in the literature. One study by Jonsson and Neuhauser (1975) found that the American physician orders three times as many tests to decide upon a simple elective surgical diagnosis as does a comparable Swedish physician. One possible explanation is that American surgeons do more testing because they are more discriminating in deciding to operate. Unfortunately, this is not consistent with the fact that the operation rate per 10,000 population is 18 percent lower in Sweden relative to the United States for inguinal hernia, and 25 percent lower for cholecystectomies and prostatectomies. The Swedish patients have the same age and diagnosis-specific mortality rates as their American counterparts, so that the additional utilization of ancillary services observed in American hospitals may not be medically necessary.

Excessive length of stay has been a central issue in the American debate about rising hospital costs. The 1972 Professional Standards Review Organization (PSRO) amendment to the Social Security Act decreed that Medicaid and Medicare services "shall be provided in the minimum duration." The PSRO program was intended to curtail hospital expenditures by controlling utilization, rather than controlling price. PSROs, working in conjunction with private utilization review efforts, are intended to help curtail the days of care utilized per episode.

Excessively long lengths of stay are a source of public concern not only because they are costly, but also because such care is often unnecessary. It has even been suggested that reduction of unnecessary or excessive amounts of care could raise the general health status of the population by decreasing the likelihood of iatrogenic complications. Reducing the length of stay minimizes the chance of exposure to antibiotic-resistant bacteria peculiar to hospitals; thus the number of difficult-to-treat infections may be lessened. Shortened lengths of stay are a morale builder for adult patients; and in the case of children, the trauma of separation from their parents is minimized, even when there are liberal visiting privileges (Innes *et al.*, 1968). One study suggests the marginal benefit of excessive days of hospitalization is negative, with 20 percent of the patients being exposed to some hazardous episode (Schimmel, 1974). Clearly, the problem of cost and iatrogenic disease played a major part in the congressional commitment to the PSRO program enacted in 1972.

Utilization patterns are not merely a function of patient characteristics and the requirement of "good medicine." Medical care requirements can be met with different amounts of resources and lengths of hospitalization. How these requirements of good medicine are met depends in some part on the physician characteristics and the hospital environment. Surgical utilization is probably affected by hospital characteristics such as the laboratory turn-around time, the availability of hospital beds, the availability of a surgical suite, and the type of hospital ownership (federal, voluntary, municipal).

Physician background characteristics are also determinants of physician behavior. The duration of stay and number of tests per patient are likely to be affected by the educational background of the surgeon and the strength of the affiliation with the local medical school (Eastaugh, 1979). The process outlined in Figure 12.1 implies a causal sequence: Differing combinations of physician and hospital characteristics lead to different styles of medicine, which in turn lead to different utilization patterns. For example, one might presuppose that medical school faculty members involved in patient care have a professional interest in curtailing inappropriate prescriptions, but it might not always be in the faculty members' interests to curtail all types of excessive utilization. Faculty members and attending physicians might have an interest in maximizing revenues for new equipment because of their interest in technology. Lave and Leinhardt (1976) have examined length of stay in considerable detail, but omit consideration of hospital characteristics from the analysis because their sample consists of individuals from only one hospital. These authors conclude that the major reason why length of stay is so long and costs are so high in the urban teaching hospital they studied is because residents, due to their comparative lack of experience, order more tests. Foreign medical graduates (FMGs) might also be expected to require more tests per case because their training is not as extensive or as diagnosis-oriented as that provided by the typical American medical school. Presumably, an inferior education is associated with greater uncertainty in affirming a differential diagnosis and the need for more time between sequential decisions and perhaps the need for more information (more tests).

Other interpretations may account for the unnecessary utilization described here. For example, one explanation for increasing lab utilization is that the American surgeon is coerced by the threat of a malpractice suit into ordering more tests. However, a survey of

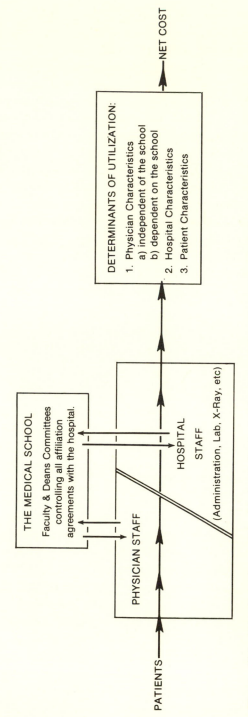
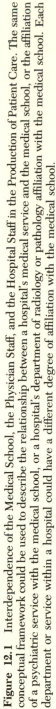

Figure 12.1 Interdependence of the Medical School, the Physician Staff, and the Hospital Staff in the Production of Patient Care. The same conceptual framework could be used to describe the relationship between a hospital's medical service and the medical school, or the affiliation of a psychiatric service with the medical school, or a hospital's department of radiology or pathology affiliation with the medical school. Each department or service within a hospital could have a different degree of affiliation with the medical school.

physician attitudes conducted by the staff of the *Duke Law Journal* suggests that the threat of malpractice had a minuscule effect on what they called positive defensive practices, that is, ordering excessive laboratory tests (Duke Law Journal, 1971). The study by Scitovsky (1976) cited previously suggests that a technological inflation in the quantity of tests and price of the procedures predates the so-called malpractice "crisis" by twenty years. The problem in interpretation here is that a number of variables, some related to the patients, some to the hospital, and some to the physician, all tend to influence utilization. The way in which that interaction occurs is most complex and demands further research. A more recent survey of 284 California physicians (Spath, 1977) suggests that when clinicians faced five hypothetical cases they ordered $47–$139 fewer lab tests per patient in a pooled-risk no-fault situation compared to the current environment of individual liability. Most individuals respond in an exaggerated fashion when confronted with such hypothetical situations; the actual behavioral change would be less pronounced.

Pertinent Empirical Studies

A number of studies have examined the question of whether length of stay is a function of physician and hospital characteristics. The studies vary with respect to hypotheses, methodology, and findings. The previously mentioned study by Lave and Leinhardt (1976) cites Ro (1969) as providing one of the few studies utilizing the individual as the unit of analysis. Ro studied a sample of 9,000 Blue Cross Plan patients admitted to twenty-two Pittsburgh hospitals during 1963. Hospital staffing ratio had a downward impact on length of stay, while medical school affiliation had an upward impact. Ro concluded that the greatest handicap in applying data to this model was "the lack of information on physicians' characteristics" (Ro, 1969). This handicap has been a barrier to better empirical work throughout the 1970s.

As overspecialization became a source of public concern in the 1970s, more researchers began collecting information on the effect of board certification on patient utilization. Garg and Mulligan (1977) have found that patients of subspecialists have shorter lengths of stay than do those of their less credentialed colleagues, after controlling for diagnosis and differences in case mix. The study concluded that specialists produced a higher quality product in a shorter period of time. Garg and Mulligan used the physician performance index (PPI) developed by Payne (1976) as the process measure of quality. Garg and Mulligan end on the optimistic hope that we could one day "discover the behavioral characteristics of cost-effective physicians so that by undergraduate, graduate, and continuing medical education, more students and physicians can learn the desired attitudes, knowledge, and skills."

Physicians are influenced to some degree by the policy and climate of the hospitals in which they work. In one early study, Gertman (1974) reported that 54 percent of inappropriate patient days of stay in Baltimore were related to delays in performing or receiving diagnostic test results, and two-thirds of the inappropriate days occurred in patients with total lengths of stay of fewer than thirteen days. One recent investigation of a utilization review project that reduced postoperative cholecystectomy length of stay by one day expressed surprise at the high level of consumer satisfaction and the high prevalence of the back-to-work disposition in their outcome analysis (Mitchell *et al.*, 1975). No patient died when he or she was released sooner. The surgeons had expected more of those patients who went home sooner to be symptomatic and bedridden, but the results were not consistent with the American physicians' conservative attitudes against shortening the length of hospitalization. The American style of medicine seems to provide a fair amount of room to be stringent on length of stay before damage will be done. One carefully controlled British study showed that patients discharged one day after hernia or varicose vein surgery did as well as those discharged after six days (Morris *et al.*, 1968).

Cross-sectional variation in average length of stay has received much attention in the literature. A 1976 Social Security Administration report prepared by Gaus found preoperative lengths of stay varying from an average of 1.9 days in four western PSRO areas to 3.9 days in two eastern PSRO areas (Gaus, 1976). The average total length of stay varied from 7.2 days in the West to 13.8 days in the East. This study corroborates the finding by Gornick of a large differential between East and West Coast Medicare patients in average length of stay (Gornick, 1975).

Interest in curtailing excessive lengths of stay was stimulated by a number of independent studies in the early 1960s. McNerney (1962) and Riedel and Fitzpatrick (1964) provide good examples of the early studies linking physician characteristics to the duration of hospitalization. Riedel and Fitzpatrick utilized bivariate statistical methods to confirm McNerney's findings that the patients of either (1) specialists, or (2) board-certified physicians, or (3) physicians in practice less than ten years had longer lengths of stay than did patients served by Michigan physicians lacking those traits. Levin (1964), however, came to exactly the opposite conclusions on all three points in his replication of the Riedel and Fitzpatrick study, controlling for patient case mix across a number of surgical diagnostic categories. Levin demonstrated that Blue Cross of Indiana patients treated by specialists or board-certified physicians had shorter lengths of stay than did any other group of patients.

A large volume of more consistent descriptive studies that correlate patient variables to the length of hospitalization is available. Lower income groups, for example, tend to have longer lengths of stay (Richardson, 1969). Patients without any hospital insurance coverage are reported to have longer lengths of stay. Unfortunately, the five studies cited thus far are suspect because the approach is always bivariate and limited to a simple comparison of group means. In a recent study by Goldfarb *et al.* (1980), diagnostic-specific length-of-stay equations were developed from a sample of sixty-four hospitals in forty-one areas. The three significant factors positively affecting length of stay were fraction insured, general hospital beds per capita, and an index for the scope of services available at the hospital.

Most of the previous multivariate hospital cost regression studies emphasize the effect of insurance coverage on various hospital output and cost measures (cost per diem, laboratory charges per episode, length of stay). These studies vary with respect to objectives and methodology. The customary approach involves an aggregate cross section of individual state or hospital observations, for each of a number of years. Davis (1971) found a positive relationship between insurance and the length of hospitalization and cost per episode. Feldstein (1971) and Hu and Werner (1976) provide corroborative evidence that more highly insured areas have higher costs per episode and longer stays, on the average. Feldstein estimated an average length of stay equation from a cross section of the fifty states, for each of ten years. Hu and Werner studied hospital and demographic characteristics in seventy hospital regions in Pennsylvania. Price per diem and mean patient income had no effect in the Hu-Werner length-of-stay equation, but insurance has a length-of-stay elasticity of 0.41 measured at the sample mean. The finding of a positive insurance effect disagrees with the results reported by Lee and

Wallace (1973) in a study of Medicare patients' length of stay within multi-hospital regional catchment areas.

Two more recent studies by Huang (1976) and by Freiberg and Schutchfield (1976) provide persuasive evidence that insurance does not affect length of stay. The "moral hazard" argument advanced by Freiberg and Schutchfield suggests that the more highly insured patients should have more tests and longer lengths of stay, because demand is less constrained by cost considerations. However, their econometric evidence rejects this hypothesis and suggests statistically insignificant negative coefficients. The findings in the literature pertaining to the effects of insurance on utilization per episode are somewhat mixed. Overall, the preliminary evidence indicates that insurance does not affect length of stay but that it is a contributory factor to rising costs.

Huang (1976) provides an example of a multivariate study of the effect of physician and hospital characteristics on utilization, with the individual patient as the unit of analysis. Huang applied data on 27,210 patients discharged from six Washington hospitals in 1975 to analyze the effects of hospital characteristics on length of stay and costs per episode. For eighteen medically homogeneous diagnoses Huang estimated equations for length of stay and found the dummy variable for insurance to be statistically insignificant, but three factors with significant positive impacts on length of stay and laboratory charges were whether the hospital had (1) a medical student teaching program, (2) a professional nursing affiliation, and (3) an internship program. Huang's findings concerning the influence of affiliation on utilization corroborates earlier findings by Salkever (1970). Salkever used a principal components analysis to delineate case-mix variables for the seventy-three New York hospitals sampled and found that interns and residents per episode had statistically significant positive impact on length of stay and costs per case episode.

In addition to the foregoing econometric studies, a number of the early industrial engineering studies have suggested a number of practical ways to contain costs and length of stay. Much of the literature of the 1960s suggested that better discharge and admission planning could reduce length of stay. One such suggestion was to eliminate elective admissions on weekends or Fridays. This was supported by McCorkle (1970) and Gustafson (1968), who studied the effect of day of the week admission on pre-operative and total length of stay.

Other recent studies have analyzed the impact of occupancy rate on the average length of stay and admission rates of various hospitals. Rafferty (1971) examined data from Indiana hospitals to estimate the length of stay elasticity and probability for admission elasticity, by diagnosis, with respect to hospital occupancy rate. The author found that the less serious medical conditions and the elective surgical cases have negative elasticities, that is to say, when the occupancy is higher the length of hospitalization or chance of admission is lowered. A few studies focused on the actual labeling of unnecessary ("misutilized") days of stay. Querido (1963) studied a sample of patients admitted to ten teaching hospitals and concluded that one-quarter of the misutilized hospital days (as judged by implicit physician review of medical records) were associated with bottlenecks (delays) in the laboratory and x-ray departments.

In summary, the studies reviewed above provide a fair amount of empirical evidence about the influence of a number of physician and hospital characteristics on tests, costs, and length of stay. Teaching variables are the most frequently studied medical staff characteristics in the foregoing empirical investigations, and occupancy rate and bed size are the most frequently studied hospital characteristics. From the point of view of public policy, additional information is needed on the impact that each of these factors has on cost and utilization of hospital services. Previous studies have utilized crude case-mix indices and aggregate data.

The approach taken in the remaining half of this chapter is to perform a more disaggregate analysis of differential cost and utilization patterns across matched patient pairs from different hospitals. By analyzing matched patient data for a limited number of diagnoses, the study reported in this chapter avoids the need for any crude case-mix index. The mathematical problems with relying on a single-valued scaler case-mix index have been reviewed elsewhere (Klastorin and Watts, 1980). The problem in interpretation with our matched pairs approach is that a number of factors—some related to patient characteristics, some to hospital inputs, some to the physicians—all tend to influence total cost, tests, and length of stay. Multiple regression analysis will provide the tool to splice out the degree of impact that each factor exhibits on cost and utilization of hospital services.

Study Design

The data for the analysis were drawn from 780 records obtained at nineteen hospitals for elective herniorrhaphy, prostatectomy, and cholecystectomy patients. The twelve VA hospitals in the study represented a 9 percent random stratified sample of VA hospitals performing surgery (National Research Council, 1977). The patient pairs were drawn from among two samples: 360 VA patients from twelve VA hospitals, and 420 nonfederal patients from seven nonfederal hospitals. The 360 VA patients were drawn as a random sample, but the 420 non-federal patients were selected in order to have patient characteristics that were as nearly similar to the federal patients as possible (Cochran and Rubin, 1973). The research rationale was to minimize the variance in patient case-mix characteristics in order to measure the effects of staff and hospital characteristics on utilization and cost.

The first step in the matching process was to select the covariables on which the two samples were to be matched. The six patient characteristics under consideration were age, sex, primary diagnosis, secondary diagnosis, socioeconomic status, and distance from the hospital. The first stage in the matching process was to have nurse abstractors of patient records enter the non-federal facility with information on the already selected federal patient pool and select a nonfederal sample that had the same sex, primary diagnosis, and welfare status. Stage two in the matching process was to apply Caliper matching methods based on predefined ranges of what constitutes an acceptable match, for example, any non-federal partner had to be within four years, plus or minus, of the federal patient's age (Rubin, 1970).

Stage three in the sampling design involved using nearest available matching methods after the data collection stages were completed, for final pairing of the non-federal and VA patient groups on the basis of age, secondary diagnosis, and five-digit zip code number (McKinley, 1974). Two of the eleven patient characteristics were different in the nearest available matched sample (258 pairs) relative to the original onsite data (720 patients). Matched patients tended to be less complex cases with fewer secondary diagnoses; they also tended to reside in zip code regions closer to the hospital (Table 12.1). Patients with a pre-admission visit to the hospital (9 percent) had their medical record abstracts coded with a −1, so that in the matching process, only patients with equivalent pre-admission workups were matched with one another. One of the explanations

Table 12.1   Mean Values for 11 Characteristics of the Matched Sample and the Original Data

	Matched Pairs After Three Stages of Matching Mean	Original Onsite Data[1] Mean
Sample Size	516 (258 pairs)	720
Fraction of Surgeons Who Are FMGs	0.27	0.28
Fraction of Surgeons on Faculty	0.08	0.08
Fraction of School's Students Doing Required Clerkship at Hospital	0.11	0.10
Lab Turnaround Time (hours)	18	19
Occupancy Rate	76%	77%
Number of Beds	412	420
Patient Census	313	323
Adult Admissions per Year	5,335	5,186
Distance Home-Hospital (miles)[2]	12	18
Number of Secondary Diagnoses[2]	1.1	1.7
Patient Age	54	51

SOURCE: Reprinted with permission of the Blue Cross Association from Eastaugh, S.R. (1980). "Organizational Determinants of Surgical Lengths of Stay," *Inquiry* 17:1 (Spring), 85–96. Copyright © 1980 by the Blue Cross Association. All rights reserved.

[1] After the second stage of matching, onsite Caliper matching.
[2] The differences between matched and unmatched samples are significant at the 0.05 level.

for the tendency of private insurance patients to have fewer tests and days of pre-operative stay is that their admission was preceded by a preadmission visit, but 91 percent of the patients in our sample entered the hospital without any pre-admission tests. In the final analysis, 102 VA patients remained unmatched, compared to 162 unmatched non-federal patients, and 258 VA–non-federal patient pairs were formed (Eastaugh, 1980).

The multiple regression approach was designed to determine how much of the variation in tests, length of stay, and cost per case are patient related, hospital related, or staff related. The sixteen dependent variables studied were:

1. Ratio between pairs in prostatectomy pre-operative length of stay.
2. Ratio between pairs in herniorrhaphy pre-operative length of stay.
3. Ratio between pairs in cholecystectomy pre-operative length of stay.
4. Ratio between pairs in pre-operative length of stay for all surgical patient pairs cited above.

5. Ratio between pairs in prostatectomy length of stay.
6. Ratio between pairs in herniorrhaphy length of stay.
7. Ratio between pairs in cholecystectomy length of stay.
8. Ratio between pairs in total length of stay for all surgical patient pairs.
9. Ratio between pairs in number of elective tests ordered pre-operatively (PT) for prostatectomy patients.
10. Ratio between pairs in PT for herniorrhaphy patients.
11. Ratio between pairs in PT for cholecystectomy patients.
12. Ratio between pairs in PT for all surgical patient pairs.
13. Ratio between pairs in costs (charges reimbursed or costs imputed in the case of hospitals lacking a patient-based accounting system) for prostatectomy patients.
14. Ratio between pairs in costs for herniorrhaphy patients.
15. Ratio between pairs in costs for cholecystectomy patients.
16. Ratio between pairs in costs for all surgical patient pairs.

Implicit in this analysis is that to do more tests or to require higher costs for producing the same product was inappropriate or wasteful behavior; the behavior was unnecessary in that the marginal benefits of more tests or days of hospitalization are minimal.

The definition of an unnecessary test in this context is one that did not make the partner better off relative to his match, undergoing the same operation, with the same outcome. Operationally, an unnecessary test is one that was provided to only one member of the pair and that Payne (1976) defines as unnecessary for a partner with given case-mix characteristics, that is, age, sex, and diagnoses. Pauly (1979) has provided a more stringent definition of what is unnecessary in the context of surgery relative to "a potential partner who has at least as much knowledge and understanding of possible costs and consequences as the physician." It should be emphasized that, in the study reported in this chapter, the criteria used to define unnecessary tests and days of stay were both professional, as Payne suggested, and normative, relative to the matched patient pair.

Operationalization of the Variables

Product definition is a most complex problem in the field of medical economics. An operational definition of a required intermediate product would be a test that was required in nearly 100 percent of the patients in the diagnostic category under study. For example, cholelithiasis is almost always confirmed in our sample of chole-cystectomy patients by radiologic evidence of single or multiple gallstones, or by evidence of a nonfunctioning gallbladder by ob-serving the movement of concentrated amounts of gallbladder dye. Some tests are elective, such as a serum amylase assay, because the majority of clinicians do not believe that this test is necessary to rule out the possibility of pancreatitis (Payne, 1976).

The information on costs came in two forms, depending on whether or not the hospital had a patient-based system of charges. For example, four hospitals in the sample had patient-based ac-counting systems for billing purposes; thus one only needed to ask for the costs and charges. Costs were assigned to the surgical de-partment by means of the multiple apportionment algebraic method of cost allocation (Berman and Weeks, 1979). However, twelve VA hospitals and three municipal hospitals in the sample had no need for itemized billing, and thus had no need for a price list or a charge-to-cost ratio. Consequently, a relative value scale* for as-sessing imputed charges was developed (Table 12.2).

All patients sampled were middle-aged males eligible for Medicaid and free VA hospital care. Three patient characteristics are included in the regression analysis as independent variables:

P_1 Distance from hospital to home in miles.
P_2 Dummy variable for lack of unmatched secondary diagnoses, between pairs.
P_3 Patient age.

The independent variables selected for inclusion in this study were chosen for reasons of either past performance in other studies or future relevance for public policy. For example, a dummy variable for affiliation with a medical school and the percentage of physicians with more than ten years of clinical experience were omitted from this study because they were considered poor proxy measures for our medical school student and faculty variables.

The list of independent variables, which will also be expressed as

---

* The hospital and ancillary costs were reduced to a relative value scale by averag-ing prevailing hospital charges in the region. Then the surgeon's fee for the area was taken from the Social Security Administration Survey of Prevailing Charges (Insti-tute of Medicine, 1976). Finally, in the case of the twelve federal hospitals and three municipal hospitals, the resources utilized in the elective surgical episode were multiplied by the relative value scale and multiplied by the conversion factor mea-sured in dollars per relative scale unit to obtain dollars per episode (Eastaugh, 1979).

Table 12.2 **Relative Value Scale for Costing Out Elective Surgical Services at the 12 VA Hospitals and 3 Municipal Hospitals without a Schedule of Charges**

	Relative Value Scale
I. Fixed Charges	
Surgeon's Fee:	
Incisional Prostatectomy	5.6
Cholecystectomy	4.2
Unilateral Inguinal Hernia	2.5
Anesthesiologist	1.75
Operating Room	1.2
Recovery Room (2–4 hours)	0.5
Anesthesia	0.26
II. Variable Charges[1]	
Basic Room Rate (per day)	0.75
Pulmonary Function Test	0.60
Cholecystogram	0.47
Cystourethrogram	0.40
Intravenous Pyelogram	0.35
Upper Gastrointestinal Series	0.32
Barium Enema	0.29
Sigmoidoscopy (Proctoscopy)	0.22
Chest X-Ray	0.16
Serum Amylase Assay	0.14
Creatine Clearance	0.11

SOURCE: Eastaugh, S.R. (1979). "Cost of Elective Surgery and Utilization of Ancillary Services in Teaching Hospitals," *Health Services Research* 14:4 (Winter), 290–308.

[1] Excluding tests necessary for admission at all 15 hospitals and the 4 voluntary hospitals.

a ratio of the non-federal patient's value for the data item divided by his matched federal partner's value, includes the following three physician-staff characteristics:

S_1 Fraction of surgeons (excluding anesthesiologists) at the facility who are FMGs.

S_2 Fraction of the attending physicians on the surgical service with actual teaching faculty appointments at the local medical school who receive salary from the school (intended as an index of the hospital's dependence on the medical school for physicians).

S_3 Fraction of the affiliated medical school's students who did their required core clinical clerkship on the hospital surgical service (intended as an index for the school's dependence on the hospital as a training ground).

As described in the literature review, Huang (1976) and Salkever (1970) have suggested a strong positive association between the teaching function and more frequent utilization of tests and hospital days. The fraction of the medical school's students depending on the individual hospital as a source of clinical education is intended as a proxy measure of the school's dependency on the hospital. One might suggest that if the school is highly dependent on a hospital for teaching cases, the students, interns, residents, and attending physicians, acting as agents of the school's interest, would have added reason to increase length of stay or tests ordered in order to maximize the number of teaching days available and to maximize tests and cost per case in order to serve a technological interest in maximizing revenues for new equipment.

Three hospital characteristics included in the list of independent variables are

H_1 Laboratory turn-around time on the average for seven basic tests.

H_2 Hospital occupancy rate.

H_3 Federal ownership of the hospital (in this specification, the equation intercept).

Overutilization of tests and unnecessary days of stay presumably may be due to the inadequacies of the hospital in providing ancillary laboratory support or surgical suites. Inappropriate utilization can be attributed to both a "systems" failure of the institution and/or a staff behavior problem. The research question then becomes one of asking how much staff improvement can be expected for a given change in the independent variables holding the following factors constant: patient age, sex, primary and secondary diagnoses, welfare status, distance from the hospital (six patient characteristics), bed availability (occupancy), and lab turn-around time. Unless one considers all these factors simultaneously, one really is not measuring the variance truly attributable to staff characteristics.

The model is estimated by the ordinary least squares method. The sixteen equations were developed for the sixteen dependent variables mentioned earlier, where *VA* denotes Veterans Administration patient member of the pair and *NF* denotes non-federal hospital patient member of the pair, under the following log-linear multiplicative specifications:

$$\ln(LOSVA/LOSNF) = \ln(P_1VA/P_1NF)$$
$$+ \ln(P_2VA/P_2NF)$$
$$+ \ln P_3$$
$$+ \ln(S_4VA/S_4NF)$$
$$+ \ln(S_5VA/S_5NF)$$
$$+ \ln(S_6VA/S_6NF)$$
$$+ \ln(H_7VA/H_7NF)$$
$$+ \ln(H_8VA/H_8NF)$$
$$+ \ln(H_9VA/H_9NF)$$
$$+ \ln(E).$$

This log-linear form, sometimes called the double log form, implies that the effect of the error term (E) is multiplicative, as are the effects of the independent variables. The intercept term is X_3.

Results of the Cost and Test Regressions

The results of the regression analysis for cost per case, displayed in Table 12.3, indicate that federal ownership had the largest elasticity. The dummy variable coefficient implies that federal hospital cost per matched surgical case was 52.3 percent higher than non-federal hospital care, *ceteris paribus* [the estimated coefficient is 0.4231 which equals $\ln(1 + 0.523)$]. The average total cost per case was \$3,174 in federal hospitals, \$1,980 in municipal hospitals, and \$2,217 in voluntary hospitals (Table 12.4). The average per-diem cost was \$198 in federal hospitals, \$187 in municipal hospitals, and \$216 in voluntary hospitals. The finding that the voluntary hospital per diem is 9 percent higher than the federal per diem is consistent with a National Academy of Sciences study finding, using almost the same group of hospitals, and 1975 prices. The NAS study group found that on the average the nursing costs per diem for voluntary hospital surgical patients exceeded federal surgical per diems in nursing by 19.8 percent (National Research Council, 1977). Expressed in terms of nursing costs per surgical case, the federal hospitals were \$262 more costly than voluntary hospitals. Nursing costs represented only 30 percent of total per-episode costs.

The following five findings summarize the results obtained in comparing utilization efficiency between different hospitals producing the same product.

1. The federal ownership hospital characteristic was consistently the most significant variable in explaining the variance between

Table 12.3   Cost Equation Regression Results (*t* values in parentheses)

Type of Surgery	Transurethral Prostatectomies	Unilateral Inguinal Hernias	Cholecystectomies	Elective Surgery (columns 1–3)
Type of Surgeon	Specialist	Generalist	Generalist	Specialist or Generalist
Sample Size (patient pairs)	109	99	50	258
R-Squared	0.8145	0.5199	0.7300	0.6441
Elasticity Coefficients for the Following 9 Independent Variables:				
Staff Characteristics				
1. Fraction of Surgeons Who Are FMGs	−0.117[1] (4.09)	−0.081[1] (2.02)	−0.088[1] (2.04)	−0.097[1] (4.25)
2. Fraction of Surgeons with Faculty Appointments at a Medical School	0.198[1] (5.72)	0.076[1] (1.99)	0.167[1] (2.69)	0.063[1] (4.74)
3. Fraction of the Medical School's Students Doing Their Core Clinical Clerkship in Surgery at the Hospital	0.311[1] (11.31)	0.108[1] (2.89)	0.285[1] (5.48)	0.213[1] (9.70)
Hospital Characteristics				
1. Laboratory Turnaround Time (hours)	0.073[1] (7.74)	0.105[1] (7.70)	0.083[1] (3.16)	0.092[1] (11.69)
2. Occupancy Rate	−0.207[1] (4.85)	−0.064[2] (1.70)	−0.100[1] (1.10)	−0.063[1] (2.05)
3. Federal Ownership of the Hospital[3]	0.134[1] (3.43)	0.696[1] (7.01)	0.721[1] (1.98)	0.523[1] (8.17)

Table 12.3 (continued)

Type of Surgery	Transurethral Prostatectomies	Unilateral Inguinal Hernias	Cholecystectomies	Elective Surgery (columns 1–3)
Type of Surgeon	Specialist	Generalist	Generalist	Specialist or Generalist
Sample Size (patient pairs)	109	99	50	258
R-Squared	0.8145	0.5199	0.7300	0.6441
Elasticity Coefficients for the Following 9 Independent Variables:				
Patient Characteristics				
1. Distance from Hospital to Home (miles)	0.073[1]	0.044[1]	0.055[1]	0.060[1]
	(6.55)	(3.13)	(2.48)	(6.87)
2. Lack of Unmatched Secondary Diagnoses, Present or	−0.085[1]	−0.079[2]	−0.044	−0.049[2]
Absent, Between Pairs	(2.04)	(1.79)	(0.54)	(1.65)
3. Patient Age	0.009	0.339	0.044	0.155[2]
	(0.07)	(0.99)	(0.14)	(1.69)

SOURCE: Eastaugh, S. R. (1979). "Cost of Elective Surgery and Utilization of Ancillary Services in Teaching Hospitals." *Health Services Research* 14:4 (Winter), 290–308.

[1] $p < 0.05$, two-tailed test.
[2] $p < 0.10$, two-tailed test.
[3] The coefficients imply a VA/non-federal percentage differential of 14.3%, 69.6%, 72.1%, and 52.3%, respectively.

Table 12.4 Average Number of Elective Tests Done, Cost per Case, and Average and Preoperative Lengths of Stay, by Hospital Ownership (sample size in parentheses)

Type of Surgery / Type of Surgeon	Transurethral Prostatectomies / Specialist	Unilateral Inguinal Hernias / Generalist	Cholecystectomies / Generalist	Elective Surgery (columns 1–3) / Specialist or Generalist
I. Average Number of Elective Pre-operative Tests				
a. VA Patients	5.1 (109)	1.8 (99)	6.0 (50)	4.4 (258)
b. Municipal Hospital Patients	4.2 (47)	0.6 (41)	2.2 (23)	2.5 (111)
c. Voluntary Hospital Patients	4.4 (62)	0.7 (58)	2.4 (27)	2.9 (147)
II. Average Cost (in dollars)				
a. VA Patients	$3,299	$2,628	$3,469	$3,074
b. Municipal Hospital Patients	2,823	1,456	1,758	1,930
c. Voluntary Hospital Patients	2,932	1,660	2,021	2,117
III. Average Length of Stay (in days)				
a. VA Patients	17.0	13.2	18.1	16.0
b. Municipal Hospital Patients	14.5	8.0	11.3	10.6
c. Voluntary Hospital Patients	14.2	7.6	10.8	10.3
IV. Average Pre-operative Length of Stay				
a. VA Patients	7.1	5.6	7.2	6.6
b. Municipal Hospital Patients	4.6	2.2	3.8	3.1
c. Voluntary Hospital Patients	4.4	1.9	3.6	2.8

matched patient pairs in tests utilized (Table 12.5) and cost per case (Table 12.3). On the average, VA patients had 104 percent more preoperative elective tests performed per case, all else being equal in the equation. VA patients also had 52 percent higher costs per elective surgical case for the same operation, *ceteris paribus*. One policy implication of these results is that shifting surgical patients from federal to non-federal facilities may be cost effective and may also prove quality-beneficial according to the National Research Council (1977) study of VA hospitals.

2. The size of the coefficient for the federal ownership variable was much smaller when the surgery is done by a specialist, compared to the sample of surgical cases treated by nonspecialists. However, the federal ownership variable was still the most statistically significant variable in all the regressions. The finding that the federal ownership coefficient was five to nine times larger in cases of non-specialty surgery, compared to specialty surgery, suggests that the specialist was more independent of the effects of working in a federal facility than his nonspecialist colleague. In other words, the specialist was more likely to exhibit the same utilization patterns, independent of whether he operated in a federal, municipal, or voluntary institution. The issue of professional autonomy is a vast and complicated problem, but some descriptive observational studies suggest that the nonspecialist is much more likely to adjust his style of medicine to reflect the more predictable, slower-paced, federal schedule for getting things done (Lindsay, 1975). Our findings suggest that the specialist is also affected, but to a lesser extent, by working within the framework of a federal institutional base.

3. The fraction of the medical school's students doing their required clinical clerkship in surgery at the hospital proved to be the second most significant factor in the regressions and had the expected positive impact on excessive utilization. One possible explanation for this finding is that as dependency of the school on the hospital for teaching beds increases, the school's need to help the hospital maximize patient days, admissions, and revenues (or budgets in the case of VA hospitals) also increases. The coefficients suggest that a 25 percent decline in students would be associated with a 6.2 percent decline in elective tests per case, and a 5.3 percent decline in cost per case.

4. The third and fourth most significant variables in the regressions were, respectively, the percentage of FMGs and faculty mem-

Table 12.5   Number of Tests Regression Results (*t* values in parentheses)

Type of Surgery	Transurethral Prostatectomies	Unilateral Inguinal Hernias	Cholecystectomies	Elective Surgery (columns 1–3)
Type of Surgeon	Specialist	Generalist	Generalist	Specialist or Generalist
Sample Size (patient pairs)	109	99	50	258
R-Squared	0.7655	0.6256	0.7239	0.6374
Elasticity Coefficients for the Following 9 Independent Variables:				
Staff Characteristics				
1. Fraction of Surgeons Who Are FMGs	0.322[1] (6.48)	0.211[1] (3.16)	0.232[1] (2.88)	0.255[1] (6.26)
2. Fraction of Surgeons with Faculty Appointments at a Medical School	−0.157[1] (2.61)	−0.200[1] (2.30)	−0.213[1] (2.15)	−0.218[1] (4.43)
3. Fraction of the Medical School's Students Doing Their Core Clinical Clerkship in Surgery at the Hospital	0.359[1] (7.54)	0.070[2] (1.83)	0.512[1] (6.14)	0.244[1] (6.23)
Hospital Characteristics				
1. Laboratory Turnaround Time (hours)	0.073[1] (4.51)	0.236[1] (10.42)	0.104[1] (2.48)	0.156[1] (11.02)
2. Occupancy Rate	0.197[1] (2.66)	0.271[1] (3.04)	0.342[1] (2.36)	0.029[1] (0.48)
3. Federal Ownership of the Hospital[3]	0.165[1] (2.52)	0.609[1] (11.10)	0.769[1] (2.40)	0.712[1] (6.83)

Table 12.5 (continued)

Type of Surgery	Transurethral Prostatectomies	Unilateral Inguinal Hernias	Cholecystectomies	Elective Surgery (columns 1–3)
Type of Surgeon	Specialist	Generalist	Generalist	Specialist or Generalist
Sample Size (patient pairs)	109	99	50	258
R-Squared	0.7655	0.6256	0.7239	0.6374
Elasticity Coefficients for the Following 9 Independent Variables:				
Patient Characteristics				
1. Distance from Hospital to Home (miles)	0.032[2]	0.030[2]	0.013	0.017
	(1.67)	(1.78)	(0.36)	(1.09)
2. Lack of Unmatched Secondary Diagnoses, Present or Absent, Between Pairs	−0.295[1]	−0.361[1]	−0.375[1]	−0.295[1]
	(3.88)	(3.22)	(2.91)	(4.57)
3. Patient Age	0.963[1]	1.008[2]	0.752[2]	0.382[1]
	(4.24)	(1.89)	(1.77)	(2.07)

SOURCE: Eastaugh, S. R. (1979). "Cost of Elective Surgery and Utilization of Ancillary Services in Teaching Hospitals," *Health Services Research* 14:4 (Winter), 290–308.

[1] $p < 0.05$, two-tailed test.
[2] $p < 0.10$, two-tailed test.
[3] The coefficients imply a VA/non-federal percentage differential of 18.2%, 184%, 116%, and 104%, respectively.

bers on the surgical service. If the values of these coefficients were confirmed on a broader scale, and over a more complete collection of diagnoses, the predicted impact of a 10 percent increase in faculty participation on the surgical service would be a 2.2 percent decline in tests performed, but a 1.3 percent increase in cost per case. It is indeed heartening to learn that the most educated manpower category, the board-certified full-time teaching faculty member, had some propensity to emphasize parsimony in the utilization of ancillary tests. Faculty may have required fewer tests to treat the same matched case, but they had a significantly higher demand for longer periods of patient hospitalization in the post-operative phase of care. The percentage of FMGs was also an important variable in explaining the variance in tests and cost per case. There might have been some within-hospital selection bias, for example, specialist FMGs got easier cases than nonspecialist USMGs. Problems of intrastaff-class correlation remain a subject for future research. The issue of FMG utilization of hospital resources has received somewhat less attention than the more emotional debate about the quality of FMG care. The estimated impact of a 25 percent decline in FMGs on the typical surgical service would be a 6.5 percent decline in the average number of tests, but a 2.4 percent increase in costs per case. In contrast to the highly educated faculty members, the FMG manpower pool of attending surgeons utilized more tests, but fewer days of hospitalization for the same case mix, with the net effect being a slightly lower average cost per case. The FMG and faculty staff characteristics explained nearly 40 percent of the variance in tests and costs per case.

5. Age was the most significant patient characteristic in the analysis. Age had its predicted positive impact on utilization. On the average, the 60-year-old man also had 19 percent more preoperative tests than his 40-year-old counterpart with the same condition. It has been suggested that older men need more testing per admission. Some of the elective tests are recommended by the Payne (1976) process criteria standards on a non-elective basis if the patient is over the age of 50. For example, Payne considers ECG to be necessary for a cholecystectomy patient over the age of 50.

Results of the Length of Stay Regressions

The results of the regression analysis for preoperative length of stay displayed in Table 12.6 indicate that federal ownership is the most significant variable. The dummy variable coefficient implies that federal hospitals have 158 percent longer pre-operative lengths of stay, *ceteris paribus* [the estimated coefficient is 0.9496, which equals ln(1 + 1.58)]. This is consistent with an average preoperative duration of stay that is 6.6 days in federal hospitals, 3.1 days in municipal hospitals, and 2.8 days in voluntary hospitals (Table 12.4). Again we find empirical support in Tables 12.6 and 12.7 to suggest that specialists appear to be increasingly autonomous of the institutional variable of federal ownership. If this finding is confirmed in different settings and for different sets of diagnoses, it would suggest that the specialist is more independent of the effects of working in a federal facility than his or her nonspecialist colleague. Nevertheless, both nonspecialists and specialists are affected by working within the framework of a federal institutional base, with consequent poor utilization of staff time, patient time, and federal money.

Empirical support for the expectation that a tight bed supply results in a lower average length of stay is provided by the statistically significant negative coefficient for occupancy rate.* This is a particularly relevant variable for policy discussions (Stuart and Stockton, 1973) because the occupancy rate seems headed toward a severe upturn. If national health insurance is ever enacted, the resultant demand could increase average occupancy rates by 5–10 percent (Newhouse *et al.*, 1974). Occupancy rates also could be increased if supply were artificially reduced by some form of public utility regulation. A recent Institute of Medicine (1976) study recommended a 10 percent reduction in the supply of acute hospital beds. A 10 percent reduction in bed supply, all other things remaining equal, translates into a 11.1 percent increase in average occupancy rate nationwide. The regression coefficients imply that an 11.1 percent increase in occupancy rate would reduce preoperative length of stay by 2 percent and total length of stay by 1 percent.

The fraction of the medical school's students doing their required clinical clerkship in surgery at the hospital proved to be a significant positive factor in the regressions. The size of the coefficients for this student affiliation factor was not especially dramatic. The coefficients suggest that a 25 percent decline in students would

---

* Multicollinearity is not much of a problem in this analysis, since only two items in the zero-order correlation matrix have absolute values of greater than 0.30. The largest negative correlation is between laboratory turn-around time and occupancy rate ($R = -0.3831$); high occupancy hospitals have quicker lab turn-around. The highest positive correlation is between FMGs and occupancy rate; high occupancy hospitals have a higher percentage of FMGs in this sample ($R = 0.6$).

Table 12.6 Preoperative Length of Stay Regression Results (t-values are in parentheses)

Type of Surgery	Transurethral Prostatectomies	Unilateral Inguinal Hernias	Cholecystectomies	Elective Surgery (columns 1–3)
Type of Surgeon	Specialist	Generalist	Generalist	Specialist or Generalist
Sample Size (patient pairs)	109	99	50	258
R-Squared	0.8403	0.6680	0.6346	0.676
Elasticity Coefficients for the Following 9 Independent Variables:				
Staff Characteristics				
1. Fraction of Surgeons Who Are FMGs	−0.138[1] (3.61)	−0.017 (0.26)	−0.048 (0.60)	−0.056[2] (1.82)
2. Fraction of Surgeons with Faculty Appointments at a Medical School	0.186[1] (4.01)	0.028 (0.33)	0.143[2] (1.79)	0.063[2] (1.69)
3. Fraction of Medical School's Students Doing Their Core Clinical Clerkship in Surgery at the Hospital	0.405[1] (11.03)	0.153[1] (2.45)	0.319[1] (3.88)	0.259[1] (7.31)
Hospital Characteristics				
1. Laboratory Turnaround Time (hours)	0.114[1] (9.10)	0.227[1] (12.21)	0.113[1] (2.72)	0.182[1] (14.30)
2. Occupancy Rate	−0.454[1] (7.98)	−0.162[1] (2.01)	−0.300[1] (2.09)	−0.147[1] (2.70)
3. Federal Ownership of the Hospital[3]	0.785[1] (4.86)	2.381[1] (12.51)	1.623[1] (2.38)	1.577[1] (5.74)

Table 12.6 (continued)

Type of Surgery	Transurethral Prostatectomies	Unilateral Inguinal Hernias	Cholecystectomies	Elective Surgery (columns 1–3)
Type of Surgeon	Specialist	Generalist	Generalist	Specialist or Generalist
Sample Size (patient pairs)	109	99	50	258
R-Squared	0.8403	0.6680	0.6346	0.676

Elasticity Coefficients for the Following 9 Independent Variables:

Patient Characteristics

1. Distance from Hospital to Home (miles)	0.045[1] (3.00)	0.034[2] (1.74)	0.012 (0.36)	0.043[1] (3.05)
2. Lack of Unmatched Secondary Diagnoses, Present or Absent, Between Pairs	−0.341[1] (5.84)	−0.312 (0.25)	−0.021 (0.17)	−0.228[1] (3.91)
3. Patient Age	0.504[1] (2.87)	0.248 (0.43)	0.064 (0.13)	0.480[1] (2.33)

SOURCE: Reprinted with permission of the Blue Cross Association from Eastaugh, S. R. (1980). "Organizational Determinants of Surgical Lengths of Stay," *Inquiry* 17:1 (Spring), 85–96. Copyright © 1980 by the Blue Cross Association.

[1] $p < 0.05$, two-tailed test.
[2] $p < 0.10$, two-tailed test.
[3] The actual coefficients for this intercept term are 0.580, 1.219, 0.964, and 0.950, respectively.

Table 12.7 Total Length of Stay Regression Results (t-values are in parentheses)

Type of Surgery	Transurethral Prostatectomies	Unilateral Inguinal Hernias	Cholecystectomies	Elective Surgery (columns 1–3)
Type of Surgeon	Specialist	Generalist	Generalist	Specialist or Generalist
Sample Size (patient pairs)	109	99	50	258
R-Squared	0.4911	0.4202	0.5457	0.4592
Elasticity Coefficients for the Following 9 Independent Variables:				
Staff Characteristics				
1. Fraction of Surgeons Who are FMGs	−0.053[2] (1.76)	−0.033 (0.78)	−0.041 (0.87)	−0.042[1] (1.98)
2. Fraction of Surgeons with Faculty Appointments at a Medical School	0.059[2] (1.73)	0.071[2] (1.81)	0.039 (0.66)	0.066[1] (2.17)
3. Fraction of the Medical School's Students Doing Their Core Clinical Clerkship in Surgery at the Hospital	0.112[1] (2.98)	0.081[1] (2.07)	0.057[2] (1.75)	0.088[1] (3.71)
Hospital Characteristics				
1. Laboratory Turnaround Time (hours)	0.057[1] (4.45)	0.094[1] (6.62)	0.107[1] (4.28)	0.074[1] (8.70)
2. Occupancy Rate	−0.196[1] (3.36)	−0.010 (0.18)	−0.018 (0.22)	−0.082[1] (2.26)
3. Federal Ownership of the Hospital[3]	0.270[1] (2.97)	0.879[1] (7.36)	0.842[1] (3.97)	0.690[1] (7.50)

Table 12.7 (continued)

Type of Surgery	Transurethral Prostatectomies	Unilateral Inguinal Hernias	Cholecystectomies	Elective Surgery (columns 1–3)
Type of Surgeon	Specialist	Generalist	Generalist	Specialist or Generalist
Sample Size (patient pairs)	109	99	50	258
R-Squared	0.4911	0.4202	0.5457	0.4592
Elasticity Coefficients for the Following 9 Independent Variables:				
Patient Characteristics				
1. Distance from Hospital to Home (miles)	0.003	0.008	0.004	0.007
	(0.22)	(0.55)	(0.18)	(0.24)
2. Lack of Unmatched Secondary Diagnoses, Present or Absent, Between Pairs	-0.080^2	-0.234^1	-0.054	-0.115^1
	(1.73)	(3.34)	(0.71)	(2.95)
3. Patient Age	0.314	0.038	0.040	0.185^2
	(1.99)	(0.10)	(0.13)	(1.71)

SOURCE: Reprinted with permission of the Blue Cross Association from Eastaugh, S. R. (1980). "Organizational Determinants of Surgical Lengths of Stay," *Inquiry* 17:1 (Spring), 85–96. Copyright © 1980 by the Blue Cross Association. All rights reserved.

[1] $p < 0.05$, two-tailed test.
[2] $p < 0.10$, two-tailed test.
[3] The actual coefficients for this intercept term are 0.239, 0.630, 0.609, and 0.524, respectively.

produce only a 2.2 percent decline in total length of stay, and a 6.5 percent decline in pre-operative stay. Another independent variable for strength of affiliation, whether or not the hospital was a member of the Council of Teaching Hospitals, was omitted from the analysis because this variable was insignificant and interacted with the student and faculty variable to make each less significant (0.10 level).

FMGs have a slight, negative (downward) impact on pre-operative and total length of stay. The effect of laboratory turnaround time on the duration of patient stay also is statistically significant. The expected impacts of a 25 percent improvement in turnaround time would be a 4.6 percent decline in average pre-operative length of stay and a 1.8 percent decline in total length of stay.

Age is the most significant patient characteristic in the analysis. All other factors being equal, for the three surgical conditions studied, a 60-year-old man will have a pre-operative length of stay that is 24 percent longer than that of a 40-year-old man, both having the same condition and surgery within the same facility.

One final caveat must be introduced in the discussion. The study design would need to be adjusted if it ever were applied to private patients in the voluntary hospital sector, since the majority of private patients would have been admitted with a preadmission diagnosis already established. Balintfy (1962), for example, found a median pre-operative length of stay in his sample of only one day. The comparison of utilization patterns in private/voluntary hospitals versus federal/municipal hospitals typically ignores the differences in operational style between the two systems. In the governmental sector, the patient tends to enter the hospital without prior examination and testing. The private hospital patient tends to have fewer tests and days of pre-operative stay, because the admission was preceded by preadmission visit(s) and tests (Dumbaugh and Neuhauser, 1976). Consequently, in this study, all the public patients (Medicaid or VA) with a pre-admission visit to the hospital (9 percent) had their medical record abstracts coded with a −1; thus, in the aforementioned matching process, only patients with equivalent pre-admission workups were matched with one another.

Policy Implications

Multiple regression analysis provided considerable insight into the roles of specific independent variables in explaining differences between hospitals along the four utilization measures (pre-operative length of stay, total length of stay, tests, and costs). The increasing concern for curtailing rapidly rising hospital costs, and renewed interest in reducing the number of hospital beds, makes it increasingly important for health services researchers to learn more about how to affect physician behavior in a direction that enhances hospital efficiency. To counterbalance the potential inflationary impact of PSRO quality assurance activities requires a targeting of resources to those facilities with the highest chance of benefiting from the programs. The study results indicate that PSRO utilization review efforts might be targeted to those surgical services in federal hospitals, or in non-federal teaching hospitals that provide over 10 percent of the local medical school's students with a required clinical clerkship in surgery. A continuing education program that emphasizes reduced ancillary utilization might best be targeted to surgical services with a high percentage of FMGs or high percentage of students. Although PSROs do not specifically fund continuing education programs, the facilities with an abundance of excessive utilization relative to the norms would seem most in need of continuing education programs.

The basic premise of the economic model emerging from this study is that the physician is influenced in patient management decisions by the economic advantage of actions to him, or his hospital, or perhaps to his medical school. We should guard against overutilization that results from physician pursuit of less explicit forms of economic advantage than income maximization tendencies under a fee-for-service system of reimbursement. The subtle incentives to overutilize are much more insidious and affect salaried and private entrepreneur physicians equally. For example, surgeons may overtly or subconsciously overutilize in pursuit of any number of economic and personal objectives: to win favor with the surgical service chief, to win prestige, to maximize revenues or budgets to the surgical service. The incentives are certainly interrelated, and they favor overutilization as a means of accomplishing other objectives. The surgeon has an interest in increasing utilization as a way to maximize budgets so as to maximize the capital funds available for the tertiary care equipment, so as to maximize the individual surgeon's future income.

If we presume that the surgeon wishes to maximize prestige or popularity within the profession, rather than overutilize for the sake of overutilization, then the problem for policy makers becomes one of framing a set of incentives that makes prestige maximization incompatible with overutilization. Federal and voluntary hospital reimbursement incentives do not favor cost-effective clinical decision making. In fact, any education program that tries to reduce cost per case or number of tests is doomed to fail because of reimbursement incentives. One can expect only professional intransigence in the face of a federal PSRO plan that asks hospitals to reduce their budgets by curtailing utilization. If the reimbursement incentives were changed, so that a hospital was provided with a fixed dollar amount for a given diagnostic group, then the physician who minimizes unnecessary care maximizes the capital funds that are useful in the pursuit of prestige maximization. The physician would still not have an incentive to underutilize, because any form of underutilization that has a detrimental effect on quality would injure the physician's prestige and image among his peers.

Three sets of dynamic, interacting interest groups seem to affect utilization patterns: the physician staff, the medical school faculty, and the hospital staff. The hospital is not an institutional island unto itself. Hospitals are influenced by a second multi-product institution: the local medical school. Conventional wisdom has it that the affiliation is mutually beneficial. The school, for example, depends on the hospital for teaching sites, while the hospital depends on the school as a source of manpower. It also is the style of some hospital administrators to drop subtle hints to physicians, such as: (1) The hospital occupancy rate is too low, consequently start increasing lengths of stay; or (2) Laboratory utilization is too low to cover costs, consequently increase the average number of lab tests. Both of these statements are indications of how a physician might shift his or her decision at the margin, without being provided with a dictum as to how to treat a given patient.

One might like to think that physician faculty members are too professional to be affected by pressures from within the hospital. Any relationship of mutual dependence implies vulnerability: the greater the degree of dependence between hospital and school, the greater the vulnerability. Resources and teaching beds obtained from the hospital therefore may not represent a large portion of the school's budget, but may in the short run be perceived by the school as necessities that are critical. Patient care revenues also play a part in the medical school's objective function, because such funds can be used to purchase future tertiary care equipment. New and better equipment always is considered by the medical school dean's committee to be a critical requirement for teaching the increasingly technological style of American medicine.

The high statistical significance of both affiliation measures suggests that it is conceptually false to view the school, hospital, and physician staff as independent entities providing services in functionally segmented medical markets. The fact that the coefficients for the faculty variable are inelastic and negative for tests per surgical case suggests that dispersal of faculty members to less affiliated hospitals would decrease the average amount of excessive testing. However, the surgical student variable has a positive inelastic coefficient, suggesting that it is better to concentrate students on surgical rotation in as few hospitals as possible in order to minimize the regionwide impact that this factor has on tests per case and costs per case. For example, if a medical school shifts 1 percent of the surgical clerkships from a hospital serving 20 percent of their students to a hospital serving 5 percent of their students, the marginal increase in utilization (tests, dollars, days) at the hospital going from 5 percent to 6 percent students is greater than the marginal decrease in utilization at the hospital going from 20 percent to 19 percent.

Future research might consider whether physicians operate under the norms hypothesis (Pauly, 1977), making length-of-stay decisions based upon the average or modal staff characteristics within their hospital, and their region, rather than handling these decisions on an individual basis. In particular, a fair test of the norms hypothesis would be to take a sample from teaching and nonteaching hospitals and compare staff characteristics for one surgeon to characteristics of everyone who made decisions about a given patient. From there, the study would proceed to characteristics of surgeons in the surgical service of a given hospital, to characteristics of all surgeons in the health service area, for a sample of both teaching and nonteaching hospitals.

One of the basic strengths in this study design was the assignment of staff characteristics to the entire surgical service. Previous studies have treated the individual patient and one individual physician as the unit of analysis; consequently, little variation has been explained. All of the phases of care from admission to discharge are not in the hands of one physician. The decisions are in the hands of a group of physicians in a teaching hospital.

The objective of the surgical study has been to discover some of the factors contributing most to excessive utilization of hospital beds. The foregoing analysis was intended to advance our understanding of the problem of unnecessary utilization and clarify the need for and nature of particular policy alternatives. Two areas for further investigation have been suggested by the regression results. The two fundamental public policy issues raised in the study involve changing the hospital reimbursement incentives, and changing the content of medical school education.

One might try reimbursing some hospitals on a per episode basis, because that policy would reverse the present incentive to lengthen stays. The profession soon may find that more is not necessarily better—and often may be worse, as in the case of the previously cited British experiment when hernia length of stay was decreased from an average of six days to one day (Morris *et al.*, 1968). This policy option, however, does carry a risk for the health services research community. Methods would have to be developed to quantify case-mix complexity if the per episode reimbursement scheme were to have any credibility, and thus impact on the hospital sector. Hospitals would have to be reimbursed more per episode for a less healthy patient case mix, or a more complex diagnostic case mix. For example, an urban teaching hospital might receive $3,000 per hernia, whereas a suburban nonteaching hospital might receive $1,500 per hernia.* The AUTOGROUP method, used for assessing case-mix complexity at Yale, partitions hospital episodes into medically meaningful classes that have similar patterns of average length of stay (Mills *et al.*, 1976). The problem with the AUTOGROUP approach is that it still provides the physician with an incentive to extend hospital stays or report "extra" diagnoses found in each episode of care. The information-theoretic-based complexity measure, developed by Evans and Walker (1972) in Canada, and Horn and Schumacher *et al.* (1979) in Maryland, uses the diagnostic mix proportions to define the information measure and the degree of concentration to define the case-mix complexity measure. The advantages of this approach are that it can be made independent of average length of stay figures. Furthermore, the mathematics are complex enough to discourage physician manipulation of the system.

Physicians have not been encouraged to address themselves to cost-containment efforts, cost-effectiveness analysis, or clinical ap-

---

* The shortcoming of the New Jersey DRG (Diagnostic Related Groups from the AUTOGROUP program) experiment is that it does not tie in the doctors. Only the hospitals are reimbursed by DRG, not the physicians. Under the scheme, the physician can prosper as the hospital loses money because physicians control the admission and discharge process. No hospital administrator has the power to discharge patients at the economically rational point, that is, when the hospital payment per DRG covers costs. One would hope that New Jersey physicians recognize the financial health of their hospital as a component in their utility function, and discharge patients more efficiently, but the learning process might take time.

plications of decision analysis. Because physicians' decisions generate a majority of medical care costs, it would seem logical to suggest that motivation for cost containment must begin in the minds of the physicians. Formal training in decision analysis and economics should yield more rational decisions and perhaps better patient outcomes. If some of the principles of cost-effective clinical decision making would seep into the subconscious cognitive processes of American physicians, a less costly style of medical care might result. Continuing education programs may affect practicing physicians' behavior, but the experiences related in Chapter 4 suggest that it might be more cost-beneficial to bring formal discussion of these issues to medical students and help them reflect upon their developing role as generators of medical costs. To help understand the scope of the problem, remember that the average clinician in 1980 will generate approximately $500,000 in medical care costs.

References

BALINTFY, J. L. (1962). "Mathematical Models and Analysis of Certain Stochastic Process in General Hospitals," unpublished dissertation, Engineering Department, Johns Hopkins University.

BELL, R. M., and SLIGHTON, R. L. (1975). "The Total Cost of Medical Care in Teaching and Nonteaching Settings." Santa Monica, Cal.: RAND Corporation.

BERG, R. L., BROWNING, F. E., and CRUMP, S. L. (1979). "Bed Utilization Studies for Community Planning," *Journal of the American Medical Association* 207:13 (March 31), 2411–2413.

BERMAN, H., and WEEKS, L. (1979). *The Financial Management of Hospitals*, 4th rev. ed. Ann Arbor: Health Administration Press.

BERRY, R. (1974). "Cost and Efficiency in the Production of Hospital Services," *Milbank Memorial Fund Quarterly* 52:3 (Summer), 291–313.

DAVIS, K. (1971). "Relationship of Hospital Prices to Costs," *Applied Economics* 3:2 (June), 115–121.

Duke Law Journal (1971). "The Medical Malpractice Threat: A Study of Defensive Medicine," *Duke Law Journal* 40:11 (November), 939–950.

DUMBAUGH, K., and NEUHAUSER, D. (1976). "The Effect of Pre-admission Testing on Length of Stay," in S. Shortell and M. Brown (eds.), *Organizational Research in Hospitals*. Chicago: Inquiry–Blue Cross Association.

EASTAUGH, S. R. (1977). "An econometric model for predicting the future VA patient census," unpublished appendix to the study *Health Care for the American Veteran* performed by the National Academy of Sciences, presented to the U.S. Congress, pursuant to Section 201 (c) of Public Law 93–82, to the Committee on Veterans' Affairs, United States Senate, June 7, 1977.

EASTAUGH, S. R. (1980). "Organizational Determination of Surgical Lengths of Stay," *Inquiry* 17:2 (Spring), 85–96.

EASTAUGH, S. R. (1979). "Cost of Elective Surgery and Utilization of Ancillary Services in Teaching Hospitals," *Health Services Research* 14:4 (Winter), 290-- 308.

EVANS, R. G., and WALKER, H. D. (1972). "Information Theory and the Analysis of Hospital Cost Structure," *Canadian Journal of Economics* 5:3 (August), 398–418.

FELDSTEIN, M. (1971). "Hospital Cost Inflation: A Study of Nonprofit Price Dynamics," *American Economic Review* 61:5 (December), 853–865.

FREIBERG, L., and SCHUTCHFIELD, F. (1976). "Insurance and the Demand for Hospital Care: An Examination of the Moral Hazard," *Inquiry* 13:1 (March), 54–63.

GARG, M., LOUIS, D., GLEIBE, W., SPIRKA, C., SKIPPER, J., and PAREKH, R. (1978). "Evaluating Inpatient Costs," *Medical Care* 16:3 (March), 191–201.

GAUS, C. R. (1970). "Hospital Use Prediction Based on Population and Medical Resource Factors," unpublished Sc.D. thesis, Johns Hopkins School of Hygiene and Public Health.

GAUS, C. R. (1976). "Hospital Costs, Stays Vary Widely Across U.S.," *American Medical News* 19:12 (March), 10–12.

GERTMAN, P. (1974). "Hospital Length of Stay," in D. Bernstein and R. Egdahl (eds.), *Perspectives on Health Policy, Peer Review Conference*, Boston University Medical Center (May), 54–60.

GIBSON, R. M. (1980). "National Health Expenditures, 1979," *Health Care Financing Review* 2:1 (Summer), 1–20.

GOLDFARB, M., HORNBROOK, M., and RAFFERTY, J. (1980). "Behavior of the Multi-product Firm: A Model of the Nonprofit Hospital System," *Medical Care* 18:2 (February), 185–201.

GORNICK, M. (1975). "Medicare Patients: Regional Differences in Length of Hospital Stays 1969–1971," *Social Security Bulletin* 38:7 (July), 16–33.

GUSTAFSON, D. H. (1968). "Length of Stay: Prediction and Explanation," *Health Services Research* 3:1 (Spring), 12–34.

HENDRICKSON, L., and MYERS, J. (1973). "Some Sources and Potential Consequences of Errors in Medical Data Recording," *Methods of Information in Medicine* 12:1 (January), 30–39.

HORN, S. D., and SCHUMACHER, D. N. (1979). "An Analysis of Case Mix Complexity Using Information Theory and Diagnostic Related Grouping," *Medical Care* 17:4 (April), 382–389.

HU, T., and WERNER, J. (1976). "The Effects of Insurance on Hospital Utilization and Costs: A Simultaneous Equation Model," Paper presented at the Econometric Society Meetings, Atlantic City, New Jersey, September 17.

HUANG, L. (1976). "An Analysis of the Effects of Demand and Supply Factors on the Utilization of Health Services in Shortstay General Hospitals," paper presented at the American Economic Association Meeting, Atlantic City, New Jersey, September 17.

INNES, A., GRANT, A. J., and BEINFIELD, M. S. (1968). "Experience with Shortened Hospital Stay for Postsurgical Patients," *Journal of the American Medical Association* 204:8 (May 20), 647–652.

Institute of Medicine (1976). *Medicare-Medicaid Reimbursement Policies*, February Policy Report. Washington, D.C.: National Academy of Sciences.

Institute of Medicine (1976). *Controlling the Supply of Hospital Beds*, October Policy Report, Washington, D.C.: National Academy of Sciences.

KLASTORIN, T. D., and WATTS, C. A. (1980). "On Measurement of Hospital Case Mix," *Medical Care* 18:6 (June), 675–685.

JONSSON, E., and NEUHAUSER, D. (1975). "Hospital Staffing Ratios in the United States and Sweden," *Inquiry* 12 (Supplement), 128–135.

KELLEY, D. C., WENG, J., and WATSON, A. (1979). "Effect of Consultation on Hospital Length of Stay," *Inquiry* 16:2 (Summer), 158–161.

KLARMAN, H. E. (1963). "Effect of Prepaid Group Practice on Hospital Use," *Public Health Reports* 78:11 (November), 955–965.

LAVE, J. R., and LEINHARDT, S. (1976). "The Cost and Length of a Hospital Stay," *Inquiry* 13:4 (December), 327–333.

LEE, M. L., and WALLACE, R. L. (1973). "Problems in Estimating Multiproduct Cost Function: An Application to Hospitals," *Western Economic Journal* 11:3 (July), 350–359.

LEVIN, P. J. (1964). "Physician Characteristics and Use of Hospital Services," unpublished doctoral thesis, Johns Hopkins School of Hygiene and Public Health.

LINDSAY, C. M. (1975). *Veterans Administration Hospitals.* Washington, D.C.: American Enterprise Institute.

MASSELL, A., and HOSEK, J. (1975). "Estimating the Effects of Teaching on the Costs of Inpatient Care: The Case of Radiology Treatments." Santa Monica, Cal.: RAND Corporation.

MCCORKLE, L. P. (1970). "Duration of Hospitalization Prior to Surgery," *Health Services Research* 5:2 (Summer), 114–131.

MCNERNEY, W. J., and study staff (1962). *Hospital and Medical Economics,* Volume 2. Chicago: Hospital Research and Education Trust.

MILLS, R., FETTER, R. B., RIEDEL, D. C., and AVERILL, R. (1976). "AUTOGRP: An Interactive Computer System for the Analysis of Health Care Data," *Medical Care* 14:7 (July), 603–615.

MITCHELL, J. H., MARDAORE, J. M., WENDEL, F. J., and LOHRENZ, F. N. (1975). "Cholecystectomy Peer Review: Measurement of Four Variables," *Medical Care* 13:5 (May), 409–416.

MORRIS, D., WARD, A., and HANDYSIDE, A. (1968). "Early Discharge after Hernia Repair," *The Lancet* 1:7544 (March 30), 681–685.

National Research Council (1977). *Health Care for American Veterans.* Washington, D.C.: National Academy of Sciences.

NEWHOUSE, J. P., PHELPS, C. E., and SCHWARTZ, W. B. (1974). "Policy Options and the Impact of National Health Insurance," *New England Journal of Medicine* 290:24 (June 13), 1345–1359.

NEWHOUSE, J., and MARQUIS, M. S. (1978). "The Norms Hypothesis and the Demand for Medical Care," *Journal of Human Resources* 13 (Supplement), 159–182.

PAYNE, B. (1976). *The Quality of Medical Care: Evaluation and Improvement.* Chicago: Health Research and Education Trust.

PAULY, M., and REDISCH, M. (1973). "The Not-For-Profit Hospital as a Physicians' Cooperative," *American Economic Review* 63:1 (March), 87–100.

PAULY, M. (1978). "Medical Staff Characteristics and Hospital Costs," *Journal of Human Resources* 13 (Supplement), 77–111.

PAULY, M. (1979). "What Is Unnecessary Surgery?" *Milbank Memorial Fund Quarterly* 57:1 (Winter), 95–117.

PHILLIP, P. J., JEFFERS, J., and HAI, A. (1976). "Indexes of Factor Input Price,

Service Intensity, and Productivity for the Hospital Industry," in *Nature of Hospital Costs*, pp. 201–262. Chicago, Ill.: Hospital Research and Educational Trust.

QUERIDO, A. (1963). *The Efficiency of Medical Care: A Critical Discussion of Measuring Procedures*. Amsterdam: Leiden Stenfert Knoose.

RAFFERTY, J. A. (1971). "Patterns of Hospital Use: An Analysis of Shortrun Variations," *Journal of Political Economy* 79:1 (January-February), 154–165.

REDISCH, M. (1978). "Cost Containment and Physician Involvement in Hospital Decision Making," in M. Zubkoff, I. Raskin, and R. Hanft (eds.), *Hospital Cost Containment: Selected Notes for Future Policy*. New York: Prodist.

RICHARDSON, W. C. (1969). "Poverty, Illness and Uses of Health Services in the United States," *Hospitals* 43:35 (July 1), 34–40.

RIEDEL, D. C., and FITZPATRICK, T. B. (1964). *Patterns of Patient Care*. Ann Arbor: University of Michigan Press.

RO, K. K. (1969). "Patient Characteristics, Hospital Characteristics and Hospital Use," *Medical Care* 7:4 (July-August), 295–312.

ROSENFELD, L. S., GOLDMAN, F., and KAPRIO, L. A. (1957). "Reasons for Prolonged Hospital Stay: A Study of Need for Hospital Care," *Journal of Chronic Disease* 6:2 (August), 141–152.

RUBIN, D. (1970). "The Use of Matched Sampling and Regression Adjustment in Observational Studies," unpublished dissertation, Statistics Department, Harvard University.

SALKEVER, D. S. (1970). "Studies in the Economics of Hospital Costs," unpublished dissertation, Economics Department, Harvard University.

SCHIMMEL, E. (1964). "Hazards of Hospitalization," *Annals of Internal Medicine* 60:1 (January), 100–110.

SCITOVSKY, A. (1976). "Changes in the Costs of Treatment of Selected Illnesses 1951–1964–1971." Rockville, Maryland: National Center for Health Services Research, Research Digest Series.

SPATH, R. (1977). "Impact of Current Malpractice Insurance Policies on the Utilization of Clinical Laboratories," unpublished dissertation, School of Public Health, University of California, Berkeley.

STIGLER, G. (1946). *The Theory of Price*. New York: Macmillan.

STUART, B., and STOCKTON, R. (1973). "Control Over the Utilization of Medical Services," *Milbank Memorial Fund Quarterly* 51:3 (Summer), 341–394.

TWADDLE, A. C., and SWEET, R. H. (1970). "Characteristics and Experiences of Patients with Preventable Hospital Admissions," *Social Science and Medicine* 4:1 (July), 141–145.

Part Four

FUTURE POLICY OPTIONS

Chapter 13

POTENTIAL FOR EFFECTIVE COST CONTAINMENT IN THE 1980s

> *An economist can tell you what will happen under any conditions. And his guess is liable to be just as good as anybody else's.*
>
> —WILL ROGERS

> *Our current problems are past solutions.*
>
> —JOHN D. THOMPSON

Compared with other countries, America has a schizophrenic attitude concerning the production and financing of medical services. Some liberals would go so far as to argue that medical services are a merit good, so crucial to preserving the general welfare of society that the services should be financed by government even if they are not cost-beneficial.* Such an attitude is maintained in the Netherlands and Sweden, where medical care is produced and financed as if it were a public good—a social service too important to be rationed on

---

* A classic example of this thinking would be the Netherlands. The Netherlands has the highest medical cost inflation rate of any OECD member (OECD, 1980). By contrast, England takes the viewpoint that certain medical services are not cost-beneficial and should not be included in the National Health Service. The American tradition is to seldom support the classic externalities argument for supporting medical services as a public good. There are few services where one can demonstrate that the society as a whole earns more if the co-workers are kept healthy through preventive medicine (Yankauer, 1981). However, most medical dollars go to curing and caring, not prevention.

market principles. Other countries, like Japan, France, and Switzerland, produce and finance medical services as if they were normal
consumer goods. Insurance is available for expensive medical services, but the coinsurance rates range as high as 30–50 percent.

However, the United States has one of the most inconsistent
policies toward medical service: We produce it as a consumer good,
finance it as a public good, and complain when providers react in a
rational way, promoting excess demand and behaving in a hyper-
inflationary "quality is all important" style of care for the subsidized
service. Some analysts argue that it would be irrational for providers
to persevere in cost containment efforts except possibly as a long-
term strategy to prevent total government control of the industry.
Advocates of competition health plans have been quick to label the
hospital industry's Voluntary Effort to contain costs as a program of
slow "voluntary suicide," that is, containing costs to the point of
contracting operating margin and/or depleting assets will lead to a
slow institutional death. While such a label is an overstatement,
anticipatory attempts to inflate cost-profiles before the advent of a
more regulated hospital economy is certainly one rational strategy
for survival.

Most liberal advocates of expanding access and promoting health
insurance did not anticipate any of the inflationary side effects that
have arisen. Expansion in the depth and scope of our health insurance options has not resulted in a simple relabeling of who pays the
bill for the same stable aggregation of contingent claims. Growth in
insurance has stimulated more claims and higher unit cost per claim.
The next effect, higher total health care expenditures, is frequently
characterized by economists with the rather misleading term,
"moral hazard." When consumers and providers consume more
when dealing with other people's money (the insured group's funds),
such behavior is better characterized as rational rather than im-
moral. The intent of competition health plans is to reduce the
myopic way in which we all spend health care dollars at the point of
consumption, by making us more price conscious at the less stressful
point of selecting an insurance option. Price competition at the point
of consumption allows less time for shopping and is liable to result in
such inequities as reduction in access for dollar-poor individuals.
Competition among insurers at the point of annual consumer enrollment might convince some consumers to select the less costly
insurers such as HMOs. If this were to occur, other insurers would
have an economic incentive to select the less costly providers if they

want to stay in business. In theory a less inflationary health care system would result. As we have seen in other sectors of the economy, only a few consumers need be well informed and willing to shop, and only a few firms need initially care about the competition to foster a highly competitive market.

Three themes have been dominant throughout this text: (1) providers should question new and unproven technologies, (2) consumers should begin to shop for the best buy, and (3) regulators should adequately reimburse institutions. Currently we have providers who seldom adequately question unproven equipment and techniques, consumers who do not have the desire or wherewithal to shop for the best buy on the basis of price and quality, and frequently inadequate reimbursement for some institutions. Health plans and providers will increasingly have to rely on such unfamiliar concepts as marketing and cost-benefit analysis to survive in the 1980s. We shall examine some of these emerging concepts, potential solutions, and resulting problems in the next three sections.

Marketing

The growing interest in marketing activities and cost-containment strategies will probably be received by physicians with either disdain, indifference, acquiescence, or creative action. Marketing in a traditionally non-profit industry will be fraught with a number of technical and political pitfalls. Some critics may argue that the academic advocates of marketing and competition have substituted benevolent descriptions of success stories for critical analysis. Future health marketing evaluation studies may conclude that the assumptions that were basic to the competition health plan argument fail to hold in all smaller communities and many larger communities. But competition health plans deserve a chance, whether they work in 15 percent of the nation or 85 percent. The process of doing market surveys may help on a national scale to convince providers that we should aggressively market caring services and demarket or decrease the marginal curing services that seldom "cure," for example, heart transplants or heroic medical procedures that prolong for months suffering in a hospital bed.

In regard to this last problem of devoting excessive resources to the hopelessly ill patient, the Critical Care Committee of Massachusetts General Hospital (MGH) has provided an excellent classification system for making the tough ethical choices of whether to send the individual to the Intensive Care Unit (ICU) or to provide minimal care (MGH, 1976). In developing the classification system, the MGH physicians were reacting less to cost containment pressures than to the pressures of irate family members who complained that a relative was constantly being shipped back to ICU and saved, rather than being allowed to die with dignity. The eventual transition from an acute care–dominated medical care system to a more balanced and caring health services system will be costly and slow.

The most popular current trend in health marketing is diversification, or the expansion and "unbundling" of services. Restructuring the organization is one form of diversification that is becoming increasingly popular. Restructuring involves spinning off a segment of the hospital into a separate for-profit corporation or non-profit foundation. Restructuring is not a new idea, but the reasons for restructuring have changed dramatically in recent years. In the 1970s restructuring was designed to share services, improve production volume, and consequently decrease unit costs. In 1981, 5–10 percent of the hospitals are already in the process of restructuring (Brown, 1981) for purposes of maximizing reimbursement and sheltering assets from erosion (caused by inflation or under-reimbursement by state rate setting commissions).

There are risks involved in restructuring. If the hospital establishes a foundation for whatever purpose (for example, preservation of assets), it faces the risk of having the IRS and rate setters question the legality of sheltering the hospital's resources through the foundation. The degree to which one non-profit institution may be held responsible for the obligations of another tax-exempt foundation, sometimes labeled the "separate corporateness" dilemma, has yet to be decided in the courts (Whitney, 1981). The separate corporateness issue is also a problem if the hospital places the profit making services in a separate for-profit corporation. One can also maximize reimbursement by spinning off services that are not reimbursed by cost payers and therefore would accumulate a high share of overhead (that is, unreimbursed overhead). Restructuring may not prove cost effective for services that lack high growth potential. The legal and consulting costs for producing the multitude of financial statements for all the separate mini-corporations may exceed the marginal benefits in improved reimbursement.

Care for the elderly will be the biggest future growth market for most health care providers. Most hospital administrators are aware

Table 13.1 **Annual Growth Rates in Total Hospital Admissions and in Admissions of Those Over 65, 1969–1980**

Year	Hospital Admissions	Admissions by Individuals Age 65+
1969	+2.1%	+6.1%
1970	6.3	2.6
1971	0.4	3.4
1972	2.6	6.1
1973	3.5	5.7
1974	3.7	6.0
1975	0.3	4.5
1976	3.4	7.0
1977	2.5	4.4
1978	0.4	4.9
1979	2.7	5.3
1980	2.0	5.8

SOURCE: American Hospital Association (1980), *Annual Survey.*

that since 1970 Medicare admission growth rates have exceeded those of the general population (Table 13.1). The medical care system must become more efficient and cost conscious in preparation for the coming geriatric burden. The two fastest growing population groups are the over-75 and the 65–74 year group, respectively. The aging population will substantially increase the proportion of GNP devoted to health care (home care, nursing care, hospice care, hip replacements, chemotherapy, and rehabilitation aids).

Somers (1980) has recently reported a number of excellent policy proposals designed to stimulate more comprehensive and equitable treatment for the elderly. All too often we have seen politicians concentrate on nursing home abuse and fraud, ignoring the fact that only 5 percent of the elderly are in nursing homes. A much larger group, estimated at 15 percent of all citizens over age 65, are seriously functionally impaired. We can simultaneously contain costs and improve patient satisfaction by providing services that keep these impaired individuals out of institutions.

Cost-Benefit Analysis

Cost-benefit analysis will become an increasingly important field of inquiry in the 1980s. Health services delivery will have to be justified in terms of the indirect and intangible benefits that it provides through reduction in pain or functional impairment. Most policymakers are now convinced that medical resources have a minuscule effect on traditional health benefit measures, such as mortality and morbidity. For example, a recent report by HEW (1979) attributed the vast majority of early (premature) mortality to factors outside the health economy: unhealthy life styles (50 percent of the deaths), genetic factors (20 percent), and environmental factors (20 percent). There is very little room to improve the most tangible aggregate health status measures of Americans through better and more accessible personal health services. Even with better measures on the benefit side, the conclusions may be equally pessimistic. Newhouse and Friedlander (1980) concluded that medical resources have a very small marginal effect on health outcomes, even in the case of more sensitive measures of improved health status. Perhaps the forthcoming results of the $35 million RAND Corporation Health Insurance Experiment (Newhouse 1974) may conclude, after examining additional outcome indices, that certain modes of health services delivery provide better marginal benefits.

Cost-benefit and cost-effectiveness studies have not proven to be useful in the case of macro-resource decisions. Because physicians' everyday micro-decisions generate the vast majority of medical care costs, it would seem logical to argue that cost containment must begin in the mind of the physician. Whether one leans toward the political right or left, real control of the cost problem requires convincing a large number of physicians of the value of cost-effective clinicial decision making.

Physicians have basic doubts about the need for cost-related evaluations for two basic reasons. First, many physicians argue that a given medical technology is a moving target that cannot be subject to evaluation until after it evolves into a mature technology. Unfortunately, mature technologies seem to develop a constituency of clinicians that are unwilling to subject their techniques to "irrelevant" cost considerations or marginal effectiveness considerations. The more prudent public policy would be to have an early evaluation of most evolving technologies with a commitment by the researchers to update the results as the technology improves. Second, many physicians lack confidence in the cost-benefit and cost-effectiveness analyses produced by their local Health Systems Agency (HSA). The overwhelming majority of such studies performed by HSAs are very poorly done. Frequently the costs are inappropriately apportioned and the benefits are almost never disaggregated into patient subgroups according to signs, symptoms, and other risk factors. We argued in Chapters 3 and 4 that there was a large potential role for government in supporting better benefit and effectiveness studies. Physicians should not be expected to read and act on such poorly designed studies. The urgency of the need for better research and evaluation has been increasing each year as the useful lifetime of a technique or machine becomes an increasingly smaller fraction of the original development lead time. As the errors of judgment in adopting unproven medical technology become more expensive, the value of technology assessment activities will rise.

The most radical proposal in this text probably is the suggestion that we pursue full-scale experimentation with a number of consumer information disclosure proposals. Such faith in consumers probably reflects the economist's traditional distaste for paternalism. Many individuals feel that consumers will make the right buy if they are only provided with more information concerning provider quality, price, and accessibility. Each individual has an opinion concerning the value of such attributes as time cost, dollar cost, survival probability, and bedside manner "quality." However, one should not allow the accuracy of information provided to consumers to go unquestioned. Without substantial external monitoring for accuracy, more free and open information disclosure could be a fine idea on paper that proves counter-productive or ineffective in practice. One cannot simply assume that competing providers would police the accuracy of their own or others' claims.

Incentive Structures

Politicians frequently seek headlines by claiming that the bulk of the medical cost problem is caused by the fraud and abuse of a few providers. This contributes to piecemeal attention being given to such infrequent problems as Medicaid kickbacks and HMO scandals, rather than the more insidious problem of inflationary incentive structures. In this section we shall review the "small" cost containment strategies that third parties can pursue by adjusting current reimbursement incentives.

There are a few marginal improvements that third parties can make by tinkering with the reimbursement formulas. More states will begin to pay hospitals on the basis of case-mix measures, such as the DRG-based reimbursement experiment in New Jersey.* The payers may soon create incentives for hospitals to await lower interest rates before financing new capital projects. More aggressive regulatory approaches, such as local pooling of depreciation payments and allocation by local planning authorities, are likely to be costly and ineffective. The best short-term reimbursement strategy might simply involve setting some reasonable ceiling on interest rates that are fully reimbursed and allowing a small 3 or 4 percent surplus of revenues over operating expenses for new capital. To underfinance all hospitals in the name of fighting excess capitalization across the entire industry risks negatively affecting productivity in all hospitals. If management is too tightly reimbursed, hospitals will typically be able to afford the big capital items that doctors demand but unable to afford the "little ticket" capital acquisitions (for example, minicomputers) that could improve productivity and cut operating costs.

If third parties wanted to create disincentives to unnecessary testing, they could link reimbursement of all tests in inverse proportion to the percentage of routine tests found to be normal. Hospitals producing a high proportion of routine tests (apart from preventive screening program tests) on health individuals would be reimbursed only 80 or 90 percent of allowable costs. This would create a financial incentive for the hospital or the independent group practice to perform fewer unnecessary tests. One could also consider reimbursing physicians for only necessary surgery. In other words, a surgeon would not be reimbursed for removing tissue that was found to be healthy. For example, the much-publicized surgeon in Boone County, Arkansas who removed over fifty "cancerous" growths that turned out to be healthy tissue would not be reimbursed for

---

* DRGs are based on isolength of stay groupings of patients with a given primary diagnosis at discharge. There are other experimental methods of grouping patients and describing case-mix differences among hospitals. Garg *et al.* (1978) have utilized disease stage levels as a method of grouping patients based on physician judgment of clinical severity. Horn and Schumacher (1979) are developing a modified form of the DRGs based on isocost clusters of patients with similar costs per hospital episode. Horn (1981) has developed an AS-SCORE system for measuring severity of illness within a diagnostic group. The acronym AS-SCORE represents the five major attributes of the severity index: age, systems involved, stage of disease, complications, and response to treatment. The index was found to have a high level of content validity, that is, as the index increased there was a concomitant increase in costs, length of stay, consultations and probability of mortality. Recently, Young *et al.* (1980) developed the first admission-focused case-mix cluster scheme, grouping cases by presenting symptoms rather than on the basis of final diagnosis.

these "services." This board-certified surgeon was removing "tumors" that the clinical pathologists found to be healthy fat tissue. In one case the tumor turned out to be a two-month-old fetus. As an example of how physicians monitor their peers, this board-certified surgeon still practices surgery three years after these abuses were uncovered. Blue Cross/Blue Shield of Arkansas still reimbursed the surgeon for "nonservice": removing the healthy uterus of a 22-year-old woman.

The way in which rate regulation is being conducted is bound to become more of an issue in the 1980s. The New York State version of command and control regulation generates tension and forces the majority of hospitals into bottom-line deficit positions. The New York approach invokes formulas which attempt to straight-jacket the individual hospitals. In addition to straight-jacketing institutions, the formula approach all too frequently stresses the negatives in decision making, such as punitive screens for increasing length of stay, increasing cost per diem, or decreasing occupancy rate. The combined effect of these punitive incentives are often antithetical to cost-effective management decision making techniques. For example, if an institution reduces average length of stay, cost per case will decline, but the hospital will be penalized for raising the cost per diem.

Maryland provides a major alternative to the brand of regulation practiced in New York State. Rather than inviting antagonism, the basic premise of the Maryland approach centers on cooperation and compromise. In Maryland the hospitals are provided with positive incentives to control costs gradually over a number of years. The Maryland approach is to pressure the hospitals incrementally to contain costs, and let the individual managers manage. The Maryland rate commission monitors the rate of change in cost per case and total expenditures, and leaves it to the 54 individual institutions to manage as they please within these constraints. In the interest of public relations, the Maryland commission has relabeled the revenue "cap" per admission as a revenue "guarantee" (that is, connoting the positive elements of the cap as a constraint). The Maryland system is not without problems. For example, a clear incentive exists to inflate the number of admissions, but the state attempts to reimburse for those "extra" admissions only at marginal cost (rather than at the higher level of average cost).

A third alternative approach to rate regulation is being developed in Rochester, New York. This three-year prospective reimbursement experiment, called the "minicap" program, attempts to elimi-

nate any incentive for inflating the number of admissions in Rochester. The nine facilities in the Rochester program have agreed to
share a fixed global regional budget; that is, there will be no incentive to inflate admissions, days of stay, tests, or procedures. In other
words, the incentives are to reduce costs rather than assure the
hospitals they will be paid whatever their costs turn out to be.

One infrequently tested cost containment idea that holds
significant promise is the concept of double-capitation payments for
both consumers and hospitals. All third-party carriers collect capitation payment from consumers, but seldom have insurance carriers
negotiated a totally capitation basis of paying hospital and other
suppliers. Pure prospective reimbursement through capitation
payments to all suppliers and capitation collections from all buyers
is the basic incentive strength of American HMOs and most
nationalized health plans. The insurance industry has experimented
with capitation reimbursement of hospitals on a very limited one-
shot basis. Colorado Blue Cross implemented the double-capitation
concept for both hospitals in rural Yuma County in the early 1960s
(Tierney and Sigmond, 1965). The authors pointed out that this new
idea of capitation payment was really the original method of reimbursement promulgated by Blue Cross and Baylor University Hospital in 1931. The advantage of the capitation payment method was
that it gave the hospital an incentive to serve the public with only
the necessary number of inpatient days. The hospitals could not
unnecessarily "dump" patients on other hospitals on a referral basis
because that patient care would have to be financed out of the
original hospital's capitation fund. However, patients still retained
complete freedom of choice to visit any hospital or physician. The
number of beneficiaries assigned to each hospital in Yuma County
would vary according to shifts in utilization patterns and shifts in
beneficiary response to the question: "Which facility do you visit for
routine hospitalization?" Any individual or family who did not designate a hospital was assigned for payment purposes to the hospital
nearest their home.

The Hartford Foundation and Blue Cross are currently supporting
a hospital capitation reimbursement experiment in two states. Eight
hospitals in North Dakota will be reimbursed on a fixed capitated
sum starting late in 1981. Hopefully, four Massachusetts hospitals
will join the capitation experiment in 1982. In addition to reducing
unnecessary inpatient days, it is hoped that the hospitals will respond
to the capitation incentives by expanding preventive medical pro-

grams to contain future costs by decreasing the future demand for inpatient care per capita. The innovation of this double-capitation scheme is the fact that payment is made on the basis of individuals served, rather than number of services produced. Capitation reimbursement eliminates incentive to inflate the provision of extra or unnecessary services, and creates new incentives to contain operating costs. Under fee-for-service reimbursement of costs, management has little or no incentive to contain costs.

The double-capitation reimbursement plan can result in some administrative savings, since the hospital need not submit individual bills for reimbursement. The hospital is presented with an economic incentive to keep consumers loyal to their hospital, implement internal cost-savings activities, and contain lengths of stay and admission rates. The chief problem with capitation reimbursement is that unless the physicians are also reimbursed on a capitation basis or are highly concerned with the financial health of their hospital, they can continue to make patient care decisions that hurt the hospital. Excess utilization benefits providers under the prevailing system of reimbursement per unit-of-service. However, the capitated hospital clearly does have an incentive to select physicians with an interest in cost-effective clinical decision making. Currently, hospital management has little incentive to exert influence on the physician committee that assigns hospital privilege rights to community physicians.

There will be a number of problems in implementing a hospital capitation program. Who is to decide what hospitals require extra subsidy payments? For example, teaching hospitals* and hospitals in high-wage areas should receive somewhat higher capitation payments. In order to encourage industry participation in capitation reimbursement programs, the hospital could be guaranteed against loss (relative to projected revenues under prior reimbursement conditions) in the initial one or two years of implementation. If the hospital gained excessively from the capitation method of reimbursement, some fraction of the gain, agreed upon by all parties, could be returned to the public in the form of lower premiums and less taxes. In summary, two-sided capitation from buyer-to-insurer

---

* Teaching hospitals currently receive higher reimbursement. For example, current Section 223 regulations for reimbursement of routine costs allow 4.7 percent higher reimbursement for every resident per ten beds. Prior to the onset of this adjustment in 1979, the members of the Council of Teaching Hospitals were receiving slightly more than half of the penalties for excessive routine costs under Medicare.

and insurer-to-hospital has potential to contain costs. However three-sided capitation, including insurer-to-physician capitation payments, may be the best cost-containment strategy for the future.

The Road Ahead

The American tradition in health policy making has been to move on an *ad hoc* piecemeal basis. In keeping with that tradition, the period 1981–1985 will probably be one in which we embrace competition health plans, decrease federal subsidies to health care, increase state government support for health services, initiate tougher local rate regulations on routine hospital costs, and initiate a program of negotiated physician fees. This last point has not been adequately considered in the text. A system of negotiated fees has two potential benefits: (1) containment of annual increases in physician expenditures* and (2) elimination of the incentives to locate in overdoctored areas and specialties. This is not to suggest that we could eliminate all substantial variations in specialty fees, but at least we should make reimbursement policy more consistent with manpower policy. Currently physician fees are based on a tradition of reimbursement for any price that is "usual, customary, and reasonable." Operationally, if the bill seems unusually high to the bill processors, they may go through the extra effort of comparing the charges on the claim to prevailing prices for that condition in the region, and reimburse the lower figure (billed or prevailing). Claims intermediaries would rather maximize short-term profit than implement an automated information system that questions too high a fraction of physicians' claims, which would cause political problems, legal suits, and reduced profit margins for the intermediary.

Health care providers should not belittle what many label a current overemphasis on cost containment and narrow financial concerns. If the nation can contain the medical cost inflation rate within reasonable limits, we might have the financial slack to extend and improve

---

* Huang and Koropecky (1973) have suggested that physician fee inflation can be reduced if we regulate or negotiate a more narrow dispersion of fees. The authors report that inflation rates are higher when the dispersion of fees is wider, and suggest that the lower priced physicians are more aggressive in "catching up" with their peers. Some analysts argue that county medical societies already support a tight system of price fixing through the use of relative value scales. However, Hsiao *et al.* (1978) have reported wide variations in fees that are inconsistent with the price-fixing hypothesis.

health services delivery. If the health economy can develop a stronger management orientation and demonstrate an improved ability to steward public funds, new national commitments to the health care sector may be forthcoming. For example, we might then be able to do something concerning the unmet health service demands of the 12.6 percent of the civilian population that has no health insurance coverage.

Balancing Economic and Financial Management Concerns

One of the popular current themes in hospital financial management meetings is that capital financing and reimbursement incentives must change in the 1980s to prevent the rapid aging and deterioration of plant and equipment. The danger is that the current policy of slightly underpaying all hospitals will eventually be detrimental to the quality of patient care and the productivity of our facilities. More thoughtfully designed reimbursement policies, accompanied by increased reliance on scientific management decision-making techniques, may result in a delicate balancing of cost-control and quality-control goals.

The neophyte in the field of health services administration may detect two seemingly inconsistent sentiments in the text: the call for a somewhat higher fair rate of institutional reimbursement for hospitals, HMOs, and medical schools on the one hand, and the call for cost containment on the other. There is some obvious trade-off between institutional financial health and cost containment. In many northern industrial states, regulators have taken the position that if we cannot close unnecessary facilities, we can pursue cost containment by slight across-the-board inequities in reimbursement (for example, by not recognizing the need for short-term working capital* or the need for modernization of plant and equipment). One can

---

* Hospital administrators have recently been forced to control the expansion of working capital due to increasingly restrictive reimbursement policies and rising interest rates. Working capital data has only been collected by the American Hospital Association for four years, but one is impressed by the fact that working capital increased by only 5.5 percent to $9.5 billion in 1979. In 1979 the bank prime interest rate rose by 3.75 points and only Washington state recognized full reimbursement for working capital. The elasticity of the prime rate on total interest expense has been found to be small (-0.04), but statistically significant (Tway, 1980). This finding is not surprising given that interest expenses are an allowable cost.

sympathize with the regulators' dilemma. Third-party payers and regulators can either be slightly unfair to all institutions or be equitable to all providers and slightly exacerbate the cost inflation problem. This book has advanced another alternative: promote competition health plans, provide consumers with more information to shop for both insurance options and providers, and increase consumer cost-sharing requirements. There is no quick-fix solution to inflation in any sector of the economy. This alternative strategy appears to have the best long-run chance of reducing the troika of problems: inflation, wasteful behavior, and inequitably low reimbursement of institutional care.

The health industry and the regulators have taken a largely defensive stand. Each party has become preoccupied with the actions and expectations of the other. However, an internal cost containment ethos and fair reimbursement of total institutional financial requirements are necessary if we are to develop a more rational national health policy; rhetoric concerning "fat" providers and mindless bureaucrats is counterproductive. Will the 1980s be a period of uncontrolled growth and expansion of the hospital economy? Or can the recent record of poor performance and sluggish productivity be reversed? The public has come to recognize that the key problem for health policy is now cost containment, not access to care. The solution to containing costs may be found in better implementation of management strategies and better research in the areas of finance and health economics. In our pluralistic society, better information is a necessary, but not sufficient, condition for achieving a more healthy health economy.

Some health policy makers have tended to reduce health economics to the level of a forensic science, full of rhetoric and devoid of research results. A main objective of this book has been to engage the interests of policy makers and managers in the research results of academicians. Policy makers, like institutional managers, are too occupied with putting out daily brush fires and reacting to symptomatology to adequately keep abreast of the health services research literature.

The challenge to health providers will be to carry on one shoulder life-saving technology and the concomitant financial burden and, on the other shoulder, the will and imagination to apply modern management techniques. If we do not improve management incentives and capability, the possibility for future improvements in our health care system will be strangled by the inevitable retrenchment that will follow the past three decades of uncontrolled expansion.

References

BROWN, M. (1981). "Systems Diversify with Ventures Outside the Hospital," *Hospitals* 55:7 (April 1), 147–153.

Department of Health, Education and Welfare (1979). *Surgeon General's Report on Health Promotion and Disease Prevention*, Publication 79-55071. Washington, D.C.: U.S. Government Printing Office.

GARG, M., LOUIS, D., GLIEBE, W., SPIRKA, C., SKIPPER, J., and PAREKH, R. (1978). "Evaluating Inpatient Costs: The Staging Mechanism," *Medical Care* 16:3 (March), 191–201.

HORN, S., and SCHUMACHER, D. (1979). "An Analysis of Case Mix Complexity Using Information Theory and Diagnostic Related Grouping," *Medical Care* 17:4 (April), 382–389.

HORN, S. (1981). "Validity, Reliability, and Implications of an Index of Inpatient Severity of Illness," *Medical Care* 19:3 (March), 354–362.

HUANG, L., and KOROPECKY, O. (1973). "The Effects of the Medicare Method of Reimbursement on Physicians' Fees and on Beneficiaries' Utilization," Volume II, DHEW Report S.S. 92-73 (October), part I. Washington, D.C.: U.S. Government Printing Office.

HSIAO, W., LURIE, P., SCHOENHERR, J., and SERRIANSKI, S. (1978). "Profile of Physicians' Charges: A Statistical Analysis," DHEW Report SSA 600-76-0058. Washington, D.C.: Health Care Financing Administration.

Massachusetts General Hospital Critical Care Committee (1976). "Optimum Care for Hopelessly Ill Patients," *New England Journal of Medicine* 295:7 (August 12), 362–364.

NEWHOUSE, J., and FRIEDLANDER, L. (1980). "The Relationship Between Medical Resources and Measures of Health: Some Additional Evidence," *Journal of Human Resources* 15:2 (Spring), 200–218.

NEWHOUSE, J. (1974). "A Design for a Health Insurance Experiment," *Inquiry* 11:1 (March), 5–27.

Organization for Economic Cooperation and Development (1980). *National Accounts of OECD Countries 1950–1979*. Paris: OECD.

SOMERS, A. (1980). "Rethinking Health Policy for the Elderly: A Six-point Program," *Inquiry* 17:1 (Spring), 3–17.

TIERNEY, T., and SIGMOND, R. (1965). "Could Capitation Ease Blue Cross Ills?" *Modern Hospital* 55:8 (August), 103–106.

TWAY, J. (1980). "An Econometric Model of Hospital Costs," Working Paper 80-3 (October). Chicago, Illinois: Office of Research Affairs, American Hospital Association.

WARNER, K., and LUCE, B. (1981). *Cost-Benefit and Cost-Effectiveness Analysis in Health Care: Principles, Practice, and Potential*. Ann Arbor: Health Administration Press.

WHITNEY, J. (1981). "Hospital Philanthropy: Strengthening the Financial Base of Nonprofit Hospitals," *Health Care Management Review* 6:2 (Spring), 19–34.

YANKAUER, A. (1981). "The Ups and Downs of Prevention," *American Journal of Public Health* 71:1 (January), 6–9.

YOUNG, W., SWINKOLA, R., and HUTTON, M. (1980). "Assessment of the AUTOGRP Patient Care Classification System," *Medical Care* 18:2 (February), 228–244.

GLOSSARY

Accounts receivable   Amounts due from patients for services provided.

Accrual-basis accounting   An accounting system in which revenue is recorded in the accounting period in which it is earned, whether or not cash has been received. Expenses are also recorded in the accounting period in which they are used or consumed in producing revenue, whether or not the cash is disbursed for the payment of those expenses.

Adverse selection   Individuals with a perceived higher self-rated risk of needing health insurance will seek out the insurance options with more comprehensive benefits and lower copayment provisions.

Aggregate production function   Relationship between the amount used of each of the inputs and the resulting amount of potential output. The aggregate production function pertains to the entire industry (e.g., hospital industry), not a single firm (e.g., a single hospital).

Aging schedule   A report showing how long accounts receivable have been outstanding, including the percent of receivables not past due and the percent past due for under 30 days, 31–60 days, 61–90 days, and over 90 days.

Allowable charge   Maximum fee allowable by a given third-party payer for a covered patient service.

Allowable costs   Elements of cost that are reimbursable, usually under a third-party reimbursement formula. For example, allowable costs under Medicare exclude the costs of such things as new telephones or anti-unionization efforts.

Ancillary services   Services other than room, board, and other professional services provided in hospitals or other in-patient health care delivery systems (e.g., laboratory and radiology).

Assignment   Agreement by which a patient assigns a hospital or other health care provider the right to receive payment from a third-party payer. In return the provider agrees to accept payment from the third party as payment in full. This third-party payment is less than the actual charges billed to patients under retrospective cost-based reimbursement or prospective reimbursement.

Bad debts   Revenue lost by a provider because of patient nonpayment when there was an expectation that the patient had the ability to pay. Medicare and some Blue Cross plans limit reimbursement for bad debts to

325

their own patients' services that are not fully covered. If the third party deducts certain amounts from the benefits of patients, the hospital must bill the patient directly for the deductible. These deductibles often become bad debts. Also, the charges for services furnished to self-pay patients sometimes become bad debts.

Balloon payment   In a case where the debt is not fully amortized, the final payment will be larger than the preceding payments.

Benefits   A service provided under an insurance policy or prepayment plan. In the case of Health Maintenance Organizations they both insure and provide the service. In the case of Blue Cross and Blue Shield, the payments are made directly to the provider on behalf of patients who are covered. Commercial insurers make payments either to the provider or to the individual subscriber.

Bond   Debt security, usually issued for long periods of time. Examples are debenture bonds and mortgage bonds.

Bond discount   Amount by which the selling price is less than the face value of a bond.

Book value   Amounts at which assets or liabilities are recorded in the accounting records of the institution. Net book value is usually the assets' cost less any accumulated depreciation.

Budget   Detailed plan expressed in financial terms, usually for a one-year period. The budget is typically broken down along departmental lines and accounts for both revenue and expenses. Hospitals participating in the Medicare or Medicaid programs are required by law (Section 233 of Public Law 92-603) to maintain a one-year operating budget and a three-year capital budget.

Capital asset   An asset with a life of more than one year that is not acquired for purpose of resale, e.g., equipment buildings and grounds.

Capital budgeting   The process of planning expenditures on assets whose economic returns are expected to extend beyond one year.

Capital cap   A fixed limit on the annual amount of new capital that can be purchased in an area. An example would be the 1979 Carter proposal for a \$3 billion nationwide cap on new hospital capital in 1981.

Capitation   A method of payment for health services in which the provider is paid a fixed per capita amount irrespective of the services actually utilized in the coming year. HMOs use this method.

Cash flow   The summation of net income or excess of revenues over expenses plus depreciation (NI + D). This provides a measure of the availability of cash to meet financial requirements such as capital replacement or amortization of debt.

Cash inflows   Revenues actually received by the firm or provider.

Cash outflows   Expenses actually paid by the firm or provider.

Catastrophic health insurance   A type of health insurance that provides protection for severe or lengthy illnesses requiring high medical expenditures (exceeding $5000). The projected costs of catastrophic insurance programs are generally much lower than those estimated for more comprehensive national health insurance programs. However, passage of a catastrophic insurance plan might prove highly inflationary. One Harvard study demonstrated that average expenses for the high-cost 1 percent of families were increasing at a rate four percentage points higher than for the average family.

Caveat   A more complete explanation to minimize the chance for misinterpretation and prevent the reader from jumping to conclusions.

Coinsurance   The cost-sharing arrangement whereby the insurer assumes only a certain percentage of the costs of covered services, e.g., 75 or 90 percent. The individual pays the remainder of the bill, and consequently has some degree of interest in cost containment.

Community rating   A method whereby the insurer determines the premium rate based on the average costs of all subscribers in a specific industry or catchment area, and all individuals pay the same rate. Community rating spreads the cost of illness evenly over all the subscribers and does not charge higher rates to those currently less healthy than the average person.

Conditional sales contract   A method of financing new equipment by paying it off in installments over a few years. The seller retains ownership of the equipment until payment has been completed.

Copayment   Form of cost sharing whereby the insured pays a specific amount at the point of consumption, e.g., $10 per visit. This differs from a coinsurance arrangement under which payment is provided as a percentage of total cost.

Cost-based reimbursement   The reimbursement arrangement currently most popular with third-party payers. Under cost reimbursement the third party pays the hospital for the care received by covered patients at cost, not on the charges actually made for those services. There are a variety of cost formulas that specify whether or not a plus factor is allowable and what type of cost apportionment methods may be used. Medicare, Medicaid, and over two thirds of Blue Cross plans rely on this method of reimbursement.

Cost-finding techniques   A process of apportioning (allocating) the costs of the non-revenue-producing cost centers to each other and then, eventually, to the revenue-producing cost centers on the basis of utilization data that measures the amount of service rendered by each center to the other centers.

Current assets   The liquid assets that can be expected to be directly or indirectly converted into cash within one year or within the operating cycle of the firm, whichever is longer.

Current liabilities   The obligations that fall due and will be paid within one year or within the operating cycle of the firm, whichever is longer.

Debenture   A form of debt in which the only protection against non-payment is the general credit of the issuer, in contrast to loans that have the additional protection of security as specified in the loan agreement.

Deductible   A form of cost sharing in which the insured incurs an initial expense of a specified amount within a given time period (e.g., $250 per year) before the insurer assumes liability for any additional costs of covered services.

Demand curve   Graphic representation of the relation between price of a good or service and the quantity demanded, e.g., the lower the price the higher the demand.

Depreciation   A method of accounting that distributes the cost or other basic value of capital assets over their estimated useful life in a systematic manner. Depreciation for any year is a portion of the total cost or basic value that is allocated to that year. It is an arbitrary process of allocation and should not be viewed as one of valuation.

Discounting   The process of finding the present value of a series of future cash flows. The discount rate in the general economy is substantially higher than the social discount rate discussed in Chapter 3.

Dual choice   The practice of giving individuals an opportunity to select from more than one health insurance or health plan (HMOs) to pay for or provide personal health services.

Economic cost   The full cost of operations, including both tangible and intangible costs.

Economies of scale   Decreasing average cost as a function of increasing scale (size). There is modest evidence for shallow economies of scale in the production of hospital patient-days. There is some suggestion that the economies would be more substantial if one could better correct for case-mix differences. Evidence on the magnitude of scale economies in the hospital industry would be more substantial if we could better adjust for the heterogeneous product mix of patient cases. When a more homogenous unit of output at the departmental level is examined, economies of scale are more substantial in the hospital industry. Cost savings generated by economies of scale constitute a primary argument for regionalization and increased reliance on shared services.

Efficiency   Economic efficiency is a relative measure of the rate at which output is produced at least cost, e.g., patient visits produced per $1000 of expenses. Technical efficiency, or productivity, is the rate at which output is produced per unit of input, e.g., number of home visits per full time equivalent home health aide.

Endowment funds   Funds given by a donor who has stipulated that the principal portion must be maintained in perpetuity. Income from investment of these funds may be expended, however. Some hospitals have been forced to "cannibalize" portions of the principal in cases where reimbursement is not sufficient to cover the existing total financial requirements of the institution.

Equity   Net worth of the institution or firm.

Excess of revenues over expenses   Difference between revenues and expenses for a defined accounting period. This phrase is the non-profit firm's term for net income.

Experience rating   A method of pricing used by the insurance industry to determine premiums based on the average projected costs of health care for different consumer subgroups. The premiums are a function of experience of the group and subgroups and are affected by such variables as age, sex, income, and health status. Thus they are in contrast to the community rating method.

Feasibility study   Report of an independent firm of financial consultants that documents an institution's ability to repay prospective debt financing with anticipated cash flow. This document is used for purposes of securing debt financing options and negotiating with health planning agencies.

Fixed assets   Assets of a relatively permanent nature held for continuous use for operations and not intended to be converted into cash through resale.

Fixed costs   Costs that do not change as a function of the quantity of output.

Financial lease   A lease that is viewed for accounting and tax purposes as a conditional sales agreement. The FASB term is "capital lease." The usual cost of ownership and depreciation, plus the financing cost on the lease, is the recognized cost of the asset leased.

Financial requirements   Phrase authored by the American Hospital Association to designate the total need for funds for continued operation of a health care facility. Total financial requirements are frequently less than the expenses reported under cost reimbursement, e.g., allowable costs are less than full costs.

General obligation   A bond secured by pledge of the issuer's taxing power and credit.

Gross National Product (GNP)   A measure of the total amount of goods and services produced by the economy.

Health Maintenance Organizations   HMOs are organizations that provide and assure the delivery of comprehensive health services for an enrolled group of persons under a prepaid capitation arrangement. Given the constraints of a fixed capitated budget, the HMO has more of an incentive to provide preventive care and improve internal operating efficiency than more traditional insurance options. HMOs achieve cost savings per capita primarily through a 30–50 percent reduction in hospital admission rates compared to those for local control populations (e.g., Blue Cross subscribers). However, the appropriateness of the "control" group remains a major problem for health services researchers. HMOs were labeled prepaid group practices prior to 1972. Under the 1972 Health Maintenance Organization Act (P.L. 93-222) all employers must offer an HMO option to their employees whenever a qualified HMO exists in the area. In signing the Act President Nixon expressed the hope that private capital and managerial talent would be drawn into the health care field, eventually eliminating the need for federal funding and direct controls.

Hospital insurance program   Compulsory Part A portion of Medicare that automatically enrolls all persons over 65 who are entitled to benefits under the Social Security system, individuals under the age of 65 who are also eligible for benefits because of disability, and insured workers and their families who require renal dialysis or kidney transplantation (see Medicare).

Indemnity benefits   Health insurance policies that provide benefits in the form of cash payments rather than actual services. Indemnity insurance contracts typically specify maximum amounts that will be paid for services included in the benefit package. After the patient has been billed for covered services, the insurance company either remits payment to the patient or directly to the provider. This type of insurance is most popular in the automobile insurance industry.

Intermediary   Private or public organization (e.g., Blue Cross) selected by the providers of health care under the hospital insurance program to pay claims and perform administrative functions for the Department of Health and Human Services. For example, over two thirds of the hospitals have selected one of 80 Blue Cross plans as their intermediary.

Internal rate of return   The rate of return calculated by finding the discount rate that equates the present value of future cash flows to the cost of the potential investment.

Investment banker   Functions as a principal rather than an agent and initially purchases all of the bonds from the issuer. Also called an underwriter, he is the middleman between the issuer and the public market.

Lease   Contract granting possession of an asset for a period of time in return for some stated compensation. See financial lease and operating lease.

Liabilities   Debts or obligations of the provider, institution, or firm.

Liquidity   Refers to the cash position of the institution and its ability to meet maturing obligations.

Major medical insurance   A popular type of health insurance designed to provide protection for heavy (above average) medical expenses that may result from a hospitalization or chronic illness. These policies do not provide first-dollar coverage but do provide more comprehensive benefits than catastrophic insurance.

Marginal cost   The cost of an additional one-unit change in the amount of goods or services produced.

Market clearing price The price that brings demand and supply into equilibrium. One can usually remove excess demand by increasing price.

Maturity The date the principal amount of a bond becomes due.

Medicare A limited national health insurance program for individuals eligible for social security benefits (Title XVIII of the Social Security Act). Medicare expenditures are projected to increase at an annual rate of 19 percent to $49 billion in fiscal 1982. Medicare contains two separate but coordinated programs: hospital insurance (Part A) and supplementary medical insurance (Part B). Most elderly individuals pay the basic premium of $11 per month for Medicare Part B. Expenditures under Part B are expected to increase from $12.4 to $15 billion from 1981 to 1982. Medicare Part A is financed by a 1.3 percent contribution rate tax on both employees and employers. Medicare Part A recipients' benefits include hospital care, skilled nursing facility care following a hospital stay, and home health care services.

Monopoly A market where only one seller exists. Monopoly conditions seldom correspond more than approximately to actual market conditions. Duopoly, two sellers, happens more frequently in geographically distinct catchment areas. Some markets are so small or the economies of scale are so significant that competition between firms cannot be maintained, and only the natural monopolist survives.

Moral hazard Form of rational behavior whereby the consumers demand more of a good or service (such as health insurance) when they do not pay the full price. It is a misnomer to refer to such behavior in "moral" terms, as was the style of 19th-century economists.

Municipal bonds Bonds issued by states or political subdivisions such as counties, cities, or villages. In most cases, interest paid on municipal bonds is exempt from federal income taxes. The term municipal bond is usually synonymous with tax-exempt bond.

Oligopoly A market with few producers. There are pure oligopoly situations where the sellers produce an identical product (e.g., cement), and differentiated oligopoly markets where the sellers produce somewhat different products (e.g., automobiles or hospital care).

Oligopsony A market with few buyers, e.g., a two-industry town purchasing all the hospital care in the area.

Operating lease A lease that cannot be considered a transfer of ownership or conditional sale. This type of lease is not capitalized and thus the relevant measure of expense is the periodic rent specified in the lease. This lease is also called a True Lease.

Opportunity cost Maximum value that might have been attained if a resource had been used in the best possible alternative way. It is the highest return that will not be earned if the funds are invested in the proposed project. Actual dollar costs of resources are a valid measure of opportunity cost; however, amortizations of prior expenditures such as depreciation are not useful measures of opportunity cost.

Plant fund   Account group used by the institution to record the transactions involving their investment in land, buildings, and equipment.

Price discrimination   Sale by a given firm of the same good or service to different buyers at two or more different prices. The price differential is not associated with differences in production costs.

Price elasticity of demand   Percentage change in quantity demanded resulting from a 1 percent change in price, all else held equal.

Prospective reimbursement   Method of reimbursing providers on the basis of rates established in advance of the delivery of the services and independent of the amount of actual services provided. An advantage of prospective reimbursement for providers is that they can better plan and budget for the future. Payers benefit from the incentive to contain costs, rather than inflate services, under prospective reimbursement.

Relative value units   Index number assigned to various procedures based upon the relative amount of resources (labor and capital) necessary to produce the good or service.

Reasonable charge   The price defined for Medicare reimbursement to physicians—either the physician's customary charge for a given service or the prevailing charge by physicians for that service in that area, whichever is lower. Medicare will pay only up to the 75th percentile of the prevailing physician charge for that service, i.e., the high-priced one fourth of physicians on that given service will not be paid the full amount.

Reasonable cost   Maximum amount stated in most cost reimbursement formulas which third-party payers will actually reimburse.

Retrospective reimbursement   Service payment to hospitals and other providers by third-party payers or government for either charges or costs that have been incurred.

Salvage value   Value of a capital asset at the end of a specified period. The salvage value is the current market resale price of an asset being considered for replacement.

Self-insure   The assumption of risk by an organization against potential losses. Groups of teaching hospitals frequently bind together as a captive insured group, thus assuming risk collectively. Many hospitals were forced into self-insurance arrangements by the rapidly escalating costs of malpractice premiums.

Shared services   Legal arrangement whereby a number of health care facilities agree to share the responsibility for the provision of certain services. Common examples are nonclinical services such as laundry and dietary services.

Surgicenter   Ambulatory care facility providing simple elective surgical treatment.

Supply curve   Graphic representation of the relation between the market price of a good or service and the quantity supplied, e.g., the higher the price the more that will be supplied.

Tax-exempt bond   A bond upon which the interest is exempt from federal income taxes. Consequently these bonds can be sold at a lower interest rate.

Time-price elasticity of demand   Measure of the responsiveness of the quantity of a good or service demanded to a change in the time (waiting and travel) cost required of the consumers.

Third-party payer   Organization that pays for or insures health or medical expenses on behalf of its beneficiaries or subscribers. Third-party payers act as the agent between the providers and consumers. Such payers include Medicare, Medicaid, Blue Cross, Blue Shield, and commercial insurance companies.

Uniform cost accounting   Use of a common set of accounting procedures and methods for the accumulation and communication of data that relate to the financial activities of multiple sections of the institution. Seven states that have established rate-setting commissions also require uniform cost accounting or uniform reporting as a requirement for reimbursement.

Usual, customary, and reasonable charges   A physician's charges for services that do not exceed the usual charge, the customary charge by other physicians for the same service in the area, or some other judgment of reasonableness. Most private health insurance plans, including most Blue Shield plans, use the UCR approach. Usual, customary, and reasonable charges are similar but not identical to the customary and prevailing charges concept used by Medicare.

Working capital   The investment of the institution in short-term assets (cash, short-term securities, accounts receivable, and inventories). Gross working capital is defined as a firm's total current assets. Net working capital is defined as the excess of current assets over current liabilities. It is a financial requirement that is usually not recognized in most cost reimbursement formulas (except in the Washington State formula).

AUTHOR INDEX

SUBJECT INDEX

DATE DUE

NOV 4 1982			
DEC 1 5 1986			
GAYLORD			PRINTED IN U.S.A.